Library of Congress Cataloging in Publication Data

Main entry under title:

Influences of hormones in tumor development.

   Bibliography: p.
   Includes index.
   1. Carcinogenesis. 2. Tumors. 3. Hormones --
Physiological effect. 4. Adenoma. I. Kellen,
John A.   II. Hilf, Russell, 1931-
DNLM: 1. Hormones--Metabolism. 2. Neoplasms--
   Etiology. QZ202.3 I43
RC268.5.I53   616.9′94′071   78-11932
ISBN 0-8493-5351-3 (v. 1)
ISBN 0-8493-5352-1 (v. 2)

© 1979 by CRC Press, Inc.
International Standard Book Number 0-8493-5351-3 (Volume I)
International Standard Book Number 0-8493-5352-1 (Volume II)

Library of Congress Card Number 78-11932
Printed in the United States

PREFACE

The increasing awareness in recent years that our environment directly or indirectly influences carcinogenesis has focused much of our attention on external factors. What is being held as general deterioration in the quality of the environment has been widely reported on and has become an important area of social and scientific concern. This has come to outweigh our concern for the part played by the internal milieu and by genetic susceptibility. No critical assessment of the complex interplay of modifiers that finally lead to malignant growth should ignore this triad. There is no doubt that in some cancers, the influence of one or more factors seem of overwhelming importance. However, it appears reasonable that, whatever theory of primary cancerogenesis* one may adhere to, internal modulation of the exposed tissue is a necessary prerequisite for tumor induction and growth.

Hormones have traditionally been assigned an important role as modifiers of the neoplastic process. Their key role in metabolism makes them a logical target for speculation of this kind. The exquisite balance between the hormones in response to physiological needs, the minute amounts of active substances acting at the molecular level, and the continuing elucidation of the amplifying systems which translate their messages, all offer potential controls where the observed changes might be affected. Hormones are not necessarily components of mitotic mechanisms; cells can divide in their absence, but the overall regulation of cell division seems to be under their control. Hormones are also capable of affecting the genetic regulatory system by modifying gene expression.

It is accepted that hormones modify cancer risk, the response of the body to carcinogens and the biological behavior of established tumors. Some hormones seem to produce tumors directly, albeit at heroic levels. Experiments involving the removal of glands that secrete substances which stimulate or support tumor growth have destroyed the idea that all cancers were independent growths. At least some tumors, like many endocrine target tissues, can be shown to be dependent on normal control mechanisms. Our knowledge on therapeutic effects of hormones has been beneficial to innumerable patients.

Tumors of endocrine organs and of organs controlled by hormones cause some 90,000 deaths out of an estimated total number of 350,000 cancer deaths in the U.S. per year. Hormone-induced tumors, ectopic hormone production, and efforts to influence the natural history of tumors by administration of hormones in experimental animals represent a considerable share of basic research. The last decade has brought about a major qualitative step in our armamentarium with the discovery of hormone receptors which already has an increasing impact on clinical thinking.

The successful attrition of billions of malignant cells in a clinically apparent tumor — a cancer "cure" — evokes much scepticism. On the other hand, step-by-step modulation of such cells towards redifferentiation by endocrine therapy does not seem to be impossible to achieve.

We have tried to present an assessment of these uncertainties and challenges in basic research with clinical implications. We have divided the information on current views and results into sections by hormones. In these, the much appreciated work of our coauthors may be seen. It is next to impossible to cover this dynamic and wide-ranging topic comprehensively, but we hope that an updated review of relevant experimental and clinical research will contribute to the development of this promising field of enquiry.

---

* For a note on the distinction between cancerogens and carcinogens, the reader is referred to *Nature* (London), 267, 306, May 26, 1977.

The relationship of hormones to neoplasia is complex and multifaceted; it is conceivable that better understanding and manipulation of this relationship will pave the way for more rational and effective treatment of many cancers.

J. A. Kellen
R. Hilf

THE EDITORS

Dr. John A. Kellen is Associate Professor and Staff Physician in the Department of Clinical Biochemistry at the Sunnybrook Medical Centre, a teaching hospital of the University of Toronto.

His primary interest is in immunology and biochemical markers in cancer; he has over 170 scientific papers and three monographies to his credit. Dr. Kellen is also Medical Editor of *Modern Medicine of Canada*. The selection of Chapters and Authors for this book were his responsibility.

Dr. Russell Hilf is Professor of Biochemistry and of Oncology, University of Rochester School of Medicine and Dentistry, Rochester, New York. His current research interests include the study of hormone action on breast cancer in humans and rodents and the investigation of methods to predict response to therapy. Dr. Hilf has published more than 150 research papers, has served as an Associate Editor for the journal *Cancer Research* and is currently on the Advisory Board for *Cancer Biochemistry Biophysics*. Since 1976, he has been a member of the Breast Cancer Task Force Committee, National Cancer Institute, National Institutes of Health, Bethesda, Maryland.

CONTRIBUTORS

K. M. Anderson, M.D., Ph.D.
Associate Professor of Biochemistry
Rush University
Chicago, Illinois

Jacques Asselin, Ph.D.
Assistant Professor
Laval University
Quebec, Canada

William T. Cave, M.D.
Assistant Professor of Medicine
University of Rochester School of
  Medicine
Rochester, New York

Yoon Sang Cho-Chung, M.D., Ph.D.
Research Biochemist
National Cancer Institute
National Institutes of Health
Bethesda, Maryland

Victor A. Drill, M.D., Ph.D.
Professor of Pharmacology
University of Illinois College of
  Medicine
Chicago, Illinois

Bernard A. Eskin, M.D.
Director of Reproductive
  Endocrinology and
Associate Professor of Obstetrics and
  Gynecology
Medical College of Pennsylvania
Chief, Gynecologic Endocrinology
  Section, Division of Obstetrics and
  Gynecology
Albert Einstein Medical Center
Philadelphia, Pennsylvania

Edward H. Fowler, D.V.M., Ph.D.
Manager of Pathology and
  Laboratory Animal Resources
Department of Pathology
Carnegie-Mellon Institute of Research
Pittsburgh, Pennsylvania

Joan T. Harmon, Ph.D.
Postdoctoral Fellow
Diabetes Branch, NIAMDD
National Institutes of Health
Bethesda, Maryland

Russell Hilf, Ph.D.
Professor of Biochemistry
University of Rochester
School of Medicine and Dentistry
Rochester, New York

Vincent P. Hollander, M.D., Ph.D.
Professor of Medicine and Director
Research Institute, Hospital for Joint
  Diseases and Medical Center
New York, New York

John A. Kellen, M.D., Ph.D.
Associate Professor
Department of Clinical Biochemistry
Sunnybrook Medical Centre
University of Toronto
Toronto, Ontario, Canada

Paul A. Kelly, Ph.D.
Senior Member
MRC Group in Molecular
  Endocrinology and Assistant
  Professor
Department of Physiology
Laval University
Quebec, Canada

**N. A. Kerenyi, M.D., F.R.C.
  (Pathol.)**
Associate Professor of Pathology
University of Toronto
Toronto, Ontario, Canada

**Fernand Labrie, M.D., Ph.D.
  F.R.C.P.(C)**
Professor and Director
MRC Group in Molecular
  Endocrinology
Laval University,
Quebec, Canada

Robert M. MacLeod, M.D., Ph.D.
Professor of Medicine
University of Virginia School of
  Medicine
Charlottesville, Virginia

J. W. Meakin, M.D., C.M.,
  F.R.C.P.(C)
Executive Director
The Ontario Cancer Treatment and
  Research Foundation
Toronto, Ontario, Canada

B. G. Mobbs, Ph.D
Clinical Research Associate
Ontario Cancer Treatment Research
  Foundation
Assistant Professor of Surgery
University of Toronto
Toronto, Ontario, Canada

Arthur H. Rossof, M.D.
Assistant Professor of Medicine
Rush Medical College
Chicago, Illinois

N. A. Samaan, M.D., Ph.D.,
  F.A.C.P., F.R.C.P.
Professor of Medicine and Physiology
  and Chief, Section of Endocrinology
The University of Texas System
  Cancer Center
    M. D. Anderson Hospital
Professor of Medicine
The University of Texas Medical School
Houston, Texas

Samir M. Shafie, Ph.D.
Visiting Scientist
Laboratory of Pathophysiology
National Cancer Institute
National Institutes of Health
Bethesda, Maryland

John Stevens, M.D.
Head
Leukemia Section
Research Institute, Hospital for Joint
  Diseases and Medical Center
New York, New York

Yee-Wan Stevens, M.S.
Research Assistant
Research Institute, Hospital for Joint
  Diseases and Medical Center
New York, New York

TABLE OF CONTENTS

Volume I

Volume II

Chapter 1

THE INFLUENCE OF ANDROGENS ON TUMOR DEVELOPMENT

K. M. Anderson and A. H. Rossof

TABLE OF CONTENTS

I. INTRODUCTION

Before considering the influence of testosterone and its congeners on the development and subsequent growth of different cancers, ideally the structures, sites of synthesis, and some cellular and subcellular biochemical effects of male sex hormones should be discussed. In lieu of this, the reader is referred to some of the excellent recent (post-1972) reviews concerning the physiology and biochemistry of androgens.[1-14] Those whose major interests are in other fields will find these subjects examined in great detail with copious documentation; the specialist in this field is already aware of the extensive information they contain.

For the authors purposes, androgens encompass the natural and synthetic derivatives of the C19 steroid nucleus (5 α-androstane) able to maintain the secondary sexual characteristics of experimental animals. Synthetic compounds include alkylated and non-alkylated androgens and derivatives of 19-nortestosterone.[14]

The nature of the biochemical events that follow administration of androgens can vary from the induction of cell division with the wide range of new RNA transcripts that this implies, to amplification of ongoing metabolic processes during cell growth that is independent of cell division,[15] to a much more limited stimulation of specific enzymatic activity, such as β-glucuronidase in the mouse kidney by 5α-androstane-diols.[16] Many, but not all (e.g., induction of β-glucuronidase) of these events seem to require qualitative or quantitative alterations in transcription of RNA. Androgens appear to function as switches to select specific developmental pathways, to activate events leading to cell division, or to amplify ongoing differentiated metabolic processes. The relationships between these different functions are not established. Expression of major developmental pathways involves replication of specific cells leading to particular intrinsically programmed biochemical events.

Any speculations about how androgen receptors (see Mobbs, in Volume I, Chapter 2) alter transcription must incorporate recent information about the organization of chromatin into subunits or nucleosomes. According to some reports, all genomic sequences are included in the repeat structure, the particles are randomly distributed, and include both active and inactive template. Other workers believe that template active regions of chromatin consist of more open and extended regions of DNA, devoid of histone-rich, RNA-free nucleoprotein complexes sedimenting at 11 to 13S. Participation of higher order folding of chromatin and of acetylation and phosphorylation of histone and nonhistone proteins in the control of gene expression are subjects of active study, although most of this work has not been performed in androgen-sensitive tissues.

Rapid in vivo and in vitro changes in phosphorylation of nuclear acidic proteins from the ventral prostate follow the administration of testosterone,[17] and the central role of acidic nuclear proteins in mandating the response to androgens is indicated.[18] The number of nuclear binding sites for androgen receptors, the nature of the acceptor material (whether protein, DNA, or their combination), the effect of added cytosol receptor on the activity of purified RNA polymerases and the template activity of prostate chromatin,[19] the function of the DNA unwinding protein,[20] effects of androgens on protein synthesis independent of new RNA synthesis,[21] and interactions between cytosol and nuclear protein kinases, cyclic nucleotides and enzyme activity[22] all represent active areas of study. Any of them may prove to be important for understanding how androgens can modify tumor growth and development. Progesterone cytosol receptor is believed to include two subunits; the B subunit binds specifically to acidic chromosomal proteins (AP₃) while the A component associates in a nonspecific manner with DNA.[23] The extent to which androgens or other steroid hormone receptors mimic this pattern is not yet established.

II. GENETIC AND EPIGENETIC CHANGES IN CARCINOGENESIS: POINTS OF INTERACTION WITH ANDROGENS

It is widely agreed that steroid hormones are not proximate carcinogens in the manner of carcinogenic hydrocarbons and other active agents.[24-26] Their tumor-promoting activity is believed related to imbalance of normal physiological functions. Thus, increased cancer incidence due to androgens (and possibly some other steroid hormones) is not thought to be due to direct but rather indirect effects on target cells that potentiate the actions of other proximate agents.

The Ames mutagenicity test provides evidence of mutagenicity in a bacterial test system and of the presumption of carcinogenicity in metazoans.[27] With few exceptions, agents that are carcinogenic in man or animals are mutagenic in that system. For example, diethylstilbestrol is weakly mutagenic and its administration to several animal species is associated with development of cancer, while carcinoma of the vagina develops in a small percentage of young women whose mothers received the drug during early pregnancy for threatened abortion.[28] The authors have been unable to document the possible mutagenicity of androgens examined by the Ames test, but this information should provide direct evidence concerning this point. If androgens are mutagenic in this system, presumably they will be able to function as proximate carcinogens. However, inability to transform organ or tissue culture cells grown in their presence suggests that they may not function in this manner (see Section III.D). Steroids can physically associate with histones and DNA in vivo and in vitro, which could be a prerequisite for altering the function of the DNA template. Irreversible binding of norethisterone epoxide to proteins with SH groups but not to DNA and RNA has been observed, which required incubation with a superoxide generating system provided by hepatic microsomes.[29] Such reactive intermediates might bind to nuclear proteins and modify their function.

The classical two-step model of carcinogenesis in the skin, including an initiating event due to a proximate carcinogen and subsequent effects of promotion on the development of skin cancers, is well known.[30] Knudson proposed a two-mutation model of retinoblastoma involving a prezygotic (germ cell) mutation plus a postzygotic (somatic cell) mutation. Comings suggested that the double mutation released a tissue specific transforming gene.[31] Cells are thought to possess multiple structural genes capable of coding for transforming factors that release cells from normal constraints on their growth. Regulatory genes, presumably paired, would suppress these tissue-specific transforming genes.

The hypothesis that cancer arises as a consequence of two or more mutations in a single cell was examined by Nordling who suggested that the age-specific incidence, $I = kt^{r-1}$, where t reflects age and r the number of mutations.[32] Overall cancer mortality in many countries increases with age as the sixth power of time, implying that r was equal to seven. Armitage and Doll[33] concluded that the age-incidence of cancer of the stomach, colon, rectum, and pancreas was consistent with this, while cancers of the lung, bladder, ovary, endometrium, cervix, breast, and prostate were not. This latter group of cancers might be subject to varying initiating and promoting influences, such as age-dependent effects of endocrine changes, over the lifetime of the individual. When this formulation was applied to latent and clinical prostatic cancer and plotted on a double logarithmic scale, a linear relationship between frequency and age was obtained.[34] The slope of the line was greater for clinical cancers, corresponding to the seventh power of age, suggesting that latent cancer results from a smaller number of "hits" than clinical prostatic cancer. Increasing frequency of a cancer with age might be due to continued or increased exposure to a carcinogen or to some direct or indirect but unknown consequence of aging (e.g., reduced ability to repair damaged DNA, etc.).

A requirement for more than one necessary event (multiple hit theory[35]) in the development of many clinical cancers clarifies the phenomena of latency, penetrance, and pleiotropism (occurrence of cancer in more than one organ) and is compatible with the concept of tumor progression embodied by Foulds six general principles of tumor progression.[36]

However, it is not settled that the events leading to neoplastic change need to be mutations in the sense of defects in DNA (point mutations, deletion of base pairs leading to frame shifts, etc.). Clonal development of cancer from a single cell might arise from disordered functional development due to epigenetic causes.[37] Proponents of this idea suggest that critical events in carcinogenesis may involve abnormal cytoplasmic control of nuclear gene function and need not primarily depend upon altered DNA for its expression. It is argued that the basic cellular mechanisms that underlie normal differentiation and cancer are fundamentally similar, but in the latter process, expression of the cells developmental pattern is abnormal. The totipotency and normal differentiation of single teratocarcinoma cells injected into mouse blastocysts is consistent with the view that teratocarcinogenesis involved changes in gene function rather than gene structure, which was restored to normal by an appropriate environment.[38]

From one point of view, cancers, whether of genetic or epigenetic origin, can be viewed as examples of blocked cellular differentiation, with the retention of a matrix of biochemical reactions inappropriate for a differentiated cell from the tissue of origin.[39] If a program for normal development of a cell is represented as a series of multiple, interrelated, branching Markov chains with a large number of links,[40] interdiction of particular events required for normal growth and differentiation by epigenetic rather than genetic means should result in phenotypically comparable developmental defects. The problem of imagining ways that steroid hormones might directly or indirectly induce crucial epigenetic changes leading to cellular autonomy is different from suggesting mechanisms that require direct modification of cellular DNA.

Generally, experimental hormone-induced carcinogenesis has been studied by repeated administration of excess hormone to attempt overstimulation of the target organ or by creating hormonal imbalance (e.g., suppress negative feedback due to estrogen by implantation of ovaries in the spleen, etc.). Berenblum has classified seven types of cocarcinogenesis.[30] If it is unlikely that androgens serve as direct (proximate) carcinogens and as there is presently no evidence that they serve as additive, synergistic, or incomplete cocarcinogenic agents as defined by Berenblum, their participation in one of the other categories of cocarcinogenic events is possible. Permissive influences affect rates of absorbtion, metabolism, or detoxification of the active agent; preparative action renders the target organ more susceptible to a carcinogen; conditional influences modify the continued growth of a transformed cell; and lastly, enhancement of a putative effect of a virus on the target cell could occur.

Although they are not mutually exclusive, participation of androgens in mechanisms two through six can be considered (Table 1). It is also clear that alternative formulations of this problem are possible.

III. ANDROGENS AS CARCINOGENS OR COCARCINOGENS

A. Cancer Associated with Administration or Secretion of Androgens in Man
1. Clinical Observations

A variety of C_{17}-substituted androgenic-anabolic steroids have been associated with the development of hepatic neoplasms in humans (Table 2). The precise nature of these tumors varies considerably from case to case. Although frequently referred to as hepatocellular carcinomas or hepatomas, the behavior of many of these tumors bears little resemblance to typical human hepatomas.

The first case reported occurred in a 27-year-old male Caucasian with Fanconi's anemia (FA) who had been taking androgenic-anabolic steroid preparation for a number of years.[41] He died in hepatic failure and autopsy revealed "nodules...of hepatocellular carcinoma" (HCC) and postnecrotic cirrhosis. Since cirrhosis has long been recognized as a risk factor in the development of HCC, incrimination of these hor-

TABLE 1

Possible Mechanisms of Androgen-enhanced Carcinogenesis

I. Direct effects
  1. Binding to and modification of nuclear DNA or its associated proteins, or alteration of events in the cell cytoplasm which modify cell differentiation by epigenetic rather than genetic means
II. Indirect mechanisms
  2. Permissive effects, modifying the absorbtion, degradation of proximate carcinogens or their precursors
  3. Preparative actions, possibly by stimulating cell growth or cell division, rendering the target cell more responsive to carcinogenesis
  4. Enhance, by either deficient feedback inhibition or, less likely, by positive stimulation, the formation of hormonal or other growth-promoting agents which increase the development of cancer by chronic overstimulation of the target cells
  5. Conditional effects upon transformed cells, such as increasing the growth of a hormone-dependent tumor, modifying host immune resistence, etc.
  6. Conversion to another substance able to increase the incidence of tumors (e.g., androgens as precursors of estrogens)
III. Remote antecedent effects
  7. Permit the expression of cancer in an organ whose development required androgen-dependent embryonic induction with or without acquisition of phenotypic gender

TABLE 2

Androgens and Anabolic Steroids Administered to Patients Who Subsequently Developed Hepatic Tumors

Trivial name	Chemical designation
17-Alkyl-substituted compounds	
Methyl testosterone	17β-hydroxy-17-methyl-androst-4-ene-3-one
Testosterone enanthate	17β[(1-oxoheptyl)oxy]-androst-4-en-3-one
Stanozolol	17-methyl-2H-5α-androst-2-eno[3,2-c]pyrazol-17β-ol
Oxandrolone	17β-hydroxy-17-methyl-2-oxa-5α-androstan-3-one
Oxymetholone	17β-hydroxy-2(hydroxymethylene)-17-methyl-5α-androstan-3-one
Methandrostenolone	17β-hydroxy-17-methylandrosta-1,4-dien-3-one
19-Nor compounds	
Nandrolone decanoate	17β[(1-oxadecyl)oxy]-estr-4-en-3-one
Norethandrolone	17-hydroxy-19-norpregn-4-en-3-one

mones alone in the etiology or pathogenesis of HCC in this patient is in doubt. An additional patient with FA[42] developed a hepatoma on a background of posttransfusional macronodular cirrhosis and hemochromatosis, but she had never received androgenic hormone preparations.

The development of some form of hepatic neoplasia was reported in five other patients with FA who received androgenic-anabolic steroid preparations (AASP)[43-48] FA is an autosomal recessive disease characterized by microcephaly, growth retardation, skeletal malformation, brownish hyperpigmentation, occasional mental deficiency, and pancytopenia. There is also a proclivity for developing cancer both in the affected patient and his relatives.[49] The androgenic-anabolic steroid preparations are used to support the failing bone marrow. This disorder is also associated with chromosomal instability, and is manifested by enhanced transformation by SV40 of cultured fibroblasts[50] and defective DNA repair,[51] apparently the result of a deficient exonuclease.[52] Despite the reported association of HCC with ingestion of androgen-anabolic steroid preparations, these extraordinary features of Fanconi's anemia somewhat weaken the argument that AASP constitutes a carcinogen or cocarcinogen for all humans.

A 21-year-old man with a syndrome described as a Fanconi variant, lacking the congenital anomalies, developed acute myelogenous leukemia. At postmortem examination, three 2.5-cm hepatic nodules were incidentally detected and were characterized as hepatomas.[53]

An additional six patients[44,54-57] with anemia (two with paroxysmal nocturnal hemoglobinuria[56,57] treated with AASP have developed hepatic tumors. In two patients, the lesions were multiple,[44] in three they were single,[55-57] and in one there was only clinical evidence of HCC without histopathologic confirmation.[54]

Hepatic tumors also developed in three patients without anemia but with endocrine disorders. A 68-year-old man who took methyltestosterone for 30 years for impotency developed a low-grade solitary HCC.[58] A 40-year-old man developed a solitary well-differentiated HCC after taking methyltestosterone for 8 years, along with thyroxin and cortisone for hypopituitarism.[56] After taking methyltestosterone and testosterone propionate for 8 years, a 33-year-old cryptorchid man developed a solitary, well-differentiated HCC.[56] A 27-year-old female transsexual taking 150 mg of methyltestosterone daily for 37 months presented with a painful right hypochondrial mass which upon surgery was found to be a liver adenoma.[59] Hearsay evidence is available that a bodybuilder who took anabolic steroids for a number of years developed Wilms tumor at the age of 38.[60] This is a common tumor of the mesonephric kidney in children but is extremely rare in adults, suggesting a possible association of this tumor with the use of AASP.

In many cases, the clinical behavior of these tumors is not consistent with that of the usual idiopathic HCC of human beings. In three cases,[44,56] there was clinical or roentgenographic evidence of tumor regression upon cessation of therapy with AASP. In other cases,[56] there were extended periods of life after tumor diagnosis. Although some patients died quickly[47,48] (more consistent with the usual clinical behavior of HCC), almost all of the tumors have been classified histologically as low grade, well differentiated,[43-45,53,55,56,58] or benign.[47,57,59]

Regression of these tumors, the chronicity of many cases, and the frequent bland histopathologic appearance all suggest that these neoplasms are not invariably malignant. The ultimate interpretation of the nature of these lesions is further hampered because many case reports are extremely brief and histopathologic material is reproduced in only six cases.[41,44,47,53] This is further complicated by some reviewers who do not accept the original histopathologic interpretations.[61,62]

In recent years, certain human neoplasms, including HCC, have been associated with the appearance in the serum of a protein marker, alpha fetoprotein (alpha FP). This marker was sought in 12 cases, but was positive in only 1[54] and this single case lacked histopathologic confirmation. Alpha FP was also increased in the one patient with FA who developed HCC without exposure to AASP.[42] The infrequent identification of this protein in this group of patients further defines the atypical character of this lesion.

Sweeney and Evans[47] reported one patient with FA and a benign hepatoma. Distant from the neoplastic lesion, they noted other hepatic changes, such as generalized hyperplasia and hepatocytic nodule formation. They observed two additional patients who had been taking oxymetholone and prednisone for 3 months each. Their hepatic histology also demonstrated nonneoplastic hepatocytic alterations such as mid-zone hyperplastic nodules and thickening of the liver cell plates. Their observations may indicate that AASP induces a series of hepatocellular changes culminating in tumor formation. Anthony[63] has reported that liver cell dysplasia is a cytologic representation of a premalignant state. Indeed, sequential changes such as these have been observed in a variety of experimental hepatic tumors.[64]

It has been known for some time that 17-alkylated androgen-anabolic steroid preparations are hepatotoxic.[65,66] The toxicity is usually slight and is detected by abnormalities noted on routine periodic blood test. Uncommonly, jaundice or other clinical signs of hepatic damage appear.

A detailed prospective analysis of liver damage due to methyltestosterone has recently appeared.[59] Of 60 patients taking 150 mg/day of this agent, 19 had at least one abnormality of serum chemistries reflecting liver injury. Of 52 liver scans done, 33 were abnormal with either enlargement of the liver, striking irregularity of the colloid uptake, or both abnormalities. In 11 liver biopsies performed, all demonstrated periportal liver cell thickening. Sinusoidal dilatation, microcyst formation, cholestasis, and migration of hepatocytes into vascular walls were noted in some of the cases. A single large liver adenoma was found in this series.

Peliosis hepatis, a benign proliferation of intrahepatic vascular channels, has been reported in patients taking AASP.[67] Intra-abdominal hemorrhage due to rupture of the cyst can be rapidly fatal.

In summary, idiopathic hepatocellular carcinomas in North America occur more often in males, with a male to female ratio of 1.9 for Caucasian and 2.7 for black patients.[68] Of the 17 reported cases of HCC associated with ingestion of androgen-anabolic steroid preparations reviewed by the authors, 7 had Fanconi's anemia, an extremely rare constitutional disorder characterized by an increased incidence of cancer. Hepatocarcinogenesis is favored by an androgenic environment, both in man and experimental animals (Sections III.B and III.C). Androgen-anabolic steroid preparations commonly cause biochemical, histologic, and clinical evidence of hepatic damage. Consequently, great caution should be exercised in the follow-up care and management of patients receiving these drugs, and they should not be prescribed for trivial reasons to healthy individuals who desire them for their protein-anabolic effect.[69]

Since 1973, close to 100 cases of benign hepatic tumors in young women using oral contraceptives have been reported.[60,69] It is not evident whether residual androgenic activity of progestational compounds could be implicated in the genesis of these tumors. Relationships between hepatic tumors and oral contraceptives are reviewed in Volume I, Chapter 6, by Drill.

2. Incidence of Cancer and Genetic Sex

The effect of genetic sex on cancer incidence can be analyzed at several levels. Differences in rates of organ-specific cancer in males and females are striking, but the immediate biological mechanisms by which genetic sex and its attendant hormonal differences might contribute to them are not established (Table 3).[70]

At the most basic level, differences in sex-organ cancers depend upon events occurring during embryogenesis (Mechanism 6 in Table 1). Phenotypic differentiation as a male following secretion of testosterone by the fetal testes is a necessary but insufficient precondition for subsequent development of cancer in sex-hormone-dependent target organs.[71] Development of cancer at these sites is thought to require continued stimulation of hormone-dependent cells over a prolonged period of time, possibly by a trophic steroid or pituitary hormone (Categories 2, 3, 4, and 5, in Table 1). Reduced synthesis of androgens with increased pituitary secretion of hormones (Category 4, in Table 1) trophic for primary or accessory sex organs occurring over many years may be important for the genesis of some of these cancers but the details are unknown. While there are experimental models available for induction of cancer by thyroid hormones and estrogens, results of attempts to produce cancers with androgens are more ambiguous (Section III.B).

When cancers of the nonsexual organs are considered, any relationship with androgens is even more obscure. Comparison of cancer incidence in children before the onset

TABLE 3

Overall Male to Female Incidence of Cancer Based on Estimated New Cases for 1977

Site	Ratio of male to female incidence[a]
Buccal cavity and pharynx (oral)	2.46
Digestive organs	1.09
Respiratory system	3.57
Bone, tissue, and melanoma	1.01
Breast	0.008
Genital organs	0.90
Urinary organs	2.30
Eye	0.89
Brain and central nervous system	1.18
Endocrine glands	0.42
Leukemia	1.29
Multiple myeloma	1.05
Lymphomas	1.23
All other and unspecified sites	0.98

(From Silverberg, E. , *CA Cancer J. Clin.*, 27, 34, 1977.)

[a] Incidence rates are derived from the National Cancer
Institute 3rd National Survey 1969 to 1971 National
Cancer Institute, Bethesda, Maryland, 1971.

of puberty provides some insight into innate differences in cancer incidence that should
not be directly related to levels of circulating androgens or other steroid hormones.
Although the overall prepubertal incidence of bone and kidney cancer is comparable,
leukemia, malignant brain tumors, lymphosarcoma, and Burkitts lymphoma are more
frequent in males, while other connective tissue tumors occur more often in females.[70]
Presently it is not possible to sort out etiologic factors responsible for differences in
cancer incidence in either sex that may be related to gender and its attendant hormonal
milieu. Either gender might entail linkage of structural or regulatory information related or not to hormonal milieu and important for the expression of cancer in a particular organ, but until detailed mapping of genes on the X and Y or other chromosomes
is done, little can be said about this. Association of the HY antigen locus on the Y
chromosome in Tfm/Y mice is a case in point.[72] Although some human diseases with
an increased incidence of cancer are inherited in a sex-linked recessive pattern (e.g.,
testicular feminization, certain gammaglobulinopathies, Fabry's syndrome or diffuse
angiokeratomas, vitamin D-resistant rickets, acrokeratosis verruciformis, congenital
dyskeratosis, or the Zinsser-Cole-Engman syndrome), there is no evidence that the
hormonal milieu associated with gender is important for their development. Other tumors (multiple trichoepithelioma, focal dermal hypoplasia) are inherited in a sex-
linked dominant manner.

    The incidence of cancer in adult males is greater in the respiratory tract, presumably
chiefly due to smoking, and in the urinary bladder, kidney, and brain, as is the incidence of lymphoma and leukemia. Women have about 3 times the incidence of thyroid
cancer, and 130 times as much breast cancer. The overall incidence of genital and
gastrointestinal cancer is comparable, although its distribution in the latter differs for
reasons that are not known (e.g., increased esophageal and gastric cancer in males,
and more gall bladder cancer, often associated with cholelithiasis in females). If it is
true that 80 to 90% of all cancers are induced by agents in the environment, a search
for sex-related cancers becomes obscured due to the overlay of differing exposures to

environmental carcinogens. To some extent, this can be circumvented by comparisons of sex-related rates of incidence of different cultures; an incidence directly related to gender should be universally expressed. For example, a male predominance of 9:1 is seen with Kaposi's sarcoma among Jews, Italians, and Bantus in the Congo. However, for most cancers, the contribution from the environment overshadows differences due to gender, both within the same sex (e.g., U.S. males have 45 times the incidence of prostatic cancer, compared to males in Singapore) or between sexes (males in Mozambique have about 1000 times the incidence of hepatic cancer, compared with Canadian women).[73]

The much greater incidence of primary lung cancer (and others, including pancreas and bladder cancer) in males parallels their increased exposure to carcinogens and is certainly not due to any innate difference in response to these agents, as is indicated by the gradually increasing incidence of lung cancer in women who smoke regularly, related overall to the length of exposure (pack-years). This is not to say that the individual rate at which males and females or even members of the same sex develop lung cancer may not differ due to subtle differences in their ability to activate or detoxify particular carcinogens. If, for example, the inducibility of aryl hydrocarbon hydroxylase is important for the genesis of lung cancer, by virtue of converting "procarcinogens to proximate carcinogens, individual differences in the inducability of the enzyme that might be influenced by genetic sex could modify the rate of development of lung cancer.[74] (It should be noted that there is uncertainty about the role of aryl hydrocarbon hydroxylase in the genesis of lung cancer.) Such considerations probably apply to other cancers and are especially evident in animal model systems in which males are less susceptible to some but more susceptible to other carcinogens (Sections III.B and III.C).

Small renal cortical adenomas are found more frequently in males than females, while the incidence of adenocarcinoma of the kidney is twice as high in males.[75] The overall incidence of cancer is equal until the time of the female menopause, but subsequently age-adjusted rates in males are higher. Overall rates of survival are probably comparable, although a few reports that survival is greater in women have been published. In malignant melanoma, there is general agreement that women with this disease live longer than men, but the reasons for this are unknown. Approximately 25% of malignant melanomas contain estrogen receptors; their significance is obscure.[76] Even within one sex, response to a tumor can vary widely; some 25% of men with clinically diagnosed carcinoma of the prostate experience rapid clinical deterioration and die within approximately 3 years, while the rest of this population undergoes a much more indolent clinical course, frequently dying of some intercurrent disease of the elderly. We are at a loss to explain these differences in response, either within or among the sexes.

3. Cancer Associated with Abnormal Sexual Differentiation and Inborn Errors of Metabolism

The following includes an abbreviated catalogue of syndromes with an increased incidence of cancer in which, although there is no direct evidence, androgens might play some etiologic role.[77,78]

Overall, the risk of gonadal malignancy in XY-gonadal dysgenesis (Swyer syndrome) is about 25%. In gonadal dysgenesis not associated with a Y chromosome (as Turner's syndrome), gonadal tumor incidence is not increased, implying that elevated gonadotropins themselves are not carcinogenic. However, nongonadal tumors, especially of neural origin, are increased. Gonadal tumors are found in 15 to 20% of 45X/46XY mosaics, usually occurring during the 2nd and 3rd decades.

In true hermaphrodites, in 46XX sex-reversed males with both ovarian and testicular tissue, and in female pseudohermaphrodites the risk of neoplasia is not increased, suggesting that at least in these patients, neither increased ACTH nor androgenic steroids directly induce cancer. In teratogenic forms of female pseudohermaphroditism following exposure in utero to exogenous androgens or progestational compounds, the developmental defects are not associated with increased evidence of cancer. Testosterone, 6α-methyltestosterone, ethisterone, norethindrone and norethindrone acetate, and virilizing maternal tumors have all caused this disorder.

Males with persistent Mullerian duct remnants have an increased incidence of testicular neoplasms approaching that of cryptorchid testes. A syndrome of male genital ambiguity, congenital nephrosis, and Wilms' tumor has been reported.[79] None of the syndromes of male pseudohermaphroditism due to enzyme defects, such as 5α-reductase deficiency, include an increased incidence of cancer. Individuals with complete testicular feminization (46XY with bilateral intra-abdominal testes) experience an incidence of testicular malignancy comparable to those with cryptorchid testes. The disorder is inherited as a sex-linked recessive or male-limited autosomal dominant; the biochemical defect is thought to be due to absence of cytosol receptor proteins for 5α-dihydrotestosterone (DHT) in the target organs. Whether this directly contributes to increased incidence of malignancy in the cryptorchid testes which are subject to malignant change is not established. Cryptorchidism is associated with a 14-fold increase in testicular neoplasia. It is not known if the same factor(s) responsible for maldescent also induces cancer, or if the intra-abdominal environment somehow predisposes to its development. However, in 25% of cases the cancer arises in the normally descended testicle. Patients with incomplete testicular feminization, the Reifenstein syndrome, pseudovaginal perineoscrotal hypospadias, anorchia, agonadia, and syndromes due to errors in testosterone biosynthesis do not experience an increased incidence of cancer. In the Kleinfelter syndrome (XXY constitution), gonadal tumors are not increased, again suggesting that increased gonadotropins need not be carcinogenic. However, the incidence of breast cancer is 20 times that of normal males, and the incidence of leukemia may be greater. The role of androgens in the development of human breast cancer is discussed in Volume II, Chapter 8, by Meakin. Primary testicular cancers include seminomas, embryonal carcinoma, choriocarcinoma, and teratomas; 40% of these tumors contain two or more cell types. Leydig and Sertoli cell tumors usually are benign.

Burton hypogammaglobulinemia, sex-linked severe combined immunodeficiency disease, and the Wiscott-Aldrich syndrome are sex-linked immune deficiencies with an associated increased incidence of various malignancies. They are mentioned because of their sex-linkage and appearance in males; there is no evidence to implicate androgenic steroids directly in their genesis or subsequent clinical course.

4. Benign Prostatic Hypertrophy and Carcinoma of the Prostate as Paradigms of Androgen-Related Abnormalities in the Control of Cell Growth and Division

Since benign prostatic hypertrophy (BPH) and carcinoma of the prostate (CAP) do not occur in males castrated before puberty, the endocrine system and especially products such as androgens elaborated by the testes must be involved in the genesis of these disorders. In addition, regression of established BPH or CAP can occur after castration or treatment with antiandrogens, evidence that androgens can influence the progression of these disorders. The incidence of BPH increases with age, and by age 80 essentially 100% of surviving males will have histologic evidence of the disease, with an incidence of carcinoma *in situ* of 4 to 6% in different series of patients requiring surgery for clinically diagnosed BPH. Carcinoma of the prostate (17%) is the second most frequent cancer in males (after cancer of the lung) and the third (10%) most common cause of cancer death (after lung and bowel cancer). About 57,000 new cases are expected to be diagnosed in the U.S. during 1977, an incidence of 16 per 10^5 population with some 20,000 deaths yearly attributable to this cause.

Benign prostatic hypertrophy occurs in the inner periurethral glandular tissue, which includes fibromuscular tissue derived from the Mullerian ducts, responsive to estrogens. A possible role for estrogens in the etiology of BPH was suggested as long ago as 1937, by Zuckerman.[80] Lacassagne[81] demonstrated growth of the dorsal lobe and urinary retention in mice after administration of estrogen. Estrogens produce increase in fibromuscular stroma and metaplasia of the epithelium of various animals, including monkeys, dogs, squirrels, and guinea pigs. Androgens antagonized these changes, but these disorders induced in the laboratory do not closely mimic human disease. Franks has classified BPH into five main forms: stromal, fibromuscular, muscular, fibroadenomatous, and fibromyadenomatous.[82] Epithelial elements are responsive to castration, but the extent to which stromal cells regress is not settled.

Of various animal species examined, only the prostates of man and dog spontaneously enlarge with age. While there are many similarities between prostatic enlargement in these two species (age incidence, size of gland, etc.), in the dog the disease primarily involves the epithelial elements of the whole gland which enlarges posteriorly causing constipation rather than involving the peripheral gland, leading to symptoms involving the lower urinary tract as in man. In addition, androstanediols seem able to promote BPH in the dog,[83] while in man, DHT is found in the prostate in increasing amounts with age.[84]

Siiteri and Wilson[84] measured the androgen content of human normal and hyperplastic prostates, observing that DHT was at least fivefold greater ($0.6 \pm .01$ ng/100 g vs. $0.13 + 0.05$ ng/100 g) in the hyperplastic prostate. The rate of formation of DHT by the 5α-reductase in normal and hyperplastic glands was similar. Georgi and collaborators observed an increased ability of tissue from hypertrophic glands to concentrate DHT.[85] DHT was found to be more mitogenic than testosterone in organ culture.[86] In addition, in the rat, age-associated changes in the affinity of prostate cytosol receptor for testosterone and DHT were suggested.[87]

After castration, 2-year-old dogs that received pharmacologic amounts of testosterone or DHT (75 mg/week) for 18 to 24 months did not develop BPH, although it was found in several of the untreated control dogs.[88] In a subsequent study, castrated dogs were treated with DHT (25 mg/week) and estrogen (0.75 mg/week), androstanediol (75 mg/week), or androstanediol with estrogen (same doses) for 1 year.[83] The last combination produced massive enlargement of the prostate (averaging 35.8 ± 1.4 g vs. 12.5 ± 2.1 g for the control), while androstanediol increased prostatic weight to 14.7 g.

Androgen deficiency, androgen excess, and estrogen imbalance have all been considered responsible for BPH. BPH involves the ambisexual part of the prostate (middle and lateral lobes) including the inner part of the gland thought to be of Mullerian duct origin and possibly sensitive to both hormones. Enlargement of the prostate due to estrogens has been observed in patients with feminizing tumors and in the newborn as a result of maternal estrogens. On the other hand, Huggins considered that nodular hyperplasia with tall columnar epithelium represents effects of androgens on cells with a reduced threshold for their effects.[89] Characteristically, symptomatic BPH is less frequent in patients with alcoholic cirrhosis with reduced degradation of estrogens, providing indirect evidence for the important role of androgens in the process.

Carcinoma of the prostate arises from the outer prostatic glands, some 80% posteriorly or posterolaterally, caudal to the genitourinary ducts. It may be preceded by atrophy, followed by hyperplasia, the progression to neoplasia with invasion through the capsule finally occurring after a prolonged period of clinically occult disease. Extension outside of the prostate is usually associated with increased prostatic acid phosphatase in the blood serum and urine, although the concentration of the enzyme in prostatic cancer cells is less than the normal prostate. Microscopic evidence of carcinoma *in situ* is reported to be present in about 30% of males over 50 years of age, but the disease is rare before that age. Prostatic cancer in the very old seems to be more indolent clinically than in younger patients.

The relationship, if any, between BPH and CAP is debated. Some workers report no association,[90] while others find a three- to fourfold greater increase in risk of CAP in patients with BPH.[91] Since the latter becomes universal in males with increasing age, sorting out of any relationship is difficult. Reduced HLA antigen B8 and increased A28 and BW 22[92] are associated more often in patients with prostatic cancer. A three-fold increased risk to first degree relatives of affected patients affected with one of a number of site-specific cancers, including carcinoma of the prostate, is claimed.[93]

Racial differences in BPH and CAP are striking, and both appear to be clinically less frequent in members of the black and oriental races living in third world and Asian countries. Japanese men with about 1/20th the age-adjusted incidence of prostatic cancer compared with U.S. blacks are reported to have a comparable number of carcinomas *in situ*. The role of environment in clinical expression of the disease is crucial, since studies of immigrant groups to the U.S. and elsewhere suggest a rise toward the levels found in indigenous members of the population. Influences of diet, particularly those diets high in animal fat, with possible alterations in the metabolism of steroid hormones, and sexual mores with early exposure to sexually transmitted viruses are factors being analyzed with respect to the etiology of prostatic disease.[94] Several non-cancerous lesions involve the outer groups of prostatic glands and include simply atrophy (probably due to diminishing circulating androgens), sclerotic atrophy with lymphocytic infiltration (which can be produced in animals by administration or deprivation of androgens), postatrophic hyperplasia (either nodular or postsclerotic with budding of epithelium from atrophic ducts), and, finally, secondary hyperplasia. Areas of cancer can develop from postsclerotic hyperplasia; the other morphological forms are not thought to be precancerous.[82]

Several spontaneous prostatic tumors are available in animals and polycyclic hydrocarbons have been used to produce prostatic tumors (cited in Section III.B), but attempts to induce prostatic cancer in animals by hormonal manipulations have generally failed. Recently, prostatic adenocarcinomas (18.4%) were produced in aged Nb rats with a spontaneous incidence of 0.45% by prolonged treatment with pellets of testosterone propionate alone or with pellets of estrogen.[95] TP or estrogen pellets (90% hormone, 10% cholesterol) of 10 mg were implanted subcutaneously and the TP pellets were replaced every 6 to 8 weeks for approximately 60 weeks until tumors developed. Combined treatment resulted in the earlier appearance of tumors which metastasized and (with one exception) were hormone dependent. Tumors were single and arose in the dorsal lobe of the coagulating gland. Larger amounts of TP yielded a greater number of tumors with a shorter mean duration before appearance. Estrone pellets could inhibit a lower but not higher exposure to testosterone, while pretreatment with estrone markedly inhibited subsequent androgen-induced tumorigenesis. Urinary obstruction was frequent, and a few primary tumors of the other organs, including the bladder and mammary glands, also developed. Areas of prostate free of gross tumor frequently showed early lesions *in situ*. Prostatic cancer might originate from atrophic cells responding abnormally to trophic stimuli or from chronically overstimulated cells responding to increased normal stimuli. However, the primary role of androgens may be to maintain at least some cells in a form that can respond to some unidentified proximate carcinogen. These questions simply are unresolved.

a. Relative Testicular Failure as a Concomitant of BPH and Carcinoma of the Prostate

The concentration of testosterone in spermatic blood decreases from the third decade onward, and excretion of testosterone glucuronide declines from the fourth decade. A gradual decline in the apparent free testosterone and a progressive increase in testosterone steroid binding globulin occurs. Other plasma steroids of testicular origin behave in much the same way with age. Arising almost exclusively in the testes, 17-hydroxy-progesterone declines with age. Although 4-androstene-3,17-dione of adrenal origin does not show a significant decrease with age, levels of dehydroepiandrosterone and its sulfate do fall, but other adrenal steroids are not similarly affected. Elderly males also evidence a small rise in estrone and estradiol levels and a considerable increase in the estradiol/testosterone ratio. Estrone and estradiol originate chiefly from peripheral conversion of androstenedione and testosterone, respectively. The free estradiol/testosterone ratios increase from 0.32 in young males to 0.80 in elderly individuals.

Decline in Leydig cell steroid production could follow a change in hypothalamic or pituitary function. Basal levels of luteinizing hormone (LH) and follicle-stimulating hormone (FSH) in males increase with age, although much less than in postmenopausal women. Prolactin levels also increase with age. In elderly males, stimulation of Leydig cell function by human chorionic gonadotropin is less both in absolute and relative terms. The rise in LH and FSH following administration of gonadotrophic releasing hormone is retained in the elderly. However, the rise in plasma testosterone after administration of tamoxifen to elderly males was less than in younger individuals and consistent with a reduced sensitivity to sex-hormone feedback. However, this is not proven because of the lesser rise in gonadotropins and reduced sensitivity of the Leydig cell to their effects.

These results correlate with reduced Leydig cell weight as a function of age. Sommers[96] and Harbitz and Haugen[97] used a morphometric analysis of the prostate and several endocrine organs in normal men and those with BPH, carcinoma, and atypical glandular hyperplasia. A positive relationship between seminiferous tubule weight and the number of Sertoli cells was observed in CAP, CAP + BPH, BPH, and in atypical hyperplasia, suggesting that hormones from this source were important in maintaining germinal epithelium. It was concluded that both BPH and CAP are associated with progressive involution of the gonads and reduced synthesis of androgens, probably due to a relative failure of the steroid-secreting cells of the testes. The stimulus to BPH could arise from nonandrogenic hormones (possibly estrogens or pituitary gonadotropins) acting in some patients on the fibromuscular elements of the prostate. The marked decrease in numbers of Leydig cells with age, seen in patients with CAP, suggested that this disorder developed in association with longstanding progressive decline in the synthesis of androgens. Since BPH begins in the inner glands, and CAP usually develops at their periphery, there seems to be no simple relationship between these disorders arising in embryologically different sites possibly associated with different facets of a gradually changing hormonal milieu.

b. Prostatic Metabolism of Androgens in BPH, CAP, and Aging

In this section some current opinions about prostatic metabolism of androgens will be briefly summarized, adumbrating a great amount of work by many authors.[98] Both normal prostatic tissue and material from patients with benign prostatic hypertrophy incubated with testosterone convert most of the hormone to DHT.[99] The increased amounts of DHT found in prostates of patients with BPH was mentioned.[84] Tissue from patients with carcinoma of the prostate is characteristically less active, and much of the added testosterone remains unconverted.[100] Normally, with advancing age, a relative increase in prostatic formation of 5β metabolites rather than 5α compounds occurs, as does a reduction in the formation of diols. Generally, no differences in physiocochemical properties of cytosol receptors from normal and neoplastic tissue have been observed (100, with at least one exception). [87]

In rodent prostate organ culture, the major metabolite of added testosterone is

DHT, with lesser formation of 3α- and 3β-androstanediol, androstenedione, and androstanedione and androsterone.[101] DHT at 10^{-6} to 10^{-9} M is 10 times as potent as testosterone in preserving structure, and in provoking cell division at higher concentrations. Androstanediol and androsterone were less active, while 3β-androsterone maintained epithelial cell formation, but did not stimulate cell division. Thus, the intracellular concentration of particular metabolites, which could alter with age, appears capable of exerting differential effects upon prostatic cell function.

It is important, but difficult, to untangle effects of aging on the metabolism of androgens. Franks[102] reported that cultured prostatic tissue from old C57 mice was less responsive to testosterone propionate than material from younger animals, was more autonomous in the absence of androgens, and was inhibited less by estrogens. Franks and Chesterman[103] studied age-chimeras of prostatic tissue from old and young animals grafted subcutaneously in C57 mice of various ages. The epithelial atrophy with reduced secretion of old grafts was reversed in prostates residing in younger animals; however, increased mitotic activity and hyperdiploid nuclei associated with greater age persisted. Metabolism of testosterone by MA 160 cells originally derived from human prostatic tissue, was reductive from the 12th to 279th passage, but by the 400th passage the cells had shifted to an oxidative pathway, and the major metabolite was no longer DHT, but rather, androstenedione[104] (however, see Section III.D).

Thus, while a number of functional properties can be evoked in aged prostatic tissue in mice, other changes are not reversed by changes in the extracellular environment and appear to be intrinsic to the cells. Part of these intrinsic changes may involve altered metabolism of androgenic hormones but whether this should be viewed as cause or effect of BPH or CAP and the extent to which these changes are brought about by gradual alterations in concentrations of pituitary or other hormones is not known.

Since the evidence that androgens can function as proximate carcinogens is not strong, additional factors that might promote the development of BPH or CAP have been sought. Light and electron microscopic examination of normal human prostates and tissue from BPH and CAP have not revealed any generally agreed upon morphologic evidence of active virus infection.[105] Dmochowski and co-workers provided morphologic evidence of C type virus particles in some samples of human CAP. Fixed immunofluorescence studies indicated that cells from BPH and CAP contain antigens related to the oncornovirus interspecies P30 protein found in murine, feline, and simian type C viruses.[106] Both CAP and human fetal prostate released particulate matter containing 70S RNA and cellular RNA from normal BPH and CAP tissue hybridized to a limited extent with several murine viral DNAs. Centifanto et al. reported the presence of herpes virion nucleocapsids in human prostatic adenocarcinoma cells, while tumor explants showed positive immunofluorescence when stained with anti-herpes type 2 antiserum.[107] Oncornovirus-like particles have been described in human leukemia, lymphoma, sarcoma, breast cancer, melanoma, brain, lung, and gastrointestinal malignancies.[108] RNA tumor virus-like activity was observed in human prostatic tissue.[109] However, any relationship between indigenous prostatic herpes (or other) viruses and either BPH or CAP is presently conjectural, and Kochs' postulates as applied to such a potential viral carcinogen have not been satisfied.

B. Occurrence of Cancer in Animals Receiving Androgens

Although testosterone is included in some lists of substances causing cancer,[110] recourse to other standard compendia of compounds surveyed for carcinogenic activity yields few examples of cancers developing after protracted administration of excess testosterone or other androgenic hormones and many more reports of negative results.[24-26, 111-115] Studies with *cis*-androstenediol, androstenediol-3α,17α and the corresponding 3β,17β compound, androstenol-17α-one-3,Δ5-*trans*-androstendiol, Δ4-androstenedione-3,17, androsterone, dehydroandrosterone and its *trans* isomer, dihydro-testosterone, 17-ethinyltestosterone, 17-methylandrostanediol-3α,17α and the 3β and Δ^5, 3β isomers, 17-methyltestosterone and testosterone *n*-valerate, testosterone acetate 3-enolbenzoate, (and the 3-enol-*n*-butyrate, 3-enolpropionate), testosterone benzoate (and the *n*-butyrate, *n*-butyrate 3-enol acetate, enoldipropionate, formate, isobutyrate, isobutyrate 3-enolacetate, 3-isobutyrate 3-enolpropionate), and the 3-enolacetate 3-enol-*n*-butyrate of testosterone propionate, injected in various organisms (usually rodents), induced no tumors.[111] While the majority of studies with testosterone did not produce cancers, fibrous tumors at the injection sites were occasionally observed.[111]

The occurrence of mammary carcinoma in mice[116,117] and of murine post-castration adrenal tumors[118] was inhibited by administration of testosterone propionate or acetate. Uterine tumors,[118] an increased incidence of hepatic hemangioendotheliomas in male rats following *o*-aminoazotoluene,[119] and protection against estrogen- and X-ray-induced lymphoma[120,121] were observed following administration of androgens. In various other rodent strains with a spontaneous occurrence of breast cancer and leukemia, treatment with testosterone propionate reduced their incidence.[112] Additional reports that testosterone or its propionate can induce theca cell ovarian and adrenal tumors in rats,[122] renal tumors in AKR mice,[123] uterine sarcomas in mice,[124] and adrenal cortical adenomas in Syrian hamsters[125] have been considered due to a nonspecific cocarcinogenicity of the steroid, especially in those systems requiring prolonged periods of time before a palpable tumor develops.

Weekly subcutaneous injection of 1.25 mg of testosterone propionate in sesame oil to a group of irradiated rats containing equal numbers of males and females was associated with 9 and 19 local fibrosarcomas, respectively.[120] Pellets of testosterone propionate (1.2 mg) implanted twice weekly into 42 hybrid (C57B1 × DBA) female mice for 6 to 13 weeks resulted in 26 uterine tumors, thought to be of decidual origin.[126] Intraperitoneal administration of testosterone acetate for up to a year produced papillary cystic adenoma in 9 out of 34 mice.[127] Steroids were often suspended in corn oil or other solvents, which might have facilitated the occasional local formation of sarcomas. Muhlbock induced theca cell ovarian tumors in rats treated with testosterone 48 hr after birth, but did not succeed in inducing tumors in the secondary sex organs of male animals.[113] Since androgens including testosterone and 4-androstenedione are precursors of estrogens, it is certainly possible that peripheral conversion to estrogenic compounds may be important in the cancers purported due to administration of androgens, especially breast, ovarian, and uterine cancers.

As mentioned previously, although prostatic hyperplasia, (or no change at all) has been produced in the dog, rhesus monkey, and lemur by large amounts of androgenic hormones, neither benign nor malignant cancers developed. Metaplasia of the prostate in mice by sustained administration of estrogens,[128] multilayer squamous cell degeneration of prostatic epithelial columnar cells in the dog after administration of FSH, and synergistic effects of prolactin, growth hormone, and androgens on prostatic growth in culture have been noted.[101,104] However, prostatic cancer did not develop. These additional effects of estrogen and pituitary polypeptide hormones on prostatic cells, whether direct or indirect, suggest in man that simple causal relationships between any putative carcinogenic agent and prostatic cancer are unlikely.

Inability to induce prostatic hypertrophy in dogs with testosterone and DHT[84] and the success observed after the use of androstenediol[83] (combined with estrogen or not) has been noted. Administration of testosterone propionate with or without estrone to Nb rats increased their low spontaneous incidence of prostatic cancer some 40-fold.[95]

This recitation of primarily unsuccessful attempts to induce cancer in various species with androgenic hormones provides little evidence for the direct carcinogenicity of androgens, at least in amounts that could be considered physiologic. Peripheral conversion of testosterone to estrogenic compounds, and the lack of reports of carcinogenicity of an androgen such as DHT, believed to be incapable of serving as an estrogen precursor, reinforce this view. Indeed, Kirschbaum,[129] after reviewing the literature to 1957, felt that there was no evidence that androgens were primary carcinogens, and other experts seem to share this view.[24-26]

C. Ability of Androgens to Inhibit or Promote Development of Cancers in Animals Receiving Estrogens and Other Agents

Although the evidence for direct carcinogenicity of androgens is not strong, these agents and progestational steroids can reduce the incidence of virtually all types of cancers that follow administration of estrogens to various animal species.[112] Androgens antagonize the development of estrogen-induced cancers in the ovary, adrenal, testis, hypophysis, uterus, mammary gland, and lymphoid tissue, but can act synergistically to increase estrogen-induced tumors of the kidney. For example, a number of androgens including 5-androsten-3β,17β-diol, 5-androsten-3β-ol-17-one, methyltestosterone, testosterone, *cis*-testosterone, and 4-androstene-3,17-dione are all reported to prevent estrogen-induced mammary tumor development. Testosterone and estrogen are both required for induction of benign uterine endometrial tumors, leiomyosarcoma of the ductus deferens-epididymal tail, and basal cell epithelioma, which also occur spontaneously. In addition, Bischoff observed a 34% incidence of local sarcoma in 34 male Marsh mice receiving 20 mg of 4-cholestrene-3,6-dione in sesame oil; in castrated male mice only one sarcoma occurred.[130]

Progesterone acts synergistically with estrogens in forming tumors of the hypophysis, mammary gland, and kidney, but under different experimental conditions can antagonize tumor formation in the breast, testis, uterus, and lymphoid tissue. Progesterone pellets implanted in 2-month-old BALB mice resulted in from 25 to 50% of the animals developing ovarian granulosa cell tumors. Norethindrone (17α-ethinyl-19-nor testosterone) and 19-norprogesterone induced tumors in 50% of the animals, but norethynodrel (17α-ethinyl $\Delta^{5,10}$-19 nortestosterone) did not. Androgenic or antiandrogenic activity of progestational compounds might be implicated in some of these effects (see Drill, Volume I, Chapter 6).

Hepatic tumors occurring spontaneously in C3H and CBA strains of mice develop more often in males.[131] This incidence can be reduced by castration or increased in females with exogenous androgen. Characteristically, hepatomas are more readily induced in male mice by hepatic carcinogens, such as para-dimethylaminoazobenzene, N-hydroxy-N-fluorenylacetamide, acetylaminofluorene, and diethylnitrosamine, but probably excluding aflatoxin.[132] Splenic implants of testosterone did not increase the incidence of hepatomas. Castration only reduced tumor formation while thyroidectomy or hypophysectomy abolished it, suggesting that its effect is indirect. Effects of thyroidectomy on hepatic carcinogenesis may be mediated via the pituitary, or even the hypothalamus (for which there are known sex-related differences in function) may be implicated. However, a role for neuroendocrine control of hepatic carcinogenesis has not been demonstrated.

The metabolic "sex" of the liver is determined largely by the hormonal environment during fetal and neonatal life, and male types of hepatic enzymes can be induced in female rats by suitable exposure to androgens.[133] Administration of testosterone to newborn female rats increases the incidence of 2-hydroxy-2-fluorenylacetamide-induced hepatic tumors, and by the same token, estrogen administrated to newborn male rats reduces their incidence.

It is well established that a number of hormones including thyroid, growth hormone, adrenal steroid, and sex organ hormones modify the growth and function of liver cells and that frequently their effects are additive.[134] In hepatic carcinogenesis, in addition to stimulating cellular proliferation, hormones may alter the metabolic activation of carcinogens and so limit or facilitate the development of tumors. Phenobarbital, given for 100 days to rats first fed acetylaminofluoroene for 21 days caused a high incidence of hepatic tumors from 3 to 8 months later.[135] If phenobarbital was given concomitantly with the carcinogen, overall tumor incidence was reduced. Effects on cell proliferation and induction of drug or hormone metabolizing enzymes are among various mechanisms of action that have been considered. For example, esterification of N-hydroxy-N-2-acetylaminofluroene is stimulated by male hormones and decreased by adrenalectomy or hypophysectomy.[136] On the other hand, a stimulus to cell proliferation associated with exposure to a carcinogen frequently can increase the yield of tumors. Tumors develop in rat liver, normally resistant to 4-dimethylaminoazobenzene carcinogenesis by preceding partial hepatectomy and subsequent exposure to the carcinogen.[137] Cells undergoing rapid cellular proliferation may be more susceptible to fixation of the transforming event.

Sex differences in the activity of various enzymes have been reviewed,[138,139] as have those related to the metabolism of carcinogens, steroids, and drugs, and the effects of sex differences on carcinogenesis have been reviewed even more recently.[133,140] These reviews provide an access to this very extensive literature.

D. Response of Cultured Prostate Cells to Androgens

Culture of prostatic cells in vitro with androgens has not resulted in autonomous growth of cells.[26,101,104] Explants of ventral prostate from young mice or rats grown in the presence of testosterone propionate (at about $10^{-6}M$) retain their structural differentiation and secretory ability, while the proliferation of connective tissue seen when explants are grown in hormone-free media is prevented. Culture with estrone produced hyperplasia and metaplasia; older glands responded with atrophy and flattening of the alveolar epithelium and hyperplasia of the fibromuscular stroma. Vitamin A deficiency caused squamous metaplasia, and insulin induced irregular proliferation of prostatic epithelium. Rat ventral prostate was comparable, except larger amounts of androgen induced cell division, cortisol maintained epithelial height, and low concentrations of estradiol had a slight androgenic effect, but higher concentrations caused regression. Ovine ventral prostate was weakly stimulated by low concentrations of prolactin, inhibited by higher concentrations, unaffected by growth hormone, inhibited by estradiol, and stimulated by cyproterone.

Baulieu et al.[86] observed that dihydrotestosterone (DHT) was a more potent stimulus for cell division, while testosterone and 5-α-androstan-3β,17β-diol preferentially maintained cellular height and secretion. Subsequently, it was reported that DHT was more potent in maintaining both functions, depending upon its concentration.

Human prostatic adenoma and carcinoma cells can grow in vitro without added androgens, but respond to added hormone with increased RNA synthesis, acid phosphatase activity, and most interestingly, increased morphologic differentiation in some samples of carcinoma.[141] Effects in vitro are complex and depend upon the use of physiologic or pharmacologic amounts of steroid hormones and a host of other variables.[101,104,142]

Methylcholanthrene increased mitoses in mouse ventral prostate epithelial cells with a loss of differentiation leading to squamous metaplasia and inhibition of the growth of connective tissue.[143] Rat ventral prostate was less responsive to the carcinogen. Estradiol increased MCA-induced cell proliferation; if the hormone followed treatment with the carcinogen, widespread destruction of the hyperplastic epithelium ensued. Testosterone or hydrocortisone reduced the incidence and extent of hyperplasia due to MCA. Comparable studies with other carcinogens including 7,12 dimethylbenzanthracene and 1,2-benzanthracene have led to similar results. However, attempts to directly transform prostate cells in organ culture with polycyclic hydrocarbons were unsuccessful. Dispersion of treated cells in suspension culture allowed growth of lines transplantable in syngeneic mice, but they lacked controls. To circumvent this, aneuploid prostate cell lines were established which were not malignant and rarely underwent spontaneous transformation. Culture of these cell lines with methylcholathrene resulted in malignant transplantable cells which gave rise to fibrosarcomas in C3H mice.[144] Neonatal hamster prostate cells have been transformed with SV40, and permanent cell lines have been established.[145]

Several spontaneous prostatic tumors are available including the Dunning tumor (spontaneous prostatic tumor in Copenhagen rats),[146] adenocarcinoma in aged germ-free Wister rats,[147] Fortner prostatic tumor from male hamsters,[148] and a form of female prostatic tumor from a virgin female Rattus (mastomys) natalensis.[149] Malignant prostatic tumors rarely occur in aged dogs, while anecdotal examples of spontaneous prostatic cancer in monkeys have been reported.

The major value of such spontaneously developing tumors probably is in establishing permanent cell lines, as from the Dunning adenocaricnoma.[150] Cell lines have been established from human prostatic tissue, for example, the MA-160, transplantable to the hamster cheek pouch.[151] Growth of these cells is stimulated by androgens, and an acid phosphatase is present. However, contamination with HeLa cells has been suggested because of characteristic rapidly moving glucose-6-phosphate isoenzyme and chromosome markers for HeLa cells.[152] The prostatic venue of some of these cell lines is argued.

Inability of testosterone at various concentrations to directly transform prostate cells in organ culture is one important piece of evidence against androgens representing proximate carcinogens capable by themselves of inducing malignant change. Since stroma is retained in organ culture, absence of interaction between epithelial and connective tissue cells should not explain the lack of transformation. Possibly, an androgenic stimulus must be applied over more prolonged periods of time. Alternately, androgens may not be proximate carcinogens or they may require interaction with other growth factors for expression of cellular transformation. Results of the Ames test for mutagenicity of androgens are eagerly awaited, since they should help to resolve some of these questions.

IV. ANDROGENS AND ANTIANDROGENS IN CANCER THERAPY

There are few cancers for which androgens represent "first line" therapy. In women with metastatic breast cancer who are less than 5 years past the menopause and whose tumors are estrogen-receptor positive, remissions are often induced by androgens in preference to estrogens.[153,154] Many physicians use estrogens in patients more than 5 years postmenopausal with metastatic disease whose tumors contain estrogen receptors. Women who are premenopausal and include these criteria are treated by castration. After failure of the primary response to the initial hormonal manipulation, a number of these patients will subsequently respond to androgens. Overall, about 1/3 of pre- and postmenopausal patients respond to a primary hormonal manipulation. Some 2/3 of the patients with estrogen receptors greater than 3 to 8 fmol/mg protein can be expected to respond,[155] and if progesterone receptors are also present, about 80% of such patients benefit from hormone therapy. The presence of receptors for androgens (specifically dihydrotestosterone), reported present in from 30 to 80% of the patients in several series, does not appear to be predictive of response to hormonal therapy for reasons that are not apparent.[156,157] The extent to which administered androgens are converted to estrogens, their role in antagonizing estrogens in the tumor cell, the nature of responses to progestational agents, and indeed, whether breast cancer in the pre- and postmenopausal patient represents dissimilar diseases requiring a different approach to therapy are discussed in Volume II, Chapter 2 by Shafie and Hilf. Occasionally, a patient who is failing on androgen or estrogen therapy will undergo a partial remission after hormone withdrawal. Attempts to stimulate breast tumor cell growth with administered hormones and to increase the growth fraction followed closely by chemotherapy have been tried, but it seems without particular success.[158]

Both oral and parenteral preparations of androgens are available, e.g., testosterone propionate or Δ^1-testololactone (Teslac®, 100 mg i.m. thrice weekly); fluoxymesterone or Halotestin®, 10 mg p.o. twice daily; or Calusterone®, 200 mg p.o. daily. Parenteral administration may be associated with less hepatotoxicity. Side effects include masculinization with increased libido, fluid retention, gastrointestinal intolerance, and hepatotoxicity with 17α-substituted compounds. Generally, osseous and cutaneous metastases respond more often than visceral lesions. Hypercalcemia occurring with the first few weeks of therapy in the presence of bone metastases may represent stimulation of tumor growth, tumor progression unrelated to therapy, or regression of tumor. Hypercalcemia late in the course of androgen therapy most likely represents a loss of response to the hormone and progression of disease in bone.

Eventual failure of hormone therapy presumably is due to selection of resistant cells whose growth is no longer modified by a steroid hormone or its antagonist.[159] Consistent with the multistep mechanism of steroid hormone action, defects in one or more of these events have been sought. Absence of cytosol receptors, their presence in insufficient amounts, synthesis of a defective receptor unable to bind steroid and/or transfer to nuclei, or once transferred, incapable of mediating changes in transcription represent possible defects to be sought. A biologically active receptor able to function in the absence of steroid hormone is conceivable. There is evidence that the antiestrogen tamoxifen binds to mammary gland cytosol receptor and that the complex is transferred to nuclei and early events of transcription are initiated, but these are not followed by the expected later events.[160] In addition, steroid-sensitive and -insensitive cells initially may be present. There may be no obligatory coupling between cellular replication and the presence of a steroid hormone receptor, although effects on cell growth (hypertrophy) might occur. Some of these possibilities have been examined with the steroid-insensitive S49 lymphoma cells derived from a mineral oil-induced lymphoma in BALB/c mice[161] and with the Shionogi S115 mouse mammary tumor cells.[162] Related studies with human mammary cancer have been reported.[163]

Occasional patients with metastatic carcinoma of the uterus, of the kidney, and with malignant melanoma have been treated with androgens, but the incidence of response is low. Human pharyngolaryngeal mucosa and a number of epithelioma derived from those sites contain soluble receptors for androgens[164] as does normal and cancerous pancreas.[165] Whether control of cell division is modified by these receptors is not established.

In the absence of much information about how androgens and other steroid hormones bring about regression of breast cancer cells, it is usually suggested that androgens and their metabolites may directly inhibit breast cancer cells or their surrounding stroma or may alter the metabolism of estrogen. There is evidence that this may not simply involve competition for cytosol estrogen receptors, since the affinity of DHT for estrogen receptor from rat uterus and human mammary tissue is much less than estradiol. However, pharmacologic amounts of hormone normally are administered, and high concentrations of DHT (10^{-6} M) can bind to and translocate to nuclei estrogen receptor of MCF-7 breast cancer cells.[188]

A fall in gonadotrophin secretion follows treatment with testosterone propionate or methyltestosterone; administration of fluoxymesterone usually is followed by a rise in serum prolactin.

The rare breast cancer in males, possibly initiated by estrogens, is first treated by castration which removes the major source of androgens. The rate of response is about 70%. and the clinical management similar to that of breast cancer in women.

Inhibiting the effects of circulating androgens or removing their testicular source represents the primary therapy for carcinoma of the prostate. Tumors from the majority of patients contain androgen receptors and most respond, at least for a time, to endocrine manipulations. In addition, estrogen and progesterone receptors are found associated with at least some prostatic cancers, but the implications of these findings are not established. Studies cited previously concerning the lack of uptake of ^{3}H-medroxyprogesterone acetate by cytosol or nuclei from androgen-insensitive tfm/y mice are compatible with the contention that functional androgen receptors are required for the antiandrogenic actions of progestational compounds.[10,12] Uptake of labeled estrogens by the ventral prostate is not reduced by unlabeled progesterone, which is consistent with the marked specificity of these hormone receptors.

Hormonal manipulations are used in patients with stage C (local extension to adjacent structures) or D (distant metastases) disease: stages A and B (cancer confined to the gland) being treated with prostatic surgery and/or external or interstitial radiation.[166,167] Disease outside the prostatic capsule is usually treated with transurethral resection to relieve any obstruction and castration, administration of estrogen, or both. Castration or administration of estrogens produces rapid improvement in bone pain in about 2/3 of symptomatic patients. Often, prostatic specific acid phosphatase falls, and measurable tumor regression occurs. Additional therapy for metastatic disease can include large intravenous doses of diethylstilbesterol diphosphate (Stilphosterol®), use of progestins, corticosteroids, adrenalectomy, hypophysectomy, radiation to affected sites, cryosurgery of the primary tumor in the hope of producing partial regression of metastases, and chemotherapy with cytoxan, fluorouracil, or adriamycin in various combinations.[168,169]

Castration destroys the main source of androgens and testicular inhibin and adrenalectomy removes a second source of weak androgens (although these androgens are secreted in large amounts), while hypophysectomy also removes polypeptide hormones such as prolactin and growth hormone that may promote growth of prostatic cancer cells. Exogenous estrogens suppress secretion of gonadotrophins including interstitial cell stimulating hormone (ICSH or LH in females) and FSH and reduce testicular synthesis of androgens. There does not seem to be a reciprocal relation between secretion of gonadotrophins and prolactin. In rats, castration is followed by compensatory adrenal hypertrophy with increased secretion of the weak androgen, dehydroepiandrosterone, that can be converted to testosterone by the prostate. In man, estrogens in therapeutic amounts also increase secretion of ACTH and prolactin and increase serum testosterone binding globulin (TBG).

Additional effects of estrogens at the cellular level include inhibition of testicular enzymes involved in androgen biosynthesis, direct inhibition of Δ^4-3-ketosteroid 5α-reductases and 3α (and 3β)-hydroxysteroid-oxidoreductases, and occupancy of prostatic estradiol receptors, but (in rats) no direct inhibition by competition of binding by dihydrotestosterone to androgen receptors, at least at near physiologic concentration. Long-term effects of estrogen suppression of androgens may reduce the concentration of prostate membrane-bound prolactin receptors, provided this expression of differentiated function was retained by tumor cells. In experimental mammary cancer, prolactin receptors are decreased by hypophysectomy, ovariectomy, antiestrogen, and androgen administration. A number of authors have stressed that estrogens (and prolactin) can potentiate the effects of androgens on the prostate and consider the ratio of androgen to estrogen to be important. Thus, administration of estrogenic compounds produces effects which seemingly could promote the growth of prostatic cancer cells with certain properties. Reports that administration of androgens to patients with carcinoma of the prostate provokes increased tumor growth in some individuals, and improvement in other patients demonstrates that we lack information necessary to rationalize these observations.

Antiandrogens, including cyproterone and its acetate,[170] and the nonsteroidal compound flutamide[171] have been used to treat metastatic prostatic cancer. Some patients with prostatic cancer resistant to estrogens respond to an antiandrogen. Generally, responses were comparable to those seen with estrogens without some of the accustomed side effects, such as sodium retention and enlargement of the breasts. These agents compete with DHT for cytosol DHT receptor proteins; cyproterone acetate also exerts central antigonadotropic effects. Although progesterone does not bind firmly to the specific B protein of rat ventral prostate cytosol, it does associate with other cytosol proteins and with various particulate fractions. Pharmacologic doses of medrogestone can inhibit 5α reduction of testosterone by microsomal preparations from the skin and the prostate. Cyproterone and its acetate reduces the accumulation in vivo of radioactive androgens by rat prostate or seminal vesicle and decreases binding of labeled DHT to cytosol β protein and the transfer of labeled DHT to cell nuclei. Neither compound seems to inhibit reduction of testosterone to DHT. Other agents which reduce the uptake of androgens (e.g., gestonorone capronate), inhibit 5α-reductase (medrogestone, SC 14207), inhibit steroid dehydrogenases (L579.229), or compete with active androgens for binding to specific cytosol receptors (BOMT, SC9420, or spironolactone) are described, but their clinical utility is not established.

Antiandrogens such as cyproterone acetate have also been used to treat benign prostatic hypertrophy, with reports of lessened obstruction and reduced epithelial height seen in prostatic biopsies.[172] With the amounts employed, libido was reduced.

Estracyt (estramustine-phosphate), in which nor-nitrogen mustard is esterified via the phenolic hydroxyl group of estradiol-17-phosphate, has been used in the treatment of advanced prostatic cancer.[173] The estradiol moiety is thought to provide some site specificity with preferential uptake by target organ cells, whereupon intracellular esterases cleave the ester linkage, releasing nitrogen mustard and estradiol-17-phosphate in situ. Prednimustine, another steroidal alkylating agent which combines prednisone and chlorambucil, has been used alone or in combination with estracyt in patients refractory to other therapy; about one quarter of some patient groups have experienced objective responses. Phosphorylated colchicine derivatives of ethanolamine and phosphate derivatives of thiocolchicine, which are also selectively cleaved by prostatic acid phosphatase, are being studied as agents that may specifically localize to prostatic cancer cells.[174]

Androgens and anabolic steroids can be employed as adjuncts to cancer therapy. Newer anabolic agents such as Durabolin® and Deca-Durabolin® are associated with less masculinization. Androgens and anabolic agents stimulate erythropoiesis, in part, by increasing erythropoietin formation by the kidney.[175] In addition, the stem-cell population may be stimulated to proliferate, increasing the number of cells responsive to erythropoietin. For example, testosterone enanthate given to patients receiving cytotoxic agents decreased the expected suppression of the white blood cell count and allowed larger amounts of cytotoxic chemotherapy to be used. The marrow-protective effects of androgens have been used as an adjunct in breast and colon cancer and in multiple myeloma, Hodgkin's disease and the treatment of other lymphomas, chronic lymphatic leukemia, and myeloid metaplasia,[176] although this practice is not widely followed. In cyclic neutropenia, androgens increased the granulocyte count and reduced that of the monocytes. Marrow-protective and anabolic effects of the anabolic agent Durabolin (nandrolone phenpropionate) has been demonstrated.[176] There is some evidence that androgens and anabolic agents may increase fibrinolysis. For example, stanazol augmented plasma fibrinolytic activity due to reduced synthesis of fibrinogen.[177] Androgens may increase immune responsiveness of lymphocytes, in part, by reducing levels of antiplasmin. Nandrolone phenylpropionate and stilbestrol both exert a protective effect on the ability of lymphocytes from breast cancer patients following surgery to respond in vitro to photohemaglutinin.[178]

In suitable situations, androgens (especially anabolic steroids) can be used to improve a patient's appetite and sense of well-being without incapacitating side effects.

V. CONCLUDING REMARKS

Many properties of cancer cells are compatible with impaired cellular differentiation and retention or acquisition of biochemical properties inappropriate for differentiated cells from the tissue of origin.[39,40] The ability of activated hormone receptors to initiate cell division is a comparatively late evolutionary event engrafted on cells previously responding to other stimuli. Expression of these biochemical mechanisms for initiating replication, which apparently is abrogated in normally differentiated target cells by the absence of activated steroid receptor, could be important for steroid independent cell division. In hormone-independent tumors devoid of steroid receptors, local intercellular controls (such as direct cell to cell contact) that normally may help to modulate cell division of hormone-dependent cells are ineffective. Since little is known about the factors promoting differentiation of prostatic cells during embryologic development, efforts to recapitulate these events during replication of cancer cells are beyond contemporary biology. Although some of the factors responsible for cellular differentiation were derived from the primitive mesenchyme,[179] this information does not aid us greatly. Conceivably, the existence of a suitably modified virus or nucleic acid-containing liposome trophic for a target cell could provide a disease vector[189,190] capable of introducing cellular information required for activation of the steroid hormone receptor mechanism, or even for initiating prostate cell regression similar to that following castration. Use of vaccination in patients with malignant melanoma, with the chief aim of increasing immune responsiveness, has been tried.[180] However, presently the occurrence in at least some tumors of prolactin receptors and cytosol receptors for estradiol, DHT, and progesterone, and their responses to administration of particular hormones provides the only known practical means of modifying prostatic and mammary cell replication by biologically active molecules intrinsic to the host.

If factors that stimulate the invasion of new blood vessels into a tumor or other tissue are tissue-specific, either directly or indirectly interdicting a response to these agents elaborated by connective tissue or cancer cells might provide a measure of local tumor control.[181] Inhibiting proteases thought to be important for local or distant extension of a cancer by natural or synthetic materials could, in principle, restrain extension of a cancer.[182] Suppressing the synthesis or function of fibroblast growth factor, perhaps by immunologic means, might represent another approach.[191] Hormone-dependent cancers may be ideal candidates for subsequent active or passive immunotherapy, once the total body tumor burden has been reduced. Surgery or irradiation to remove bulk tumor, chemotherapy to reduce the active growth fraction of both hormone-dependent and independent cells, or hormonal manipulation to induce regression in residual hormone-dependent cells, succeeded by immunotherapy in an effort to destroy remaining independent tumor cells, may represent a logical approach to the treatment of several hormone-dependent cancers. To the extent that cellular steroid receptor content can be altered by administration of a hormone to patients with hormone-independent cancer cells, these cells might differentiate after exposure to the primary stimulatory hormone (e.g., androgens in prostatic cancers resistant to estrogens). Differential stimulation of androgen, estrogen, progesterone, or prolactin receptors, alone or in combination, might prove to alter the growth of some steroid hormone-independent cancer cells.

Several patients with breast cancer metastatic to bone improved after treatment with the antibiotic, mithramycin, which is not tumoricidal for these cancers.[183] The drug can inhibit the function of host osteoclasts. At least some metastatic tumors appear able to activate host osteoclasts, presumably by synthesis of an osteoclast activating factor[184] associated with destruction of bone and extension of the cancer. Blocking the function of a tumor-elaborated product that stimulates a response in host target cells deleterious to the patient by inhibiting the host target cell is a potential means of modifying the extension of breast and prostate cancers.

Compared with normal cells, many cancer cells exhibit differential sensitivity to elevated temperature, especially evident when combined with chemotherapy.[185] It has been reported that hyperthermia increased the uptake of acidic nuclear proteins from the cytoplasm by HeLa or Chinese hamster ovary cell nuclei.[181,182] Possibly, a group of cancer patients exists with androgen or other steroid hormone receptors unable to enter their cell nuclei. Exposure to hyperthermia might circumvent such a barrier to expression of steroid hormone action and alter the response of steroid-insensitive cells.

A much broader study of events distal to the application of a hormonal stimulus with greater attention to elaboration by cancer cells and their stroma of angiogenesis and fibroblast proliferation factors, extracellular proteases and their inhibitors, and related biologically active materials may aid in further defining androgen-induced biochemical mechanisms capable of exploitation. Increasing focus on interactions between epithelial and connective tissue cells may uncover biochemical events, some of them responsive to hormones, capable of manipulation to the advantage of patients with cancer.

VI. ADDENDUM

Rereading this chapter after a lapse of time, some addtional comments are in order. It was perhaps simplistic to suggest that the question of mutagenicity of androgens would necessarily be settled by the application of the Ames test alone. In view of the approximately 30 or more different in vitro and in vivo mutagenicity assays, any assessement of androgens for mutagenicity would be more secure if a number of these techniques led to the same conclusion. In addition to the various bacterial mutagenicity assays, procedures using cultured mammalian cells and even insect and plant cells have been developed. In vivo mammalian mutagenicity assays include effects on germinal cells (mouse-specific locus, heritable translocations, dominant lethal, and germinal cytogenetic effects), while somatic cells effects include cytogenetic changes, unscheduled DNA synthesis, sister chromatid exchanges, the micro-nucleus test, the spot test, and direct observation of oncogenicity.[192] Thus, the final conclusions concerning the mutagenicity and consequently, the potential for carcinogenicity of androgens, determined by in vivo and in vitro testing will await results from a number of assays which measure biological effects of the test compound that may be produced by a number of different molecular mechanisms.

Attention should be called to the International Agency for Research on Cancer monograph 6, in which evidence of carcinogenicity of a number of sex steroids is reviewed,[193] and was not previously available to us. Results of subcutaneous injection or imlantation of testosterone are reviewed and cervical-uterine cancers in mice,[126] vaginal tumors in neonatal mice exposed to testosterone for 5 days,[194] theca-cell tumors in rats,[122] tumors induced in Syrian hamsters,[125,195,196] and leiomyomas and leiomyosarcomas in Syrian hamster uterine horns and epididymi,[197] the latter similar to those described by Kirkman and Algard,[196] are cited. Inhibition of spontaneous hepatomas in male C3H mice,[198] reduced mammary tumor incidence in C3H mice,[199,200] increased incidence of mammary cancer in MTV-bearing female BALB/cf C3H mice,[201] and reduced incidence of leukemia in ovariectomized female Rockefeller mice treated with pellets of testosterone propionate,[202] supplement the information presented in Sections IIIB and C. It was suggested that steroid hormones "precipitate" neoplasia by (a) direct carcinogenic action, (b) stimulate formation of other hormonal factors themselves causing cancer, (c) synergistically promote the growth of a tissue affected by a physical, chemical, or viral carcinogen, (d) modify the metabolism of chemical agents, to increase or reduce the formation of the proximate carcinogen, and lastly (e) alter the immune response. The four patients with aplastic anemia[44] who developed hepatocellular carcinoma after long-term therapy with androgenic-anabolic agents were not considered adequate epidemiologically to form a conclusion about carcinogenicity, in view of the frequent association of hemosiderosis and hepatitis in these patients.

Mention should again be made of the continuing series of publications concerning carcinogenicity testing from the National Cancer Institute[110,111,203] (for extensive information about carcinogenicity of steroids). An additional case report of Wilms tumor in an adult who used large amounts of androgen-anabolic steroids for years can be cited.[204]

Lastly, we have observed morphologically typical C-type RNA viruses replicating in and released from prostate epithelial cells of Sprague-Dawley and Long-Evans rats.[205] Presumably, this represents "spontaneous" release of endogenous C-type rat RNA virus, but the matter is under study.

ACKNOWLEDGMENTS

This work was supported by the National Cancer Institute Grant No. 1-RO1-CA 22246, the Charles P. Perlia Memorial Foundation, and the Wadsworth Memorial Fund. We thank Dr. S. Economou, Professor of Surgery and Associate Director of Surgery, Rush Medical College, Chicago, Illinois, for his continuing support.

REFERENCES

1. Williams-Ashman, H. G. and Reddi, A. H., Androgenic regulation of tissue growth and function, in *Biochemical Actions of Hormones*, Litwack, G., Ed., Academic Press, New York, 1972.
2. Goland, M., Ed., *Normal and Abnormal Growth of the Prostate*, Charles C. Thomas, Springfield, Ill., 1975.
3. Brandes, D., Ed., *Male Accessory Sex Organs*, Academic Press, New York, 1974.
4. King, R. J. B. and Mainwaring, W. I. P., *Steroid-Cell Interaction*, University Park Press, Baltimore, 1974.
5. Liao, S., Cellular receptor and mechanism of action of steroid hormones, *Int. Rev. Cytol.*, 41, 87, 1975.
6. Hilf, R., Mechanism of action of androgens, *Handbook of Experimental Pharmacology*, Volume 38, 2nd ed., Sartorelli, A. C. and Johns, D. G., Eds., Springer-Verlag, Berlin, 1975, 139.
7. Munson, P. L. and Diczfalusy, F. Eds., Endocrine control of the prostate, *Vit. Horm.*, 33, 1, 1975.
8. Makin, H. L. J., Ed., *Biochemistry of Steroid Hormones*, Blackwell, Oxford, 1975.
9. Grayhack, J. T., Wilson, J. D., and Scherbenske, M. J., Benign Prostatic Hyperplasia, DHEW Pub. No. (NIH) 761113, 1976.

10. Liao, S., Molecular actions of androgens, in *Biochemical Actions of Hormones,* Vol. 4, Litwack, G., Ed., Academic Press, New York, 1977, 351.

11. Bardin, C. W., Bullock, L. P., Mills, N. C., Lin Y-C., and Jacob, S. T., Role of receptors in anabloic action of hormones, in *Receptors and Hormone Action,* Vol. 2, O'Malley, B. W. and Birnbaumer, L., Eds., Academic Press, New York, 1978, 83.

12. Martini, L. and Motta, M., Eds., *Androgens and Antiandrogens,* Raven Press, New York, 1977.

13. Mainwaring, W. I. P., *The Mechanism of Action of Androgens,* Springer-Verlag, New York, 1977.

14. Brotherton, J., *Sex Hormone Pharmacology,* Academic Press, London, 1976.

15. Kadohama, N. and Anderson, K. M., Nuclear non-histone proteins from rat ventral prostate cells undergoing hypertrophy or hyperplasia, *Exp. Cell Res.,* 99, 135, 1976.

16. Ohno, S., Dofuku, R., and Tettenhorn, U., More about the x-linked testicular feminization of the mouse as a noninducible (is) mutation of a regulatory locus: 5α-androstan 3α,17β-diol as the true inducer of kidney alcohol dehydrogenase and β glucuronidase, *Clin. Genet.,* 2, 128, 1971.

17. Ahmed, K., Studies on nuclear phosphaprotein of rat ventral prostate: incorporation of ^{32}P from (γ^{-32}P) ATP, *Biochim. Biophys. Acta,* 243, 38, 1971.

18. Wang, T. Y. and Nyberg, L. M., Androgen receptors in the nonhistone protein fractions of prostatic chromatin, *Int. Rev. Cytol.,* 39, 1, 1974.

19. Davies, P., Thomas, P., and Griffith, K., The influence of steroid-receptor complexes on the stages of transcription of target tissue chromatin, *J. Steroid Biochem.,* 7, 993, 1976.

20. Mainwaring, W. I. P., Keen, J., and Stewart, M. W., Further studies on the DNA-unwinding protein of the rat-ventral prostate: evidence for local areas of denaturation, *J. Steroid Biochem.,* 7, 1013, 1976.

21. Liang, T. and Liao, S., A very rapid effect of androgen on initiation of protein synthesis in prostate, *Proc. Natl. Acad. Sci. U.S.A.,* 72, 706, 1975.

22. Singhal, R. L., Tsang, B. R., and Sutherland, D. J. B., Regulation of cyclic nucleotide and prostaglandin metabolism in sex steroid-dependent cells, in *Advances in Sex Hormone Research,* Vol. 2, Singhal, R. L. and Thomas, J. A., Eds., University Park Press, Baltimore, 1976, 325.

23. Schrader, W. T., Coty, W. A., Smith, R. G., and O'Malley, B. W., Purification and properties of progesterone receptors from chick oviduct, *Ann. N. Y. Acad. Sci.,* 286, 64, 1977.

24. Segaloff, A., Steroids and carcinogenesis, *J. Steroid Biochem.,* 6, 171, 1975.

25. Jull, J. W., Endocrine aspects of carcinogenesis, in *Chemical Carcinogenesis,* Searle, C. E., Ed., American Chemical Society, Washington, D.C., 1976, 52.

26. Bischoff, F., Carcinogenic effects of steroids, *Adv. Lipid Res.,* 7, 165, 1969.

27. McCann, J. and Ames, B. N., Detection of carcinogens as mutagens in the salmonella/microsome test: any of 300 chemicals: discussion, *Proc. Natl. Acad. Sci. U.S.A.,* 73, 950, 1976.

28. Herbst, A. L., Ulfelder, H., and Poskanzer, D. C., Adenocarcinoma of the vagina: association of maternal stilbestrol therapy with tumor appearance in young women, *N. Engl. J. Med.,* 284, 878, 1971.

29. Kappus, H. and Bolt, H. M., Irreversible protein binding of norethisterone (norethindrone) epoxide, *Steroids,* 27, 29, 1976.

30. Berenblum, I., *Carcinogenesis as a Biological Problem,* North-Holland, Amsterdam, 1974.

31. Comings, D. E., A general theory of carcinogenesis, *Proc. Natl. Acad. Sci. U.S.A.,* 70, 3324, 1973.

32. Nordling, C. E., A new theory on the cancer-inducing mechanism, *Br. J. Cancer,* 7, 68, 1953.

33. Armitage, P. and Doll, R., The age distribution of cancer and a multi-stage theory of carcinogenesis, *Br. J. Cancer,* 8, 1, 1954.

34. Ashley, D. J. B., On the incidence of carcinoma of the prostate, *J. Pathol. Bacteriol.,* 90, 217, 1965.

35. Ashley, D. J. B., The two "hit" and multiple "hit" theories of carcinogenesis , *Br. J. Cancer,* 23, 213, 1969.

36. Foulds, L., *Neoplastic Development,* Vol. 1, Academic Press, New York, 1969, 69.

37. Braun, A. C., *The Biology of Cancer,* Addison-Wesley, Reading, Mass., 1974.

38. Illmensee, K., and Mintz, B., Totipotency and normal differentiation of single teratocarcinoma cells cloned by injections into blastocysts, *Proc. Natl. Acad. Sci. U.S.A.,* 73, 549, 1976.

39. Markert, C. L., Neoplasia, a disease of cell differentiation, *Cancer Res.,* 28, 908, 1968.

40. Anderson, N. G. and Coggin, J. H., Molecular mechanisms in blocked autogeny and retrogression: paraneoplastic syndromes, *Ann. N. Y. Acad. Sci.,* 230, 508, 1974.

41. Recant, L. and Lacy, P., Fanconi's anemia and hepatic cirrhosis, *Am. J. Med.,* 39, 464, 1965.

42. Cattan, D., Vesin, P., Wautier, J., Kalifat, R., and Meignan, S., Liver tumors and steroid hormones, *Lancet,* 1, 878, 1974.

43. Port, R. B., Petasnick, J. P., and Ranniger, K., Angiographic demonstration of hepatoma in association with Franconi's anemia, *Am. J. Roentgenol. Radium Ther. Nucl. Med.,* 113, 82, 1971.

44. Johnson, F. L., Feagler, J. R., Lerner, K. G., Majerus, P. W., Siegel, M., Hartmann, J. R., and Thomas, E. D., Association of androgenic-anabolic steroid therapy with development of hepatocellular carcinoma, *Lancet,* 2, 1273, 1972.

45. Bernstein, M. S., Hunter, R. L., and Yachnin, S., Hepatoma and peliosis hepatis developing in a patient with Fanconi's anemia, *N. Engl. J. Med.*, 284, 1135, 1971.
46. Guy, J. T. and Auslander, M. O., Androgenic steroids and hepatocellular carcinoma, *Lancet*, 1, 148, 1973.
47. Sweeney, E. C. and Evans, D. J., Hepatic lesions in patients treated with synthetic anabolic steroids, *J. Clin. Pathol.*, 29, 626, 1976.
48. Mokrohisky, S. T., Ambruso, D. R., and Hathaway, W. E., Fulminant hepatic neoplasia after androgen therapy, *N. Engl. J. Med.*, 296, 1411, 1977.
49. Swift, M., Fanconi's anemia in the genetics of neoplasia, *Nature (London)*, 230, 370, 1971.
50. Todaro, G. J., Green, H., and Swift, M. R., Susceptibility of human diploid fibroblast strains to transformation by SV40 virus, *Science*, 153, 1252, 1966.
51. Sasaki, M. S. and Tonomura, A., A high susceptibility of Fanconi's anemia to chromosome breakage by DNA cross-linking agents, *Cancer Res.*, 33, 1829, 1973.
52. Poon, P. K., O'Brien, R. L., and Parker, J. W., Defective DNA repair in Fanconi's anemia, *Nature, (London)*, 250, 223, 1974.
53. Sarna, G., Tomasulo, P., Lotz, M. J., Bubinak, J. F., and Shulman, N. R., Multiple neoplasms in two siblings with a variant form of Fanconi's anemia, *Cancer*, 36, 1029, 1975.
54. Henderson, J. T., Richmond, J., and Sumerling, M. D., Androgenic-anabolic steroid therapy and hepatocellular carcinoma, *Lancet*, 1, 934, 1973.
55. Meadows, A. T., Naiman, J. L., and Valdes-Dapena, M., Heaptoma associated with androgen therapy for aplastic anemia, *J. Pediatr.*, 84, 109, 1974.
56. Farrell, G. C., Joshua, D. E., Uren, R. F., Baird, P. J., Perkins, K. W., and Kronenberg, H., Androgen-induced hepatoma, *Lancet*, 1, 430, 1975.
57. Bruguera, M., Hepatoma associated with androgenic steroids, *Lancet*, 1, 1295, 1975.
58. Ziegenfuss, J. and Carabasi, R., Androgens and hepatocellular carcinoma, *Lancet*, 1, 262, 1973.
59. Westaby, D., Ogle, S. J., Paradinas, F. J., Randall, J. B., and Murray-Lyon, I. M., Liver damage from long-term methyltestosterone, *Lancet*, 2, 261, 1977.
60. Antunes, C. M. F. and Stolley, P. D., Cancer induction by exogenous hormones, *Cancer*, 39, 1896, 1977.
61. Anthony, P. P., Hepatoma associated with androgenic steroids, *Lancet*, 1, 685, 1975.
62. Goldfarb, S., Sex hormones and hepatic neoplasia, *Cancer Res.*, 36, 2584, 1976.
63. Anthony, P. P., Precursor lesions for liver cancer in humans, *Cancer Res.*, 36, 2579, 1976.
64. Farber, E., Pathogenesis of liver cancer, *Arch. Pathol.*, 98, 145, 1974.
65. Foss, G. L. and Simpson, S. L., Oral methyltestosterone and jaundice, *Br. Med. J.*, 1, 259, 1959.
66. deLorimier, A. A., Gordan, G. S., Lowe, R. C., and Carbone, J. V., Methyltestosterone, related steroids and liver function, *Arch. Intern. Med.*, 116, 289, 1965.
67. Bagheri, S. A. and Boyer, J. L., Peliosis hepatis associated with androgenic-anabolic steroid therapy, *Ann. Intern. Med.*, 81, 610, 1974.
68. Johnson, F. L., Androgenic-anabolic steroids and hepatocellular carcinoma, in *Hepatocellular Carcinoma*, Okude, K. and Peters, R. L., Eds., John Wiley & Sons, New York, 1976, 95.
69. Liver tumors and steroid hormones (editorial), *Lancet*, 2, 1481, 1973.
70. Silverberg, E., Cancer statistics, 1977, *CA Cancer J. Clin.*, 27, 26, 1977.
71. Goldstein, J. L. and Wilson, J. D., Genetic and hormonal control of male sexual differentiation, *J. Cell Physiol.*, 85, 365, 1973.
72. Bennett, D., Boyse, E. A., Lyon, M. F., Mathieson, B. J., Scheid, M., and Yamagisawa, K., Expression of H-Y (Male) antigen in phenotypically female Tfm/Ymice, *Nature, (London)*, 257, 236, 1975.
73. Higginson, J., Annual Report, International Agency for Research on Cancer, World Health Organization, Leon, France, 1968.
74. Kellerman, G., Shaw, C. R., and Luyten-Kellerman, M., Aryl-hydrocarbon hydroxylase inducibility and bronchogenic carcinoma, *N. Engl. J. Med.*, 289, 934, 1973.
75. Bloom, H. J. G., Renal cancer, in *Endocrine Therapy in Malignant Disease*, Stoll, B. A., Ed., Saunders, W. B., London, 1972, 339.
76. Fisher, R. I., Neifeld, J. P., and Lippman, M. E., Estrogen receptors in human malignant melanoma, *Lancet*, 2, 337, 1976.
77. Simpson, J. L., Jirasek, J. E., Speroff, L., and Kase, N. G., *Disorders of Sexual Differentiation*, Academic Press, New York, 1976.
78. Mulvihill, J. J., Congenital and genetics diseases, in *Persons at High Risk of Cancer*, Fraumeni , J. F., Ed., Academic Press, New York, 1975, 3.
79. Barakat, A. Y., Popadopoulov, Z. L., Chandra, R. S., Hollerman, C. E., and Calcagno, P. L., Pseudohermaphroditism, nepthron disorder and Wilms tumor; a unifying concept, *Pediatrics*, 54, 366, 1974.
80. Zuckerman, S. and Groome, J. R., The etiology of benign prostatic enlargement of the prostate in the dog, *J. Pathol. Bacteriol.*, 44, 113, 1937.

81. Lacassagne, A., Metaplasie epidermoide de la prostate provoquee chez la souris por des enjections repetee de forte doses de folliculine, *C. R. Soc. Biol.*, 113, 590, 1933.
82. Franks, L. M., Atrophy and hyperplasia in the prostate proper, *J. Pathol. Bacteriol.*, 68, 617, 1954.
83. Walsh, P. C. and Wilson, J. D., The induction of prostatic hypertrophy in the dog with androstenediol, *J. Clin. Invest.*, 57, 1093, 1976.
84. Siiteri, P. K. and Wilson, J. D., Dihydrotestosterone in prostatic hypertrophy. I. Formation and content of dihydrotestosterone in the hypertrophic prostate in man, *J. Clin. Invest.*, 49, 1737, 1970.
85. Georgi, E. P., Meses, T. F., Grand, J. K., Scott, R., and Sinclair, J., *In vitro* studies on the regulation of androgen tissue relationship in canine normal and human hyperplastic prostate, *Mol. Cell. Endocrinol.*, 1, 271, 1974.
86. Baulieu, E. E., Lasnitzke, I., and Robel, P., Metabolism of testosterone and actions of metabolites on prostate glands grown in organ culture, *Nature, (London)*, 219, 1155, 1968.
87. Mainwaring, W. I. P., *Advances in the Study of the Prostate*, Heineman, London, 1970, 86.
88. Wilson, J. D., Gloyna, R. E., and Siiteri, P. K., Androgen metabolism in the hypertrophic prostate, *J. Steroid Biochem.*, 6, 443, 1975.
89. Huggins, C., The etiology of benign prostatic hypertrophy, *Bull. N. Y. Acad. Med.*, 23, 696, 1947.
90. Armenian, H. K., Lilienfeld, A. M., Diamond, E. L., and Bross, I. D. J., Relationship between benign prostatic hypertrophy and cancer of the prostate, *Lancet*, 2, 115, 1974.
91. Greenwald, P., Kirmiss, V., Polan, A. K., and Dick, V. S., Cancer of the prostate among men with benign prostatic hyperplasia, *J. Natl. Cancer Inst.*, 53, 335, 1974.
92. Terasaki, P. I., Perdue, S. T., and Mickey, M. R., HLA frequencies in cancer: a second study in, *Genetics of Human Cancer*, Mulvihill, J. J., Miller, R. W., and Fraumeni J. F., Raven Press, New York, 1977, 321.
93. Anderson, D. E., Familial Susceptibility, in *Persons at High Risk of Cancer*, Fraumeni, J. F., Ed., Academic Press, New York, 1975.
94. Wynder, E. L. Mabuchi, K., and Whitmore, W. F., Epidemiology of cancer of the prostate, *Cancer*, 28, 344, 1971.
95. Noble, R. L., The development of prostatic adenocarcinoma in Nb rats following prolonged sex hormone administration, *Cancer Res.*, 37, 1929, 1977.
96. Sommers, S. C., Endocrine changes with prostatic cancer, *Cancer*, 10, 345, 1957.
97. Harbitz, T. B. and Haugen, O. G., Endocrine disturbance in men with benign hyperplasia and carcinoma of the prostate, in *Endocrine Aspects of Benign Hyperplasia and Carcinoma of the Human Prostate*, Oslo, 1974.
98. Ofner, P., Effects and metabolism of hormones in normal and neoplastic prostate tissue, *Vit. Horm.*, 26, 237, 1968.
99. Voigt, K-D., Horst, H-J. and Krieg, M., Androgen metabolism in patients with benign prostatic hypertrophy, *Vit. Horm.* 33, 417, 1975.
100. Attramadal, A., Tveter, K. J., Weddington, S. C., Djoseland, O., Naess, O., Hansson, V., and Torgersen, O., Androgen binding and metabolism in the human prostate, *Vit. Horm.*, 33, 247, 1975.
101. Lasnitzki, I., The prostate gland in organ culture, *Vit. Horm.*, 33, 348, 1975.
102. Franks, L. M., Hormone excretion in prostatic cancer: an attempt to correlate urinary hormone excretion and clinical state, *Br. J. Cancer*, 13, 54, 1959.
103. Franks, L. M. and Chesterman, F. C., Irreversible cellular changes in old mice, *Nature (London)*, 202, 821, 1964.
104. Lasnitzki, I., Growth and humoral response of prostatic tumors, in *Urologic Pathology: The Prostate*, Tannenbaum, M., Ed., Lea & Febiger, Philadelphia, 1977, 215.
105. Zeigel, R. F., Arya, S. K., Horoszewicz, J. S., and Carter, W. A., A status report. Human prostatic carcinoma, with emphasis on potential for viral etiology, *Oncology*, 34, 29, 1977.
106. Dmochowski, L., Ohtsuki, Y., Seman, G., Maruyama, K., Knesek, J. E., East, J. L., Bowen, J. M., Yoshida, H., and Johnson, D. E., Search for oncogenic viruses in human prostate cancer, *Cancer Treat. Rep.*, 61, 119, 1977.
107. Centifanto, Y. M., Kaufman, H. E., and Zam, Z. S., Herpes virus particles in prostatic carcinoma cells, *J. Virol.*, 12, 1608, 1973.
108. Balda, B.-R., Hehlmann, R., Cho, J.-R., and Spiegelman, S., Oncornovirus-like particles in human skin cancers, *Proc. Natl. Acad. Sci. U.S.A.*, 72, 3697, 1975.
109. Arya, S. K., Job, L., Horoszewicz, J. S., Zeigel, R. F., and Carter, W. A., RNA tumor virus-like activities in human prostate: possible novel pharmacologic approaches, *Cancer Treat. Rep.*, 61, 113, 1977.
110. Christensen, H. E., Luginbyhl, T. T., and Carroll, B., Suspected Carcinogens, Department of Health Education and Welfare, Rockville, Md., 1975, 302.
111. Hartwell, J. C., Survey of Compounds Which Have Been Tested for Carcinogenicity, 2nd ed., National Cancer Institute, Washington, D.C., 1951, 380.

112. Gardner, W. V., Hormonal aspects of experimental tumorgenesis, *Adv. Cancer Rest.,* 1, 173, 1953.
113. Mühlbock, O. and Boot, L. M., The mechanism of hormonal carcinogenesis, in *CIBA Symposium on Carcinogenesis,* Wolstenholme, G. E. W. and O'Connor, M., Eds., Little Brown, Boston, 1959, 83.
114. Clayson, D. B., *Chemical Carcinogenesis,* J& A. Churchill, London, 1962.
115. Noble, D. B., *The Hormones,* Vol. 5, Pincus, G. and Thimann, K. V., Eds., Academic Press, New York, 1964, 559.
116. Lacassagne, A. and Raynaud, J. P., Effets, sur la souris d'enjections longtemps repetees de propionate de testosterone, *C. R. Soc. Biol.,* 130, 689, 1939.
117. Lacassagne, A., Relationship of hormones and mammary adenocarcinoma in the mouse, *Am. J. Cancer,* 37, 414, 1939.
118. Wooley, G. W., Effect of hormonal substances on adrenocortical tumor formation in mice, *Cancer Res.,* 10, 250, 1950.
119. Andervont, H. B. and Dunn, T. B., Susceptibility of strain C mice to o-aminoazotoluene, *Cancer Res.,* 7, 730, 1947.
120. Gardner, W. V. and Rygaard, J., Further studies on the incidence of lymphomas in mice exposed to X-rays and given sex hormones, *Cancer Res.,* 14, 205, 1954.
121. Gardner, W. V., Dougherty, T. F., and Williams, W. L., Lymphoid tumors in mice receiving steroid hormones, *Cancer Res.,* 4, 73, 1944.
122. Horning, E. S., Carcinogenic action of androgens, *Br. J. Cancer,* 12, 414, 1958.
123. Rudali, K. E., Desormeaux, B., and Juliand, L., *Bull. Assoc. Fr. Etude Cancer,* 43, 445, 1956.
124. Homburger, F., Borges, P., and Tregier, A., The production of uterine sarcomas in hydro-uteri of mice receiving testosterone, *Proc. Am. Assoc Cancer R.,*2, 215, 1957.
125. Kirkman, H. and Robbins, M., The carcinogenicity of testosterone propionate in the Syrian hamster, *Proc. Am. Assoc. Cancer Res.,* 2, 125, 1956.
126. Van Nie, R., Benedetti, E. L., and Mühlbock, O., A carcinogenic action of testosterone provoking uterine tumors in mice, *Nature,* (London), 192, 1303, 1961.
127. Kendrey, G., Balo, J., and Juhasy, J., Carcinogenic effect of Androfort (testosterone acetate), *Kiser 1. Orvost ud.,* 5 and 6, 531, 1958.
128. Lasnitzki, I., The effect of estrone alone and combined with 20-methylcholanthrene on mouse prostate glands grown *in vitro, Cancer Res.,* 14, 632, 1954.
129. Kirschbaum, A., The role of hormones in cancer; laboratory animals, *Cancer Res.,* 17, 432, 1957.
130. Bischoff, F., Cocarcinogenic activity of cholesterol oxidation products and sesame oil, *J. Natl. Cancer Inst.,* 19, 977, 1957.
131. Andervort, H. B., Studies regarding the occurrence of spontaneous hepatomas in mice of strain C3H and CBA, *J. Natl. Cancer Inst.,* 11, 581, 1950.
132. Pitot, H. C., Carcinogenesis and aging — two related phenomena, *Am. J. Pathol.,* 87, 444, 1977.
133. Toh, Y. C., Physiological and biochemical reviews of sex differences and carcinogenesis with particular reference to the liver, *Adv. Cancer Res.,* 18, 155, 1973.
134. Tata, J. R., Regulation of protein synthesis by growth and developmental hormones, in *Biochemical Actions of Hormone,* Vol. 1, Litwock, G., Ed., Academic Press, New York, 1975.
135. Peraino, C., Fray, R. J. M., Staffeldt, E., and Kisieleski, W. E., Effects of varying the exposure to phenobarbital on the enhancement of 2-aminoacetyl-fluorene-induced hepatic tumorigenesis in the rat, *Cancer Res.,* 33, 2701, 1973.
136. Lotikar, P. D., Effects of sex hormones on enzymatic esterification of 2-(N-hydroxyacetamido) fluorene by rat liver cytosol *Biochem. J.,* 120, 909, 1970.
137. Warwick, G. P., The covalent binding of metabolites of dimethylaminoazo-benzene to liver nucleic acids *in vivo.* The possible importance of cell proliferation in cancer initiation, in *Physio-Chemical Mechanisms of Carcinogenesis,* Bergmann, E. D., Ed., Israel Academy of Science, Jerusalem, 1969, 218.
138. Knox, W. E., Auerbach, V. H., and Lin, E. C. C., Enzymatic and metabolic adaptation in animals, *Physiol. Rev.,* 36, 165, 1956.
139. Barzilai, D., The effect of the sex hormones on liver physiology and pathology, *Acta Hepato-Splenol.,* 12, 1, 1965.
140. Gustafsson, J. A., Eneroth, P., Pousette, A., Skett, P., Sonnenschein, C., Stenberg, A., and Ahlen, A., Programming and differentiation of rat liver enzymes, *J. Steroid Biochem.,* 8, 429, 1977.
141. Prout, G. R. and Brewer, W. R., Response of men with advanced prostatic carcinoma to exogenous administrations of testosterone, *Cancer,* 20, 1871, 1967.
142. Fraley, E. E. and Paulson, D. F., Experimental carcinogenesis of the prostate, in *Male Accessory Sex Organs,* Brandes, D., Ed., Academic Press, New York, 1974, 383.
143. Horning, E. S., The effects of castration and stilbestrol on prostatic tumors in mice, *Br. J. Cancer,* 3, 211, 1949.

144. Chen, T. T. and Heidelberger, C., *In vitro* malignant transformation of cells derived from mouse prostate in the presence of 3-methylcholanthrene, *J. Natl. Cancer Inst.*, 42, 915, 1969.

145. Paulson, D. F., Rabson, A. S., and Fraley, E. E., Viral neoplastic transformation of hamster prostate tissue *in vitro*, *Science*, 159, 200, 1968.

146. Dunning, W. F., Prostate cancer in the rat, *Natl. Cancer Inst. Mongr.*, 12, 351, 1963.

147. Pollard, M., Spontaneous prostate adenocarcinomas in aged germfree Wistar rats, *J. Natl. Cancer Inst.*, 51, 1235, 1973.

148. Fortner, J. G., Funkhauser, J. W., and Cullen, M. R., A transplantable, spontaneous adenocarcinoma of the prostate in the Syrian (golden) hamster, *Natl. Cancer Inst. Monogr.*, 12, 371, 1963.

149. Snell, K. and Stewart, H., Adenocarcinoma and proliferative hyperplasia of the prostate gland in female Rattus (Mastomys) Natalensis, *J. Natl. Cancer Inst.*, 35, 7, 1965.

150. Pollard, M., Chang, C. F., and Burleson, G. R., Investigations on prostate adenocarcinoma in rats, *Cancer Treat. Rep.*, 61, 153, 1977.

151. Fraley, E. E., Ecker, S., and Vincent, M. M., Spontaneous *in vitro* neoplastic transformation of adult human prostatic epithelium, *Science*, 170, 540, 1970.

152. Gartler, S. M., Apparent HeLa cell contamination of human heterodiploid cell lines, *Nature*, (London), 217, 750, 1968.

153. Stoll, B. A., Breast cancer — endocrine therapy, in *Endocrine Therapy in Malignant Disease*, Stoll, B. A., Ed., Saunders, W. B., London, 1972, 111.

154. Horton, J. , Breast cancer, in *Clinical Oncology*, Horton, J. and Hill, G. J., Eds., W. B. Saunders, London, 1977, 366.

155. McGuire, W. L., Carbone, P. P., and Vollmer, E. P., Eds., *Estrogen Receptors in Human Breast Cancer*, Raven Press, New York, 1975.

156. Wagner, R. K. and Jungblut, P. W., Dihydrotestosterone receptor in human mammary cancer, *Acta Endocrinol. (Copenhagen) Suppl.*, 173, 65, 1973.

157. Trams, G. and Maass, H., Specific binding of estradiol and dihydrotestosterone in human mammary cancers, *Cancer Res.*, 37, 258, 1977.

158. Taylor, S. G., Pocock, S. J., Shnider, B. I., Colsky, J., and Hall, T. C., Clinical studies of 5-fluorouracil and premarin in the treatment of breast cancer, *Med. Pediatr. Oncol.*, 1, 113, 1975.

159. King, R. J. B.,Clinical relevance of steroid-receptor measurement in tumors, *Cancer Treat. Review*, 2, 273, 1975.

160. Nicholson, R. I., Davies, P., and Griffiths, K., Effects of estradiol-17-β and Tamoxifen estradiol-17β receptors in DMBA-induced rat mammary tumors, *Eur. J. Cancer*, 12, 201, 1976.

161. Yamamoto, K. R., Gehring, V., Stampfer, M. R., and Sibley, C. H., Genetic approaches to steroid hormone action, *Rec. Prog. Horm. Res.*, 32, 3, 1976.

162. Gordon, J., Smith, J. A., and King, R. J. B., Metabolism and binding of androgens by mouse mammary tumor cells in culture, *Mol. Cell Endocrinol.*, 1, 259, 1974.

163. Charreau, E. H., and Baldi, A., Binding of estradiol receptor complexes to isolated human breast chromatin, *Mol. Cell Biochem.*, 16, 79, 1977.

164. Saez, S. and Sako, F., Androgen receptors in human pharngyolaryngeal mucosa and pharyngo-laryngeal epithelioma, *J. Steroid Biochem.*, 7, 919, 1976.

165. Pousette, A., Demonstration of an androgen receptor in rat pancreas, *Biochem. J.*, 157, 228, 1976.

166. Woodruff, M. W., Zoronow, D. H., and Olson, H. W., Cancer of the urologic and male reproductive system, in *Clinical Oncology*, Horton, J. and Hill, G. J., Eds., W. B. Saunders, Philadelphia, 1977, 472.

167. Ackerman, L. V. and del Regato, J. A., Cancer of the male genital organs, in *Cancer*, 4th ed., C. V. Mosby, St. Louis, 1970, chap. 12.

168. Murphy, G. P., Current status of therapy in prostatic cancer, in *Urologic Pathology: The Prostate*, M. Tannenbaum, Ed., Lea & Febiger, Philadelphia, 1977, 225.

169. Murphy, G. P., Carcinoma of the prostate, *Sem. Oncology*, 3, 101, 1976.

170. Bracci, U. and Di Silverio, F., Role of cyproterone acetate in urology, in *Androgens and Antiandrogens*, Martini, L., and Motta, M., Eds., Raven Press, New York, 1977, 333.

171. Stoliar, B. and Albert, D. J., SCH 13521 in the treatment of advanced carcinoma of the prostate, *J. Urol.*, 111, 803, 1974.

172. Scott, W. W. and Coffey, D. S., Non-surgical treatment of human benign prostatic hyperplasia, *Vit. Horm.*, 33, 439, 1975.

173. Mittelman, A., Shukla, S. K., Welvaart, K., and Murphy, G. P., Oral estramustine phosphate (NSC-89199) in the treatment of advanced (Stage D) carcinoma of the prostate, *Cancer Chemother. Rep.*, 59, 219, 1975.

174. Paul, B. D., Serrano, J. A., Friedman, A. E., Sarlos, I. J., Sternberg, N. J., Wasserkrug, H. L., and Seligman, A. M., New agents for prostatic cancer activated specifically by prostatic acid phosphatase, *Cancer Treat. Rep.*, 61, 259, 1977.

175. Shahidi, N. T., Androgens and erythroporiesis, *N. Engl. J. Med.*, 289, 72, 1973.

176. Brodsky, I. and Rigberg, S., The role of androgens and anabolic steroids in the treatment of cancer, in *Clinical Cancer Chemotherapy,* Greenspan, E. M., Ed., Raven Press, New York, 1975, 349.

177. Davidson, J. F., Lochhead, M., McDonald, G. A., and McNichol, G. P., Fibrinolytic enhancement by stanozolol: a double blind trial, *Br. J. Haematol.,* 47, 13, 1972.

178. Pentycross, C. R., Toussis, D., and McKinna, J., Effect of hormone therapy on mitogenic responses of lymphocytes from patients with cancer of the breast, *Lancet,* 2, 177, 1973.

179. Cunha, G. R., Epithelial-stromal interaction in development of the urogenital tract, *Int. Rev. Cytol.,* 47, 137, 1976.

180. Eastern Cooperative Oncology Group Protocol 0170, Study of combination BCNU, DTIC, vaccinia virus and BCG in malignant melanoma, Madison, Wisconsin, January, 1970.

181. Folkman, J. and Cotran, R., Relation of vascular proliferation to tumor growth, *Int. Rev. Exp. Pathol.,* 16, 207, 1976.

182. Kuettner, K. E., Hiti, J., Eisenstein, R., and Harper, E., Collagenase inhibition by cationic proteins derived from cartilage and aorta, *Biochem. Biophys. Res. Commun.,* 72, 40, 1976.

183. Anderson, K. M. and Bonomi, P., Mithramycin and local control of osteolytic metastases, Paper presented at Clinical Research Society of Toronto, 1977.

184. Brockman, R. S., Myers, W. P., and Laird, W. P., Osteotropism of human breast cancer, in *Cancer Invasion and Metastases, Biologic Mechanisms and Therapy,* Day, S. B., Laird, W. P., Myers, W. P., Stansly, P., Grattini, S., and Lewis, M. G., Eds., Raven Press, New York, 1977, 431.

185. Rossi-Fanelli, A., Cavaliere, R., Mondovi, B., and Moricco, G., Eds., Selective Heat Sensitivity of Cancer Cells, *Springer-Verlag,* Berlin, 1977.

186. Tomosovic, S. P., Turner, G. N., and Dewey, W. C., Effect of hyperthermia on non-histone proteins isolated with DNA, *Biophys. J.,* Abstr. 60a, 17, 1977.

187. Roti, J. L., Cohen, S., and Lynch, M. L., Increased binding of chromosomal proteins induced by hyperthermia, *Biophys. J.,* Abstr. 60a, 17, 1977.

188. Zava, D. T. and McGuire, W. L., Androgen action through estrogen receptor in a human breast cancer cell line, *Endocrinology,* 103, 624, 1978.

189. Ostro, M. J., Giacomoni, D., Lavelle, D., Paxton, W., and Dray, S., Evidence for translation of rabbit mRNA after liposome-mediated insertion into a human cell line, *Nature (London),* 274, 921, 1978.

190. Nasmyth, K., Eukaryotic gene cloning and expression in yeast, *Nature (London),* 274, 741, 1978.

191. Gospodarowicz, D., Humoral control of cell proliferation: the role of fibroblast growth factor in regeneration, angiogenesis, wound healing, and neoplastic growth, in *Membranes and Neoplasia: New Approaches and Strategies,* Marchesi, V. T., Ed., Alan R. Liss, New York, 1976, 1.

192. Clive, D. and Spector, J. F. S., Comparative chemical mutagencity: can we make risk estimates?, *Comparative Chemical Mutagenicity,* in press.

193. Evaluation of Carcinogenic Risk of Chemical to Man, Sex Hormones, International Agency for Research on Cancer, Monogr. 6, (1974).

194. Kimura, T. and Nandi, S., Nature of induced persistent vaginal cornification in mice. IV. Changes in the vaginal epithelium of old mice treated neonatally with estradiol or testerone, *J. Natl. Cancer Inst.,* 39, 75, 1967.

195. Kirkman, H., Steroid tumorigenesis, *Cancer (Philadelphia),* 10, 757, 1957.

196. Kirkman, H. and Algard, F. T., Characteristics of an androgen/estrogen induced dependent leimyosarcoma of the ductus deferens of the syrian hamster, *Cancer Res.,* 25, 141, 1965.

197. Riviere, M. R., Chouroulinkov, I., and Guerin, M., Actions hormonales experimentales de longue duree chex le hamster du point de vue de leur effect cancerigene. II. Etude de la testosterone associee a un oestrogene, *Bull. Cancer,* 48, 499, 1961.

198. Schenken, J. R. and Burns, E. L., Spontaneous primary hepatomas in mice of strain C3H. III. The effect of estrogens and testosterone proprionate on their incidence, *Cancer Res.,* 3, 693, 1943.

199. Jones, E. E., The effect of testosterone propionate on mammary tumors in mice of the C3H strain, *Cancer Res.,* 1, 787, 1941.

200. Gardner, W. U., The incidence of mammary tumors and the structure of mammary gland of estrogen-plus-testosterone treated mice, *Cancer Res.,* 6, 493, 1946.

201. Bern, H. A., Mori, T., and Young, P. N., Preliminary report on the effects of perinatal exposure to hormones on the mammary gland of female BALB/cf. C3H mice, *Proceedings of the 8th Meeting on Mammary Cancer in Experimental Animals and Man,* Airlie House, Virginia, (1973), 12.

202. Murphy, J. B., The effect of castration, theelin, and testosterone on the incidence of leukemia in a Rockefeller Institute strain of mice, *Cancer Res.,* 4, 622, 1944.

203. Survey of Compounds Which Have Been Tested for Carcinogenic Activity, U.S. Government Printing Office, supplements in 1957, 1969, 1971, 1973, 1974.

204. Pratt, J., Gray, G. F., Stolley, P. D., and Coleman, J. W., Wilms tumor in an adult associated with androgen abuse, *JAMA,* 237, 2322, 1977.

205. Anderson, K. M., Rubenstein, M., and Seed, T. M., In vivo expression of a C-type RNA virus in rat ventral prostate epithelial cells, *Biochem. Biophys. Res. Commun.,* in press.

Chapter 2

Interrelationship of Estrogen with Prolactin, Insulin, and Progesterone in Breast Cancer

S. M. Shafie and R. Hilf

Table of Contents

I. INTRODUCTION

It is probably safe to state that if one were to ask the question "Name the class of hormones most likely to be carcinogenic", the answer would likely be estrogens. The reasons for such a response are due, at least in part, to:

1. The high incidence of cancer of the breast and the uterus, target tissues of estrogens in the female
2. The widespread use of oral contraceptives, which contain a major component synthetic estrogens (so-called combined preparations), and the uncertainities attendent to the long-term use of such preparations
3. The widespread use of estrogens as agents to ameliorate the symptoms of menopause

The publicity directed towards the potential hazards has often taken the form of articles in newspapers and magazines, in panel discussions on radio and television, and papers in a variety of scientific publications. The question still remains as to whether estrogens, as a class, or specific estrogenic substances, such as diethylstilbestrol, are truly carcinogenic agents or whether these hormones are co-carcinogens, that is, act as facilitative substances for the neoplastic transformation induced by carcinogenic agents such as chemicals, X-irradiation, viruses, etc. Berenblum, in his treatise on carcinogenesis,[1] considers hormones (in general) as permissive or modifying influences.

If we agree with such a simplification, we can illustrate such a role for estrogens as they are related to the maintenance or stimulation of the target tissue, such as the breast. In the former role, the hormone is needed to provide an appropriate cell target for the carcinogen to attack and in the latter role, the hormone influences the target cell by inducing the appropriate stage of differentiation that is susceptible to transformation by the carcinogen. Examples of each of these roles for estrogen can be cited from studies with the rat, an animal that has been extensively utilized for experiments with the polycyclic hydrocarbon carcinogens, such as 3-methylcholanthrene or 7,12-dimethylbenz(a)anthracene (DMBA). Rats intubated with single or multiple doses of DMBA demonstrate a rapid and high incidence of mammary tumors. This result can be prevented by removal of the ovaries prior to feeding the carcinogen.[2,3] However, administration of the carcinogen to prepubertal rats, or to rats in which the mammary glands have been stimulated by pregnancy, lactation, or exogenous administration of estrogens, demonstrates a significantly lower incidence of mammary cancers.[4-6] This latter behavior suggests that susceptibility to hydrocarbon-induced neoplastic transformation may be higher at certain stages of cell maturation, stages that are intermediate in the spectrum ranging from undifferentiated to fully committed. It should be noted that this suggestion may apply only to the breast; the finding of higher incidence of vagina carcinomas in young women, whose mothers received diethylstilbestrol during pregnancy to prevent abortion, would imply that differences in target cell susceptibilities exist.[7]

Another interesting aspect of estrogens regards the differences in tumor incidences found between men and women. Although women are susceptible to high tumor incidence in the accessory sex organs, the incidence of cancers of organs not part of the reproductive system is higher in males than in females.[8] This situation can be demonstrated in the laboratory in the rat or mouse for the induction of hepatic cancer by chemical carcinogens. Male rats or mice show considerably higher incidence of hepatomas after exposure to azo dyes or 2-acetylaminofluorene (see review by Toh).[9] Castration of the male rat decreased liver tumor incidence induced by 2-acetylaminofluorene and the induction of hepatomas could be restored by the administration of testosterone.[10] Further, some data were reported suggesting that the administration of diethylstilbestrol or other estrogens could reduce the carcinogen-induced hepatoma formation in the male rat.[11]

The difficulty facing the researcher in assessing the role of a single hormone in neoplasia is, first, the potential multihormonal responsiveness of the tissue undergoing neoplastic transformation, or second, the apparent lack of clear-cut evidence of hormonal influences on the target cell under study. This is further compounded by the interaction of several hormones leading to synergism or antagonism depending on the target cell examined, the level of hormone studied, or the presence of other as yet described factors. Since the occurrence of cancer is an event that takes place in the whole animal, and since the neoplastic transformation may be expressed (diagnosed) over long periods of time, it becomes extremely difficult to identify those critical events that occur in an internal milieu that is under constant change. One of the most challenging situations is that of breast cancer, which, while clinically more apparent in the postmenopausal woman, may be present and undetected for many years spanning the time period that includes premenopause, perimenopause, and postmenopause. The hormonal milieu of each of these stages is different in the sense that the balance between the hormones of the ovary and the pituitary changes at different times and, further, the event of menopause is not an abrupt one, but is a gradual alteration in ovarian function. We feel it is more expedient here to describe the interrelationships of estrogen with other hormones at the cellular level in an attempt to demonstrate that there is a need to elucidate such relationships if we are to make progress in the area of hormones and tumorigenesis. It is also probable that such an approach would shed light on the mechanisms whereby the same hormone can actually have beneficial therapeutic effects on established tumors, a fact best exemplified by the estrogens, a seemingly paradoxical situation.

II. CONCEPT OF RECEPTORS IN HORMONE ACTION

Estrogens, either steroidal or nonsteroidal in structure, are small and rather simple molecules which, nevertheless, elicit a complex array of biochemical responses in their target tissues, often leading to profound changes in growth and differentiation. Exactly how they achieve this response is only now being elucidated, but there is very good evidence that the first step of crucial importance is the specific association of the hormone with specific cytoplasmic receptors.[12]

Available knowledge strongly suggests that tumorigenesis and its prevention in estrogen target organs such as ovary, uterus, and the breast may be controlled, or at least significantly influenced, by estrogens.[13-16] Thus, over the years, evidence has accumulated in assigning a carcinogenic or cocarcinogenic role for estrogens, thereby implicating these sex hormones as etiological factors for cancers of the female reproductive organs.

The role of specific estrogen receptors in mediating the action of estrogens in target organs has received considerable attention in the last decade.[17] Macromolecular estrogen receptors initially identified in the uterus and vagina[12] have also been found in some mammary tumors, both experimental[18] and human.[19] Their presence in these normal organs is associated with a high uptake and prolonged retention of estrogen in the intact animal. The presence of these specific hormone receptors in tumors, therefore, was interpreted as indicating hormone dependence; tumor growth and function, like that of the normal cell, were potentially subject to being regulated by the hormonal environment. Consequently, hormonal control of tumor cell depends not only on plasma concentrations of hormone, but also on the presence of hormone receptor. This latter concept has strongly contributed to a more wide and general practice of selecting a course of endocrine therapy for those cancer patients in whose tumors hormone receptors could be identified.[17,19] This is best exemplified by estrogens which represent the topic of major concern in this chapter. Synthetic estrogens, and more recently anti-estrogens, have been commonly used in the treatment of advanced breast cancer.[19] The kind and degree of mammary tumor response to endocrine manipulations may thus vary according to the type of tumor (receptor positive or negative), as well as the number of receptors involved.

Experimental data suggest that the mammary gland is sensitive not only to estrogens but to a number of other hormones, including progesterone, glucocorticoids, growth hormone, prolactin, and insulin.[20] The above hormones have all been shown over the years to be necessary for the development and/or growth of mammary tissue. Receptors which bind to each of these hormones both tightly and specifically have been identified in the mammary gland (cytoplasmic receptors for the steroids and cell surface receptors for the polypeptides). These hormone receptors also have been demonstrated to occur in certain hormone-sensitive breast cancers and they are *presumed* to be important in the growth of mammary carcinoma.[21,22] Moreover, recent data indicate that the level of hormone receptors is not static but can be markedly influenced by various hormone treatments.[23-28]

The presence of estrogen receptors has been considered as the universal marker for the prediction of hormone dependence[19] and consequently to designate a breast cancer patient for endocrine therapy. Since not all breast cancer patients who demonstrate a positive estrogen receptor assay in their tumors can be helped by the practiced hormonal alterations (i.e., ablative or additive), many investigators started to focus on the fact that estrogen-responsive breast cancers are likely to depend not only on estrogen, but also on other hormonal interrelationships in which estrogen is implicated. It is the opinion of the authors that the efficacy of endocrine treatment of breast cancer may be improved by gaining a better understanding of the mechanisms of changes in levels of receptors for estrogen and other hormones to influence mammary tumor growth.

III. ESTROGEN AND PROLACTIN

The question regarding the role of prolactin in mammary tumorigenesis is still unresolved, and this is due, at least in part, to the relationship of estrogen to prolactin. A comprehensive and recent review has appeared[29] and it is our recommendation that the reader examine this paper. Estrogen acts directly on the normal mammary gland to promote growth and differentiation.[30,31] The administration of estrogen to certain strains of mice and rats sharply increases mammary tumor incidence.[32,33] Estrogens also stimulate the release of pituitary prolactin, and ovariectomy reduces the secretion of this hormone.[15,34,35] In addition to its role in stimulating mammary gland growth and development[36-38] prolactin has been described as one of the most important hormones in breast tumor growth.[39] Prolactin alone is able to reactivate mammary tumor growth after ablation of the ovaries, adrenals, and pituitary gland.[38] These functions of prolactin, coupled with the beneficial response of patients with breast cancer to hypophysectomy, have led to the generally accepted proposal that prolactin may be the single most important hormone in mammary cancer.[39] Indeed, the above observations led to the concept that estrogens are mammary oncogenic primarily because of the stimulatory effects of the steroids on prolactin secretion, and support for this concept was accumulated from results on different experimental mammary tumors.[34,35,40] Following ovariectomy and adrenalectomy, or after hypophysectomy, DMBA-induced mammary tumors in Sprague-Dawley rats regress completely and the animals live for several months without recurrence of the tumor.[37] After ovariectomy-adrenalectomy-induced regression, estradiol benzoate administration reactivates the growth of the tumor. After a hypophysectomy-induced remission, estrogen failed to reactivate tumor growth, but a prompt tumor reactivation was observed following the administration of ovine prolactin. Ovine prolactin also reactivated growth of tumors that regressed after ovariectomy-adrenalectomy.[38] These results suggested that DMBA-induced rat mammary carcinomas are prolactin dependent and that the effects of estradiol on tumor growth might be mediated through effects on prolactin secretion.[37] Brooks and Welsch[40] recently reported that chronic treatment of female C_3H mice with estrogens increased the incidence of mammary tumors. However, when concurrent prolactin suppression was induced with the ergot drug CB-154, the mammary tumor incidence was sharply reduced to a level comparable to the nonsteroid-treated animals.

Although the observations cited above strongly support the importance of prolactin in mammary cancer, major criticism of this concept included the observation that after ovariectomy-adrenalectomy, resumption of tumor growth by prolactin is temporary even though prolactin levels remain elevated[16,41] and sustained growth occurs with the addition of ovarian isografts to ovariectomized rats bearing hypothalamic lesions. Regardless of what may be the exact role of either of these hormones, it seems to be a complex one. One can, however, propose the existence of such a relationship (of whatever nature that could be) between the two hormones in certain mammary carcinomas. Furthermore, a study at the level of the neoplastic cell, in which concentrations of hormone receptor are examined as they may be influenced by the other hormone, seems to be a useful approach in the elucidation of this relationship. In fact, such data have been sought in a few laboratories and an indication that estrogens stimulate prolactin binding in rat liver has been reported by Posner et al.[23] and Kelly et al.[24]

Studies with organ culture techniques were described by Leung and Sasaki[42] and have indicated that prolactin increased the level of specific estrogen receptor in explants of both rat uterus and mammary gland, the latter being obtained during pregnancy and lactation. A relationship between the two hormones at the receptor level was also described[43] in DMBA-induced mammary tumors whereby prolactin stimulated estrogen receptor levels by three to four times in tumor explant cultures. Vignon and Rochefort[44] also showed that the concentration of estrogen receptor sites in DMBA-induced tumor tissue was increased significantly by prolactin in castrated DMBA-treated rats. Gibson and Hilf[25] also reported that estrogen binding capacity was significantly reduced in DMBA-induced tumors from animals treated with lergotrile mesylate, a synthetic ergoline compound that inhibits secretion of prolactin by the pituitary. More recently, Asselin et al.[26] reported data on the interaction of estrogen, prolactin, and progesterone in the control of receptors for these hormones in DMBA-induced mammary tumors of the rat. In their studies, prolactin stimulated the level of estrogen receptor and ovariectomy, which resulted in tumor regression, and led to a marked reduction in prolactin binding by the tumor. Treatment of ovariectomized rats with estrogen reactivated tumor growth and stimulated prolactin binding. All of the data cited above strongly indicate the importance of prolactin in regulating the estrogen receptor level and suggest an intimate interaction between estrogen and prolactin at the tumor site, which, in turn, influences tumor growth. Since the data were obtained from experiments carried out in the whole animal or in organ culture, it is not certain from the results whether prolactin brought about the stimulation of growth of receptor-containing cells or whether there was an increase in the intracellular level of estrogen receptor. In addition, the actual effect of prolactin at the cellular estrogen receptor level should be investigated in the absence of other hormones which could contribute to the observed effect. Results from such experiments were in fact reported by Shafie and Brooks[45] working on the human breast cancer cell line MCF-7, an estrogen receptor containing cell line, under strictly controlled and better defined environment, in vitro. It was shown that estrogen binding in these MCF-7 cells was doubled after 36 hr of exposure to either ovine or human prolactin.

Although no clear-cut picture has emerged as yet on a well-defined role for prolactin in breast cancer, the bulk of evidence from the data cited above appears to directly implicate an interaction between estrogen and prolactin at the tumor cell site, at least in terms of hormone receptors.

IV. ESTROGEN AND INSULIN

While most attention has been given to the role of estrogen and prolactin in mammary tumorigenesis and neoplastic growth, data are now accumulating which suggest that insulin should be considered as another hormonal factor in this disease. There seems to be little doubt that insulin alone is a critical stimulating factor in the development and growth of rodent mammary tumor models of breast cancer. In fact, it has been shown that certain of the DMBA-induced experimental mammary tumors are insulin dependent and completely regress when the tumor-bearing host was made diabetic.[46] More recently, Cohen and Hilf[47,48] have shown that all of the DMBA-induced tumors were observed to regress in estrogen-treated diabetic rats and have suggested that insulin deprival plus estrogen therapy may have additive effects. Estrogen-insulin interrelationships have also been noted by Shafie and Brooks,[49] who demonstrated that estradiol augmented the insulin-stimulatory effect on cell division of the human breast cancer cell line, MCF-7. Gibson and Hilf[25] showed that estrogen binding capacity in DMBA-induced mammary tumors was significantly reduced in regressing and static tumors from diabetic rats. Furthermore, Cohen and Hilf[50] reported that estrogen and insulin, injected simultaneously, had an additive effect to retard growth of the transplantable R3230AC mammary tumor of the Fischer rat. Thus, depending on the mammary tumor model examined, insulin may stimulate or retard mammary tumor growth and such an effect may also implicate an interaction of insulin with other hormones, especially estrogen.

There are several reports indicating the presence of abnormalities in glucose tolerance in breast cancer patients. These findings have been taken to implicate insulin as an important factor in this disease and a greater risk for breast cancer has been related to obesity. It is certainly of considerable interest that, in a recent paper,[51] Rhomberg observed that the course of disease in 30 women (advanced metastatic patients) who had diabetes was protracted compared to the 100 nondiabetic women studied with comparable disease stage. More interest in the role of insulin was stimulated by the identification and characterization of a specific receptor to insulin in experimental and human mammary tumors.[22,27,28] The importance of the latter finding is strongly supported by the concept that the hormone binding capacity of breast cancers might predict the endocrine responsiveness of the neoplasm and that the receptor concentration may vary in pathological conditions and under conditions in which the hormonal milieu of the tumor-bearing host was altered.[21,22,25-28]

The results reported above also suggested that an estrogen-insulin axis could be operative in mammary tumor growth, particularly at the cellular level, and this turned our attention to examination of insulin binding and its alteration by estrogens, an event that would be expected to precede and be responsible for the biological responses seen. Specific insulin binding to freshly dissociated cells from R3230AC tumors, a transplantable autonomous responsive adenocarcinoma with respect to estrogen, insulin, and prolactin, was measured after the tumor was allowed to grow for 2 to 3 weeks in Fischer rats. Insulin binding was two- to threefold higher[27] in these cells than the amount of insulin binding measured in cells from the same donor tumor transplanted to and growing in intact rats (control). The increase in insulin binding above control levels by tumors that had been growing in ovariectomized hosts was detectable between the first and second week after tumor transplantation and was not accompanied by any change in levels of serum insulin or blood glucose. Thus, it was concluded that removal of gonadal steroids was most probably responsible for the significant increase in insulin binding capacity in the carcinoma. Injection of tumor-bearing ovariectomized rats with 1 mg estradiol valerate brought about a decrease in insulin binding in the tumor. The amount of insulin bound by the tumor after estrogen treatment, however, remained significantly higher than that of control tumor cells (intact rats). This partial reversion in insulin binding by estrogen treatment might be explained by proposing that the selected dose of estrogen did not completely duplicate endogenous estrogen levels. Another possible explanation for the results is that after ovariectomy a more complex hormonal change including feedback and feedforward changes occurred and that estrogen alone could not completely reverse this effect, e.g., progesterone was also removed by ovariectomy. Along the same lines, estrogen binding was significantly reduced by 75% in 2- to 3-week old R3230AC tumor cells from hosts that were made diabetic 2 days prior to tumor implantation. Results from these experiments are outlined in Figure 1. Thus, this represents the first evidence at the cellular receptor level of a suggested relationship between insulin and estrogen in this mammary tumor system.

Similar studies were conducted in our laboratory with the hormone-dependent DMBA-induced mammary tumors. It was important to extend our investigation on the apparent relationships between insulin and estrogen, which we observed at the receptor level in the hormone-responsive R3230AC tumor, to another model system that demonstrates hormone dependence. It has been observed that hormonal therapy, such as diabetes or ovariectomy, resulted in differential effects on growth patterns and hormone binding of DMBA-induced tumors coexisting in the same host or in different hosts.[28] Tumors that continued to grow in ovariectomized hosts (ovarian independent) showed an increased (127%) insulin binding capacity while tumors that started to re-

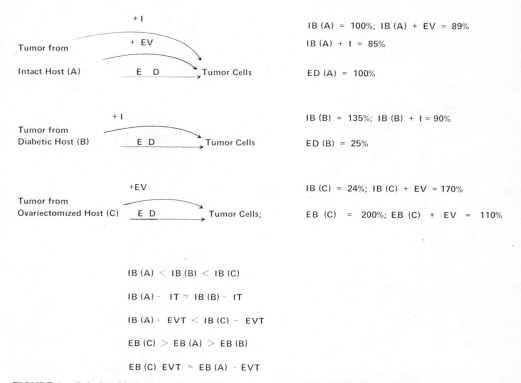

$IB (A) < IB (B) < IB (C)$

$IB (A) - IT \simeq IB (B) - IT$

$IB (A) - EVT < IB (C) - EVT$

$EB (C) > EB (A) > EB (B)$

$EB (C) EVT \simeq EB (A) - EVT$

FIGURE 1.   Relationship between insulin binding (IB) and estrogen binding (EB) in R3230AC tumors from intact, diabetic, or ovariectomized host. In certain experiments the host was injected with either 4 IU of insulin (I) or with 1 mg estradiol valerate (EV); ED = collagenase-hyaluronidase dissociation. (From Shafie, S. M., Gibson, S. L., and Hilf, R., *Cancer Res.*, 37, 4655, 1977. With permission.)

gress (ovarian dependent) demonstrated decreased (70%) insulin binding. Insulin binding capacity was unchanged in lesions that remained static after ovariectomy.

DMBA-induced mammary tumors that continued to grow after the host was made diabetic (insulin independent) demonstrated a significant increase (147%) in estrogen binding and decreased insulin binding (64%), and lesions that started to regress (insulin dependent) showed decreased (58%) estrogen levels and a significant increase binding (155%). These results are outlined in Figure 2.

Taken together, these data add further support to the proposed estrogen-insulin axis in mammary tumors and suggest that the role of insulin in mammary tumor growth and regression could be

1. A direct effect on the tumor via the receptor
2. To influence ovarian hormone receptors, at least estrogen receptor
3. To influence ovarian hormones which appear to be involved in the regulation of insulin receptor

V. ESTROGEN AND PROGESTERONE

The importance of progesterone in enhancing the induction of DMBA mammary tumors has been reported by Huggins and colleagues.[6,52,53] More recently, Jabara and co-workers[54,55] concluded from their studies on DMBA-induced mammary tumors, and in agreement with the earlier reports,[6] that progesterone enhances tumorigenesis. The mechanism of this progesterone effect is unclear but it may occur indirectly

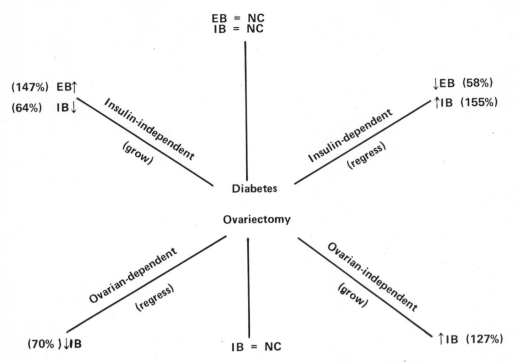

FIGURE 2.   Insulin-estrogen binding and relationship to hormonal regulation of growth of DMBA-induced mammary tumors; IB = insulin binding; EB = estrogen binding; NC = no change. (Shafie, S. M. and Hilf, R., *Cancer Res.*, 38, 759, 1978. With permission.)

through effects on prolactin secretion. Since progesterone can synergize with or be antagonistic to estrogen, depending on the dose of progesterone relative to estrogen, the effects of progesterone to enhance tumorigenesis may occur by offsetting the effects of estrogen to inhibit tumorigenesis.

The role of progesterone in the growth of established tumors is even more obscure as is the mechanism by which progestins induce tumor regression.[56] Tumor growth in the lactating, suckled rat can be prevented by ovariectomy and restored by progesterone alone.[57,58] Taken as such, and considering that the suckled ovariectomized animals had both high prolactin levels and intact adrenal glands, one cannot interpret these observations in a way that progesterone alone is responsible for maintaining tumor growth. Nevertheless, these observations strongly suggest that progesterone plays an important role in stimulating tumor growth, a process which could include other factors. Earlier reports by Huggins et al.[6] had also suggested that progesterone is a factor in stimulating tumor growth and it was shown that pregnancy (high progesterone) prompted the growth of DMBA-induced rat mammary tumors. Administration of progesterone to intact rats accelerated the appearance of tumors and increased the number and enhanced the growth rate of established tumors. Growley and McDonald[59] and Stoll[60,61] have shown that, at least in some cases, patients whose tumors have failed to regress following treatment with high doses of estrogen alone have responded to a combination of estrogen plus progesterone. McCormick and Moon[62] reported that large doses of progesterone could induce mammary tumor regression or even prevent tumor appearance, at least when combined with moderate to large doses of estrogen.

Interest has been renewed in the role of progesterone in mammary cancer following the report of Horwitz et al.[63] who attempted to seek a correlation between the presence of progesterone receptor and estrogen receptor with clinical response to hormonal therapy. These authors presented data in humans, which suggested that the percentage of patients with breast cancer demonstrating regressions to a progesterone estrogen combination was generally higher than that observed with estrogen alone or progesterone treatments alone. Stoll[60,61] reported that some of the observed progesterone-mediated DMBA-induced mammary tumor regressions required estrogen. McGuire et al.[64] suggested that this estrogen requirement for progesterone to influence tumor regression may be due to estrogen stimulation of progesterone receptor. Injection of estrogen to rats caused an eightfold increase in progesterone receptor levels in rat uterus within 24 hr.[65] This increase was prevented by administration of inhibitors of RNA synthesis, thus suggesting that estrogen induced *de novo* synthesis of progesterone receptor. The same qualitative relationship between estrogen and progesterone receptor in the uterus has been also documented in mammary tumors.[66] Tumors from ovariectomized-adrenalectomized DMBA-induced tumor-bearing rats (at proestrus) demonstrated a decreased progesterone receptor level.[66] Estrogen treatment of regressed tumors restored both tumor growth and progesterone receptor. It is noteworthy that progesterone treatment as reported by the authors failed to duplicate the effects of the estrogen treatment or to sustain tumor growth despite the initial presence of progesterone receptor. These observations strongly suggest that the synthesis of progesterone receptor is dependent upon the action of estrogen, a relationship which could prove to be of paramount significance in the biochemical evaluation of breast cancer and the endocrine therapy of patients.

In human breast cancers, progesterone receptor is rarely found in estrogen-receptor-negative metastatic tumors, but it is present in approximately 59% of estrogen-receptor-positive metastatic tumors, especially those tumors that demonstrate high estrogen receptor levels.[64] Consequently, it was reported that patient response to endocrine therapy was significantly higher if the tumor contained receptors for both estrogen and progesterone than if the tumor contained receptor for estrogen alone. The fact that progesterone receptor has been described to be under acute estrogen control and is one end product of estrogen action and the presence of receptors for both estrogen and progesterone in the tumor could indicate that tumors have maintained their hormone dependence, thus reflecting the integrity of cellular estrogen-receptor-response pathway rather than reflecting only the initial hormone binding step. While these observations could be of extreme importance in giving breast cancer patients a better chance of a rewarding endocrine therapy, it appears that the available data cannot rule out the shortcomings of this extrapolation. Horwitz and McGuire[66] reported that certain estrogen-independent DMBA-induced tumors, which continued to grow in ovariectomized hosts, also had their progesterone receptor level decreased upon removal of estradiol. This finding suggested to the authors that there was a dissociation between the estrogenic control and tumor growth and estrogen stimulation of progesterone receptor.

Although we do not yet know the exact details whereby hormones may stimulate or repress the synthesis of receptors for other hormones, and our ignorance is probably due at least in part to the complexity of the tumor endocrine environment, this aspect of regulation is certainly one of the critical problems that several laboratories have begun to explore. The exact hormonal requirement at the tumor site is unknown, but apparently, the experiments with various mammary tumors have uncovered several interesting hormonal relationships, which make it unlikely that the observed hormonal effect on tumor cells is indeed the effect of that single hormone alone. Since estradiol stimulates prolactin secretion,[35] it is reasonable to propose that the apparent stimulation of progesterone receptor attributed to estrogen is indirect and that it is the elevation of endogenous prolactin that may be responsible for stimulating progesterone receptor. This picture is complicated further when one considers the results of Leung and Sasaki[42] and Sasaki and Leung,[43] who studied the interrelationship of prolactin, estrogen, and progesterone at receptor level. It was reported that prolactin (5 μg/mℓ)

significantly increased estrogen binding in uterine and breast tissues of lactating rats maintained in organ culture and in DMBA-induced tumors in vivo. Progesterone (1 μg/mℓ) was shown to offset this stimulatory effect of prolactin. These authors concluded that progesterone could serve as a feedback control *in situ* for the prolactin-stimulated estrogen binding and they further suggested that their data could explain the many antagonistic actions of estrogen and progesterone. Along the same lines, Bohnet[67] reported that the administration of 17-hydroxyprogesterone to mother rats immediately after birth decreased estrogen binding in the mammary gland but left prolactin binding unchanged. Taken together these findings could suggest that progesterone does not influence prolactin receptor per se but, rather, the effect of progesterone occurs at a particular step prior to estrogen receptor synthesis, which eventually implicates prolactin. Asselin et al.[26] examined the same phenomenon in ovarian-dependent (regress after ovariectomy) DMBA-induced mammary tumors. These authors demonstrated that such tumors have a markedly decreased estrogen, progesterone, and prolactin binding 5 weeks following ovariectomy. Administration of estrogen (0.5 μg/day), but not progesterone (0.5 mg/day), to the tumor-bearing ovariectomized host, for 3 weeks increased tumor size and increased binding capacity for all three hormones. Administration of prolactin (2 mg/day) alone resulted in a slight increase in tumor size and increased estrogen binding, but there was no effect on progesterone binding. These results add support to the conclusions presented by Horwitz and McGuire[66] that stimulation of progesterone receptor by estrogen does not occur via an effect of prolactin, unless one wishes to consider the role of prolactin to stimulate estrogen receptor.

VI. CONCLUSIONS

Studies on the hormone-dependent nature of some human and experimental breast cancers have been discussed in light of available data on hormone action and hormone receptors. Historically, hormone dependence in this disease has been taken to mean estrogen dependence, but partial response, or even lack of response, to estrogen therapy has been reported in a significant number of cases. These results have led many investigators to consider that other hormones such as progesterone, prolactin, and insulin are important factors in this disease. There seems to be little doubt that all these hormones interrelate with each other in a way that ultimately influences tumor growth and biochemistry. If one considers the level of cellular hormone receptors as a measure of the hormones biological potency, then the interrelationships among these hormones may be justifiably examined at the receptor level. Initiation of such studies were made following a course of observations on the hormone biological activities. Results reported by different laboratories on the relationship observed between estrogen and other hormones on the induction, maintenance, and regression of mammary tumors were frequently related at the receptor level. Estrogen stimulates progesterone receptor and progesterone offsets the prolactin stimulation of estrogen receptor in DMBA-induced mammary tumors. The estrogen receptor level has also been reported to be influenced by circulating levels of both estrogen and prolactin. Estrogen stimulates the secretion of prolactin and apparently helps in maintaining prolactin receptor. Furthermore, estrogen receptor and prolactin receptor seem to be maintained only in the presence of insulin, and estrogen and insulin appear to have a negative regulatory effect on insulin receptor. A summary of these observations is presented (Figure 3).

Thus, it appears that all these hormones are components of a complex format of exchanged and mutual effects that makes it extremely difficult to understand hormone-dependent breast cancer. An overall accounting for all these hormonal interrelationships should result from studies of each factor individually and in combination, in

	Estrogen Receptor	Insulin Receptor	Prolactin Receptor	Progesterone Receptor
Estrogen	+ [26, 68]	– [27, 28]	– [69]	+ [26, 63, 64, 66]
Insulin	M [25, 27, 28, 49]	– [27, 28]	M [69]	?
Prolactin	+ [42⁻45]	?	– [69]	?
Progesterone	– [42, 43]	?	?	?

+ = positive effect
– = negative effect
M = Maintenance
? = no data

FIGURE 3.   Relationships among estrogen, insulin, prolactin, progesterone, and their receptors as obtained from the references indicated in brackets.

vitro and in vivo, and will be required before one can assign specific cause and effect relationships. Consequently, there is a greater need for animal model tumor systems that could predict the clinical success of hormonal combinations since, as apparent, no one animal tumor can completely represent all the variations in growth potential and endocrine responsiveness encountered in the clinical disease. Furthermore, animal tumor models must have well-defined and reproducible growth patterns and reactivities to the hormones so that modifications in parameters resulting from experimental manipulations can be correctly interpreted.

There remains, however, the still greater difficulty of testing and thus applying these data from animal models to the clinical setting. Here, the experimental scientist must contend with restrictions that are of a different order of magnitude, ranging from considerations at the clinical level of quantitation of tumor burden and assessment of response or lack of response to those dealing with ethical and medicolegal issues. While the former problem has been the subject of considerable effort, which has led to the establishment of criteria that enable large collaborative clinical efforts to be mounted, the need for more exacting disease assessment is still to be resolved. Unlike the animal models, which are studied under conditions that can be controlled, the patient with breast cancer represents an outcome of a process that results from uncontrolled and indeed unknown factors including etiologic agents, hormonal variations, age at onset, and progress of disease. The ability to measure a variety of biochemical parameters in human breast cancers is hampered by size of sample, accessibility, and frequency of sampling; the data obtained are most often static in nature rather than dynamic as in animals. For example, as we have suggested above, it would appear that hormonal regulation of receptors may offer an additional approach to successful therapy, whereby one hormone may facilitate the action of a second hormone.

The studies presented above on experimental mammary tumors have provided the impetus to explore similar hormonal effects in human breast cancer. To that effect, in vitro studies with a number of organ cultures and cell cultures of human breast carcinomas (referred to in text) are being utilized towards the evaluation of tissue response to these different hormonal agents. Certainly, with the degree of complexity that the human disease represents, massive and cumulative efforts in endocrine research are needed before one can safely assign clear-cut roles and interrelationships that may have beneficial clinical applications.

ACKNOWLEDGMENTS

The studies from the authors laboratory were supported by USPHS Grants CA16660, CA12836 and, in part, by Cancer Center Support Grant 5-P30-CA 11198-09, National Cancer Institute, National Institutes of Health. Dr. Samir M. Shafie is the recipient of a National Institutes of Health Fellowship 1F32-CA 05941-01 from the National Cancer Institute.

REFERENCES

1. Berenblum, I., *Carcinogenesis as a Biological Problem,* Elsevier, New York, 1974.
2. Shay, H., Harris, C., and Gruenstein, M., Influence of sex hormones on the incidence and form of tumors produced in male or female rats by gastric instillation of methylcholanthrene, *J. Natl. Cancer Inst.,* 13, 307, 1952.
3. Huggins, C., Grand, L. C., and Brillantes, F. P., Critical significance of breast structure in the induction of mammary cancer in the rat, *Proc. Natl. Acad. Sci. U.S.A.,* 45, 1294, 1959.
4. Dao, T. L. and Sunderland, H., Mammary carcinogenesis by 3-methylcholanthrene. I. Hormonal aspects in tumor induction and growth, *J. Natl. Cancer Inst.,* 23, 567, 1959.
5. Dao, T. L., Bock, F. G., and Greiner, M. J., Mammary carcinogenesis by 3-methylcholanthrene. II. Inhibitory effect of pregnancy and lactation on tumor induction, *J. Natl. Cancer Inst.,* 25, 991, 1960.
6. Huggins, C., Moon, R. C., and Morii, S., Extinction of experimental mammary cancer. I. Estradiol-17β and progesterone, *Proc. Natl. Acad. Sci. U.S.A.,* 48, 379, 1962.
7. Adam, E., Decker, D., Herbst, A., Noller, K., Tilley, B., and Townsend, D., Vaginal and cervical cancers and other abnormalities associated with exposure in utero to diethylstilbestrol and related synthetic hormones, *Cancer Res.,* 37, 1249, 1977.
8. Silverberg, E., Cancer statistics, 1977, *CA Cancer J. Clin.,* 27, 26, 1977.
9. Toh, Y. C., Physiological and biochemical reviews of sex differences and carcinogenesis with particular reference to the liver, *Adv. Cancer Res.,* 18, 155, 1973.
10. Firminger, H. I. and Reuber, M. D., Influence of adrenocortical, adrogenic, and anabolic hormones on the development of carcinoma and cirrhosis of the liver in A × C rats fed N-2-fluorenyldiacetamide, *J. Natl. Cancer Inst.,* 27, 559, 1961.
11. Reuber, M. D. and Firminger, H. I., Effect of progesterone and diethylstilbestrol on hepatic carcinogenesis and cirrhosis in A × C rats fed N-2-fluorenyldiacetamide, *J. Natl. Cancer Inst.,* 29, 933, 1962.
12. Jensen, E. V. and Desombre, E. R., Mechanism of action of the female sex hormones, *Annu. Rev. Biochem.,* 41, 203, 1972.
13. Cutts, J. H. and Noble, R. L., Estrone-induced mammary tumors in the rat. I. Induction and behavior of tumors, *Cancer Res.,* 24, 1116, 1964.
14. Hilf, R., Biochemical studies of experimental mammary tumors as related to human breast cancer, in *Methods in Cancer Research,* Vol. 7, Busch, H., Ed., Academic Press, New York, 1973, 55.
15. Meites, J., Relation of prolactin and estrogen to mammary tumorigenesis in the rat, *J. Natl. Cancer Inst.,* 48, 1217, 1972.
16. Sinha, D., Copper, D., and Dao, T. L., The nature of estrogen and prolactin effect on mammary tumorigenesis, *Cancer Res.,* 33, 411, 1973.
17. Jensen, E. V., Block, G. E., Smith, S., Kyser, K., and Desombre, E. R., Estrogen receptors and breast cancer responses to adrenalectomy. Prediction of response in cancer therapy, *Natl. Cancer Inst. Monogr.,* 34, 55, 1974.
18. Wittliff, J. L., Steroid-binding proteins in normal and neoplastic mammary cells, in *Methods in Cancer Research,* Vol. 11, Busch, H., Ed., Academic Press, New York, 1975, 203.
19. McGuire, W. L., Carbone, P. P., and Vollmer, E. P., *Estrogen Receptors in Human Breast Cancers,* Raven Press, New York, 1975.

20. Lyons, W. R., Li, C. H., and Johnson, R. E., The hormonal control of mammary growth and lactation, *Recent Prog. Horm. Res.,* 14, 219, 1958.
21. Holdaway, I. and Friesen, H., Correlation between hormone binding and growth response of rat mammary tumors, *Cancer Res.,* 36, 1562, 1976.
22. Holdaway, I. M. and Friesen, H., Hormone binding by human mammary carcinoma, *Cancer Res.,* 37, 1946, 1977.
23. Posner, B. I., Kelly, P. A., and Friesen, H. G., Induction of a lactogenic receptor in rat liver: Influence of estrogen and the pituitary, *Proc. Natl. Acad. Sci. U.S.A.,* 71, 2407, 1974.
24. Kelly, P. A., Ferland, L., Labrie, F., and DeLean, A., Hormonal control of liver prolactin receptors, in *Hypothalamus and Endocrine Functions,* Labrie, F., Meites, J. and Pelletier, G., Eds., Plenum Press, New York, 1976, 321.
25. Gibson, S. L. and Hilf, R., Influence of hormonal alteration of host on estrogen binding in DMBA-induced mammary tumors, *Cancer Res.,* 36, 3736, 1976.
26. Asselin, J., Kelly, P., Caron, M., and Labrie, F., Control of hormone receptor levels and growth of DMBA-induced mammary tumors by estrogens, progesterone and prolactin, *Endocrinology,* 101, 666, 1977.
27. Shafie, S. M., Gibson, S. L., and Hilf, R., Effect of insulin and estrogen on hormone binding in the R3230AC mammary adenocarcinoma, *Cancer Res.,* 37, 4655, 1977.
28. Shafie, S. M. and Hilf, R., Relationship between insulin and estrogen binding to growth response in DMBA-induced rat tumors, *Cancer Res.,* 38, 759, 1978.
29. Welsch, C. W. and Nagasawa, H., Prolactin and murine mammary tumorigenesis: a review, *Cancer Res.,* 37, 951, 1977.
30. Reece, R. P., Mammary gland development and function. in *The Endocrinology of Reproduction,* Velardo, J. T., Ed., Oxford University Press, New York, 1958, 213.
31. Rivera, E. M., Maintenance and development of whole mammary glands in organ culture, *J. Endocrinol.,* 30, 33, 1964.
32. Bern, H. A. and Nandi, S., Recent studies of the hormonal influence in mouse mammary tumorigenesis, *Prog. Exp. Tumor Res.,* 2, 90, 1961.
33. Welsch, C. W., Interaction of estrogen and prolactin in spontaneous mammary tumorigenesis of the mouse, *J. Toxicol. Environ. Health Suppl.,* 1, 161, 1976.
34. Chen, C. L. and Meites, J., Effects of estrogen and progesterone on serum and pituitary prolactin levels in ovariectomized rats, *Endocrinology,* 86, 503, 1970.
35. Desombre, E. R., Kledzik, G., Marshall, S., and Meites, J., Estrogen and prolactin receptor concentrations in rat mammary tumors and response to endocrine ablation, *Cancer Res.,* 36, 354, 1976.
36. Meites, J. and Nicoll, C. S., Adenohypohysis: prolactin, *Annu. Rev. Physiol.,* 28, 57, 1966.
37. Pearson, O. H., Llerena, O., Llerena, L., Molina, A., and Butler, P. T., Prolactin-dependent rat mammary cancer: a model for man?, *Trans. Assoc. Am. Physicians,* 32, 225, 1969.
38. Pearson, O. H., Endocrine aspects of breast cancer, in *Current Research in Oncology,* Anfinsen, C. B., Potter, M., and Schechter, A. N., Eds., Academic Press, New York, 1972, 125.
39. Manni, A., Trujillo, J., and Pearson, O., Predominant role of prolactin in stimulating the growth of DMBA-induced mammary tumor, *Cancer Res.,* 37, 1216, 1977.
40. Brooks, C. L. and Welsch, C. W., Inhibition of mammary dysplasia in estrogen-treated C₃H/HeJ female mice by treatment with 2-bromo-ergocryptine, *Proc. Soc. Exp. Biol. Med.,* 145, 484, 1974.
41. Nagasawa, H. and Yanai, R., Effects of prolactin or growth hormone on growth of carcinogen-induced mammary tumors of adreno-ovariectomized rats, *Int. J. Cancer,* 6, 488, 1970.
42. Leung, B. S. and Sasaki, G. H., Prolactin and progesterone effect on specific estradiol binding in uterine and mammary tissue, *in vitro, Biochem. Biophys. Res. Commun.,* 55, 1180, 1973.
43. Sasaki, G. H. and Leung, B. S., On the mechanism of hormone action in DMBA-induced mammary tumor. Prolactin and progesterone effects on estrogen receptor *in vitro, Cancer (Philadelphia),* 35, 645, 1975.
44. Vignon, F. and Rochefort, H., Regulation of estrogen receptors in ovarian-dependent rat mammary tumors. Effects of castration and prolactin, *Endocrinology,* 98, 722, 1976.
45. Shafie, S. M. and Brooks, S. C., Effect of prolactin on growth and the estrogen receptor level of human breast cancer cells (MCF-7), *Cancer Res.,* 37, 792, 1977.
46. Heuson, J. C. and Legros, N., Influence of insulin deprivation on growth of DMBA-induced mammary carcinoma in rats subjected to alloxan diabetes and food restriction, *Cancer Res.,* 32, 226, 1972.
47. Cohen, N. D. and Hilf, R., Influence of insulin on growth and metabolism of DMBA-induced mammary tumors, *Cancer Res.,* 34, 3245, 1974.
48. Cohen, N. D. and Hilf, R., Effect of estrogen treatment on DMBA-induced mammary tumor growth and biochemistry in intact and diabetic rats, *Proc. Soc. Exp. Biol. Med.,* 148, 339, 1975.
49. Shafie, S. M. and Brooks, S. C., The relationship of insulin to regulation of breast tumor cells by 17β-estradiol, *Cancer Res.,* in Press.

50. **Cohen, N. D. and Hilf, R.**, Influence of insulin estrogen-induced responses in the R3230AC mammary carcinoma, *Cancer Res.*, 35, 560, 1975.
51. **Rhomberg, W.**, Metastasierendes Mammakarsinom und Diabetes Mellitus eine Prognostisch gunstige Krankheitskombination, *Dtsch. Med. Wochenschr.*, 100, 2422, 1975.
52. **Huggins, C. and Yang, N. C.**, Induction and extinction of mammary cancer, *Science*, 137, 257, 1962.
53. **Huggins, C.**, Two principles in endocrine therapy of cancers: hormone deprival and hormone interference, *Cancer Res.*, 25, 1163, 1965.
54. **Jabara, A. G.**, Effects of progesterone on 9,10-dimethyl-1,2-benzanthracene-induced mammary tumours in Sprague-Dawley rats, *Br. J. Cancer*, 21, 418, 1967.
55. **Jabara, A. G. and Harcourt, A. G.**, The effects of progesterone and ovariectomy on mammary tumours induced by 7,12-dimethylbenz(a)anthracene in Sprague-Dawley rats, *Pathology*, 2, 115, 1970.
56. **Stoll, B. A.**, Effect of lyndiol, an oral contraceptive, on breast cancer, *Br. Med. J.*, 1, 150, 1967.
57. **McCormick, C. M. and Moon, R. C.**, Effect of pregnancy and lactation on growth of mammary tumours induced by 7,12-dimethylbenzanthracene (DMBA), *Br. J. Cancer*, 19, 160, 1965.
58. **McCormick, C. M. and Moon, R. C.**, Hormones influencing postpartum growth of DMBA-induced rat mammary tumors, *Cancer Res.*, 27, 626, 1967.
59. **Growley, L. G. and McDonald, I.**, Delalutin and estrogens for the treatment of advanced mammary carcinoma in the postmenopausal women *Cancer (Philadelphia)*, 18, 436, 1965.
60. **Stoll, B. A.**, Progestin therapy of breast cancer: comparison of agents, *Br. Med. J.*, 3, 338, 1967.
61. **Stoll, B. A.**, Vaginal cytology as an aid to hormone therapy in postmenopausal breast cancer, *Cancer (Philadelphia)*, 20, 1807, 1967.
62. **McCormick, G. M. and Moon, R. C.**, Effect of increasing doses of estrogen and progesterone on mammary carcinogenesis in the rat, *Eur. J. Cancer*, 9, 483, 1973.
63. **Horwitz, K. B., McGuire, W. L., Pearson, O. H., and Segaloff, A.**, Predicting response to endocrine therapy in human breast cancer. A hypothesis, *Science*, 89, 726, 1975.
64. **McGuire, W. L., Horwitz, K. B., Pearson, O. H., and Segaloff, A.**, Current status of estrogen and progesterone receptors in breast cancer, *Cancer (Philadelphia)*, 39, 2934, 1977.
65. **Rao, B. R., Wiest, W. G., and Allen, W. M.**, Progesterone receptor in rabbit uterus. Characterization and estradiol-17β augmentation, *Endocrinology*, 92, 1229, 1973.
66. **Horwitz, K. B. and McGuire, W. L.**, Progesterone and progesterone receptors in experimental breast cancer, *Cancer Res.*, 37, 1733, 1977.
67. **Bohnet, H. G.**, Prolactin and estrogen binding sites in the mammary gland of the lactating and non-lactating rat, *Endocrinology*, 101, 1111, 1977.
68. **Hawkins, R., Hill, A., Freedman, B., Killen, E., Buchan, P., Miller, W. R., and Forrest, A.**, Estrogen receptor activity and endocrine status in DMBA-induced rat mammary tumors, *Eur. J. Cancer*, 13, 223, 1977.
69. **Smith, R. D., Hilf, R., and Senior, A.**, Prolactin binding to R3230AC mammary carcinoma and liver in hormone-treated and diabetic rats, *Cancer Res.*, 37, 595, 1977.

Chapter 3

PROGESTERONE AND SYNTHETIC PROGESTINS: THEIR
BIOLOGICAL ACTIVITY AND ROLE IN NEOPLASIA

E. H. Fowler

TABLE OF CONTENTS

I. INTRODUCTION

It is entirely appropriate that this chapter be prepared at the University of Rochester School of Medicine and Dentistry where Dr. George W. Corner did much of the pioneering work to describe the mammalian reproductive system. There, Dr. Corner first proposed the term "progestin" to name the hormone elicited by the mammalian corpus luteum and responsible for maintaining pregnancy, i.e., pro-gestation.[1] Allen described the hormone as one which produced characteristic changes in the rabbit uterus and maintained pregnancies which would otherwise have been doomed.[1] A crystalline though still impure substance was purified from corpora lutea in 1932,[2] and in 1935 the then-prominent workers in the field issued a joint communique in which "progesterone" was suggested as the name to be used to describe the hormone.[3]

During the past 40 or more years since the identification, purification, and initial description of progesterone, much research has been directed at the biologic and therapeutic properties of this hormone. Synthetic progestins, derivatives of both progesterone and testosterone with potent progestational activity, have been extensively produced, tested, and used in man and other animals for both contraceptive and therapeutic purposes. Many progestins, including progesterone, have been associated with and believed responsible for a host of adverse conditions, including neoplasia, in several species.

The objectives of this chapter are to review the biologic features of the progestins and their tumorigenic potential. Minimal emphasis will be placed on problems, other than neoplasia, believed to be related to the use of progestins. This review is confined almost entirely to the use of progestins in experimental animals, although some information gleaned from their use in humans will be included where applicable.

Entire books and even multiple volumes have been written concerning progesterone and other progestins, an indication of the amount of information available on the subject. This review includes selected information concerning production sites, metabolism, mechanism of action, biological activity, and their relationship to the development of neoplasia. Purposely excluded from this text is discussion of levels of progesterone found in plasma or serum of several species during the estrous cycle and pregnancy, except for how these levels are influenced by other hormones, or of the changes in blood chemistry produced with the use of these progestins, except in a few instances where other hormones are affected. Also excluded from this review are the potential role of progestins in human breast and uterine cancer or in hepatocellular carcinoma, as these will be dealt with elsewhere in this book.

II. PRODUCTION SITES

A. Ovary

Progesterone is the primary steroid hormone synthesized by the corpus luteum. In rats, the progesterone level increases as the corpus luteum develops on the afternoon of the first day of diestrus, reaches a maximum early on the second day, and is quickly followed by a precipitous fall during the same day correlating with regression of the corpus luteum.[4] Progesterone levels then remain low until the afternoon of proestrus when an increase again occurs. Cervical stimulation, which produces a corpus luteum of pseudopregnancy, results in a dramatic rise in the progesterone level considerably above that found during diestrus.[4] In the hamster, the theca interna and granulosa cells of the follicles together with the interstitial cells contribute approximately equal amounts of progesterone during the preovulatory period of the cycle.[5] Granulosa cells from human ovarian follicles in vitro more actively convert pregnenolone to progesterone than do thecal cells.[6] Levels of progesterone and 17α-OH progesterone are higher in the follicular fluid of preovulatory human ovarian follicles than they are in the plasma.[7] The progesterone level in the fluid of human Graafian follicles is 1000 to 10,000 times higher than in plasma.[8] Granulosa cells from preovulatory follicles of Rhesus monkeys when placed in cell culture become luteinized and secrete elevated levels of progestins for up to 6 days in culture.[9] If either human luteinizing hormone (LH) or follicle-stimulating hormone (FSH) is added to the cultures, the progestin secretion is prolonged to at least 27 days.[9]

Progesterone production in rabbits can be stimulated by LH in the absence of corpora lutea.[10] Luteinization of sheep granulosa cells occurs 6 to 12 hr following ovulation and is associated with a slight rise in serum progesterone concentration.[11] The principal precursor for progesterone biosynthesis, at least in the rat, is cholesterol rather than acetate.[12]

B. Other

Progesterone is also synthesized from appropriate precursors in the adrenal gland and placenta.[13-17] The concentration of progesterone is higher in the adrenal effluent plasma of rats and Rhesus monkeys (*Macaca mulatta*) during the estrous cycle than is found in the ovarian venous blood.[13,14] The level is lowest in the adrenal venous blood of rats between the first 2 to 4 hr of estrus and highest between the 14th and 16th hr of proestrus and the 10th to 12th hr of estrus. The proestrus elevation supports the hypothesis that adrenal progesterone is possibly involved in the facilitation of the preovulatory LH release.[13] The adrenal gland of female dogs secretes more progesterone than the adrenal of males, and secretion decreases following castration of either sex but can be increased by estrogen administration.[15]

III. METABOLISM

A. Liver

The major metabolic site for progesterone is the liver where the metabolites are conjugated prior to excretion by the kidneys, a process which takes about 2 days. About one third of plasma progesterone is metabolized in tissues other than liver.[18] In the mouse, the greatest amount of radiolabeled progesterone was taken up by the liver, rapidly secreted through the biliary system, and then excreted into the G.I. tract.[19] The biological halflife of radioactivity in the blood was 11 min when the labeled progesterone was given intravenously. The metabolic clearance rate of progesterone in several different species varied between 40 and 180 ℓ/day/kg, with man being between 60 and 70 ℓ/day/kg, monkeys between 40 and 50 ℓ/day/kg, rabbits between 55 and 60 ℓ/day/kg, sheep 110 ℓ/day/kg, rats 120 ℓ/day/kg, and guinea pigs 180 ℓ/day/kg.[20] The major clearance sites included liver, brain, and uterus. The specific metabolites of progesterone included 20α-hydroxy-pregnan-4-en-3-one and 5α-pregnan-3,20-dione.[20]

B. Brain

Progesterone uptake by brain and pituitary of estradiol-primed ovariectomized adult female rats is higher than found in uterus or vaginal tissues, where uptake occurs later and is followed by slower release.[21] Progesterone is metabolized by cell-free homogenates of adult rat brain and other target tissues, with 5α- and 20α-reduction being greatest in pituitary glands of males compared with epididymis, hypothalamus, cerebral cortex, and ventral prostate gland.[22] A lower rate of 5α-reduction occurs in the female rat pituitary gland.[22]

The major metabolic pathways for progesterone in the hypothalamus and pituitary are via reductive pathways to 5α-dihydroprogesterone involving a Δ4-steroid 5α-reductase, and to 3α-hydroxy-5α-pregnan-20-one involving 3α-hydroxysteroid dehydrogenase, both of which appear to be regulated by endogenous hormones and other factors, since their activity fluctuates with various physiological and hormonal states.[23] The 5α-dihydroprogesterone metabolite appears to be the primary one involved in governing progesterone-sensitive processes in the pituitary and hypothalamus.

C. Ovary and Uterus

Both the ovary and uterus are able to metabolize progesterone, thereby producing other steroids (ovary) or inactivation (uterus). Within 5 min after canine ovaries have been infused with ^{3}H-pregnenolone, the steroid is metabolized to 17α-hydroxypregnenolone, progesterone, 17α-hydroxyprogesterone, dehydroepiandrosterone (DHEA), androstenedione, testosterone, and probably estradiol.[24] During estrus, there is a high conversion of pregnenolone to testosterone and androstenedione, whereas during early pregnancy, much of the pregnenolone is converted to progesterone.[24] Progesterone is metabolized by ovarian follicles to 17α-hydroxyprogesterone, androstenedione, testosterone, estrone, and estradiol.[25] Progesterone is reported to be the final step in the steroid metabolic pathway of corpora lutea by some workers,[26] whereas others have demonstrated further metabolism to androgens and estrogens.[27,28]

Progesterone metabolism in rat uteri is primarily by a nuclear 5α-reductase which is stimulated by estradiol treatment in vivo.[29] The 5α-reductase activity in mitochondrial and microsomal fractions is not increased by estradiol treatment. Progesterone is also reduced to 20α-hydroxy-4-pregnan-3-one by an estrogen-stimulated soluble enzyme in rat uteri.[29]

The rate of progesterone metabolism in intact rat uteri varies with the hormonal status of the animal in a concentration-dependent manner. With low progesterone concentration, ring A reduction is decreased in estrogen-stimulated uteri; at high progesterone concentration, ring A reduction is increased following estrogen treatment.[30] Estrogen stimulation always increases the rate of progesterone metabolism in dilute homogenates of uterus through increased activity of ring A reductases.[30]

D. Other

The adrenal gland is capable not only of synthesizing progesterone from precursors, but also of further metabolism to androgens, estrogens, and corticoids.[31,32] Testicles acquire the capacity to convert progesterone to testosterone,[33,34] and may show striking age-dependent changes in the pattern of conversion of progesterone to androgens.[35] Human skin and vaginal mucosa are capable of actively metabolizing progesterone.[36]

IV. MECHANISM OF ACTION

A. Progesterone Binding—General

The mechanism of action of progesterone has been reviewed by Jensen and DeSombre, and the reader is referred to their treatise for a complete coverage of this subject.[37] The progestational hormones apparently act by bringing about expression of new regions of DNA template, which gives rise to different species of RNA necessary for the synthesis of differentiated cell products.[37] The mechanism by which the progestins initiate these biochemical changes in target tissues involved specific progestin-receptor complexes which will be briefly reviewed here.

In 1970, Falk and Bardin reported that uterine tissue from castrated guinea pigs retained labeled progesterone longer than did heart or diaphragm and that uptake of the ^{3}H-progesterone was blocked by unlabeled progesterone, but not by cortisol, estrogen, or testosterone, which suggested a specific binding of progesterone that was of limited capacity.[38] Falk and Bardin also discovered that estrogen pretreatment for 2 days increased the uptake of ^{3}H-progesterone sevenfold in the uterus.[38] Since this important discovery, progestin binding components, or progestin receptors, have been reported in rats and mice,[39] immature rabbit and again in the guinea pig,[40] hamsters,[41] sheep,[42] primates including both monkeys and man,[43] and in chicken oviduct,[44] to name but a few species. It is reasonably clear that progesterone and synthetic progestins exert their effect initially by complexing with specific receptors in the target tissues which initiates a series of biochemical events leading to the specific biological effect, such as cell proliferation or synthesis of some product for intracellular metabolism or secretion.

B. Characteristics of Progesterone Receptors

Progesterone receptors are synthesized in the uterus of several species in response to estrogen, and progesterone administered simultaneously with estrogen will block this synthesis.[45] Estrogen-stimulated synthesis of progesterone receptor can also be blocked by prior administration of actinomycin D or cycloheximide.[41] Pronase was effective in abolishing progesterone binding, suggesting that the binders are in part protein, and protamine sulfate and p-hydroxymercuribenzoate also obliterated the cytoplasmic binding, implying that this receptor is an acid protein containing sulfhydryl groups necessary for the binding.[41]

The progesterone receptors exist in three different classes or forms, the largest being a 7S complex which is thought to contain all the functional units, the smallest being a 4S protein which under certain conditions can be converted to the 7S complex by removal of salt, and an intermediate form with a sedimentation coefficient of 5.5 to 6.0 S, which has been implicated in nuclear binding.[45] The specificity of nuclear binding appears to reside in the cytoplasmic receptor.

Progesterone concentration was lower in the microsomal, mitochondrial, and nuclear fractions of pregnant rat myometrium than in the cytosol on the 14th day of pregnancy and thereafter increased to approach that of the cytosol; the amounts in the microsomal fraction exceeded the cytosolic concentration after the 18th day. The concentration of progesterone decreased sharply in all fractions during the last 4 days of pregnancy and was low in all fractions on the day prior to parturition.[46] The microsomal binding of progesterone in pregnant and post-partum rat myometrium is of two types; binding of high affinity and limited capacity and binding of low affinity but high capacity.[47] These binding components are specific for progesterone. Of 18 different steroids tested, only testosterone, 5α-dihydrotestosterone and 5α-pregnan-3,20-dione exhibited moderate competition with progesterone for the binding sites. Rat liver microsomes exhibited progesterone binding resembling that of myometrial microsomes, whereas striated muscle and heart microsomal preparations showed only low concentrations of nonspecific progesterone binding. The microsomal progesterone binding components were felt to be distinctly different from the cytosolic high-affinity progesterone-binding proteins found in rat myometrium.[47]

Estrogen-induced progesterone receptors in the guinea pig uterus have a halflife in vivo of about 5 days in the hormone-deprived animal, but with progesterone administration, the receptor decays more rapidly.[48] The maximum concentration of progesterone receptor in the cytosol of guinea pig uteri was present during proestrus, 40,000 binding sites per cell, followed by progressive decrease during estrus and metestrus to a level 16 times below that in diestrus.[49]

Progesterone receptors in rabbit uteri were evaluated for their affinity for a number of synthetic progestins.[50] Progesterone, 17-hydroxyprogesterone caproate, chlormadinone acetate, megestrol acetate, and cyproterone acetate had similar affinities for the progestin receptor, whereas medroxyprogesterone acetate (MPA) and DU-41164 possessed much higher affinities. Of the nortestosterone derivatives, norethisterone equalled progesterone in affinity for the progestogen receptor while *d*-norgestrel and WY-4355 were more active. Norethynodrel and ethynodiol diacetate had much lower receptor affinities than progesterone. Only norethynodrel and ethynodiol diacetate showed marked affinity for the estrogen receptor.[50] In contrast to the high affinity of the rat uterine progestin receptor for medroxyprogesterone acetate, the guinea pig uterine receptor was unique because of its low affinity for biologically potent 17α-substituted progestins such as medroxyprogesterone acetate.[51] It was concluded that the potent biological activity of MPA relative to progesterone in the guinea pig uterus was due in part to its slower rate of metabolism and longer nuclear retention.[51]

V. BIOLOGICAL ACTIVITY

Progestins exert an effect on nearly every endocrine or steroid hormone target organ in the body. These are manifested as morphologic or functional changes, including stimulation or inhibition of intracellular and extracellular products. No attempt is made to completely cover all of the biological actions of these steroids, but rather a brief review will be presented, designed to include some of the many and varied effects in the different organs to indicate the magnitude of the situation. Some changes in target tissues result from the direct effects of the progestins, while others occur indirectly because of the interrelationship between progestins and other hormones. An attempt will be made later in this chapter to describe some of the hormonal interrelationships that occur and the changes that result.

The biological effects of progesterone are basically related to uterine function, gonadotropin production and/or release, ovulation, sexual behavior, lactation, sleep patterns-anesthetic effects, blood formation-erythropoiesis, thermogenesis, and protein metabolism.[52] Further characterization of the biological activities includes inhibition of ovulation during pregnancy and the normal cycle and induction of ovulation in certain species such as the cow, rat, chicken, and rabbit; stimulation of tubal contractions during passage of sperm and ova; inhibition of fertilization in vivo at higher dosage levels; supporting the implantation of the fertilized egg; maintenance of the fetus and normal pregnancy; inhibition of parturition and prolonged pregnancy; mucification of the vaginal epithelium; progestational proliferation of the uterine endometrium; growth and development of the deciduoma; inhibition of uterine contractility and prevention of contractility following exposure to oxytocin; inhibition of the release of pituitary gonadotropins; in conjunction with estrogen, the stimulation of growth of the lobulo-alveolar system of the mammary gland; stimulating atrophy of the adrenal gland; in high doses, acting as the anesthetic agent; inhibition or potentiation of the action of estrogen, especially in the uterus, oviduct, mammary gland, and behavior; influencing electrolyte balance; inducing slight rise in body temperature; acting synergistically with estradiol to induce psychic or sexual heat in the female; necessary for maternal behavior such as care of the young; inhibition of the action of relaxin on the pubic ligament of the mouse; and stimulation of the release of relaxin.[53] Zarrow pointed out that not only should the relationship of progesterone to estrogen be kept in mind when characterizing its action, but also the interaction with estrogen since progesterone can synergize or antagonize estrogen depending on the ratio of the two hormones.[53]

A. Anterior Pituitary and Hypothalamus

One of the principal mechanisms whereby high doses of progesterone and the synthetic progestins exert their contraceptive action is by depressing the gonadotropic hormones, primarily LH, thereby inhibiting ovulation. Progesterone administered to Rhesus monkeys for 8 days beginning 12 days after the peak concentration of serum estrogen resulted in a prolonged luteal phase of progesterone in 6 of 10 animals, and length of time between LH peaks differed significantly between animals treated with progesterone and those treated with cholesterol. Progesterone did not alter the concentration of FSH in the stages of the cycle.[54] Progesterone and one of its metabolites, 20α-hydroxyprogesterone, caused enzyme changes in the hypothalamus of female rabbits which could be correlated with a known pattern of gonadotropic hormone secretion, further substantiating the hypothesis that there is a relationship between enzyme levels in the hypothalamus and gonadotropic hormone secretion.[55]

Increased ovarian progesterone appears to play an important role in controlling the timing and duration of the LH peak,[56] but some investigators refute this hypothesis.[57] However, the majority of studies have shown that LH levels are directly influenced by progesterone and progestin administration in several different species, including rats,[58,59] hamsters,[60] monkeys,[61] dogs,[62] and women.[63] Even though mean LH levels may not be significantly altered with some low-dose progestins, the pattern of excretion is usually altered, particularly in the midcycle peaks.[64] The response of the rat anterior pituitary to luteinizing-hormone releasing-factor (LHRF), measured by LH output, increased significantly when progesterone was administered during proestrus to ovariectomized rats and treated with estradiol benzoate during the previous diestrus.[65] Follicle-stimulating hormone, on the other hand, did not respond to LHRF in rats treated with either estradiol benzoate or progesterone immediately after ovariectomy, but did increase significantly after sequential administration of estradiol benzoate and progesterone.[65,66]

Progesterone and progestins also influence other anterior pituitary hormones. Peak plasma growth hormone concentrations after glucose and insulin administration were significantly blunted in all individuals after progesterone administration.[67] Progesterone also impaired somatotropic hormone (STH) responses to arginine. These results suggested that placental production of progesterone and rising concentrations in the maternal plasma contribute to the inhibition of pituitary release of STH and to the hyperinsulinemia observed during late gestation.[67] Medroxyprogesterone acetate reduces growth hormone levels in acromegalic people,[68] while the acromegalic-like changes in beagles receiving progestins such as chlormadinone acetate are felt to be due to stimulated anterior pituitary activity and presumably increased growth hormone.[69] Medroxyprogesterone acetate suppresses the adrenal cortex in man[70,71] and dogs (unpublished observations) presumably because of its glucocorticoid properties and depression of ACTH secretion and/or excretion from the pituitary. Progesterone produces a dose-related decrease in prolactin production on rat pituitary cells in vitro reaching 60% of control value.[72]

Striking quantitative morphologic variations were found in the hypothalamic-adenohypophyseal system of cattle receiving chlormadinone acetate and norethisterone acetate.[73] The cyclic variation in activity of the FSH cells and cells in the medial preoptic and infundibular nuclei in the hypothalamus were abolished by the gestagens. The metabolic activity of the FSH cells were inhibited and activity of the hypothalamic neurons was slightly elevated.[73]

The morphology of the baboon pituitary gland was evaluated after administration of progesterone and several synthetic progestins.[74] Progesterone did not affect pituitary cytology but did appear to depress the thyroid gland and adrenal cortex. MPA resulted in the greatest cytologic alteration of the anterior pituitary after 5 months of treatment; the chromophobic and acidophilic cells were unaffected, but the basophils appeared almost entirely degranulated, enlarged in diameter, and practically unstainable either by the periodic acid Schiff (PAS) method or the paraldehyde-fuchsin technique. All basophilic elements resembled chromophobes and any evaluation of the percent ratio among different cell types was impossible.[74] Two of the other synthetic progestins did not alter pituitary cytology, indicating that the action was directly on the genital tract without being mediated through the pituitary gland.[74]

In ovariectomized rats, MPA was the only one of three progestins implanted in the anterior pituitary which failed to alter the morphology of either the prolactin or LH cells.[75] The other two progestins, both possessing estrogenic activity, caused hypertrophy of prolactin cells in a region that spread laterally, ventrally, and caudally from the pellet, and the LH cells were reduced in size.[75] Subcutaneous administration of MPA to rats (0.5 to 1.5 mg/100 gm body weight per day for 14 to 28 days) caused marked reduction in the size of prolactin cells and enlargement of growth hormone cells which were also increased in relative number.[76] The response of the gonadotropic cells was variable, some being enlarged and more intensely stained in certain rats.[76]

Melengestrol acetate increased the number of chromophobes, presumably originating from gonadotropin-secreting cells, in the anterior pituitary gland of cattle.[77] No alterations were found in the cells secreting prolactin, somatotropin, or corticotropin.[77]

B. Ovary

Progesterone is capable of slowing down follicular growth in the ovary of female Wistar rats if injected at the appropriate time during the estrous cycle. The investigators believed that exogenous LH slowed down follicular growth by increasing the production of endogenous progesterone which they found elevated in the ovarian venous blood.[78] When progesterone is administered to guinea pigs on days 2 through 5 or on days 4 through 7, it fails to alter the length of the estrous cycle.[79]

Fifteen progestins, including progesterone, dihydroprogesterone, and 13 synthetic progestins used in oral contraceptives, were evaluated for their ability to suppress pubertal ovulation in the Charles River strain of CD® rat.[80] All progestins except ethynodiol diacetate inhibited initial ovulation. The synthetic progestins tested included MPA, megestrol acetate, melengestrol acetate, chlorsuperlutin, ethisterone, dimethisterone, norethynodrel, lynestrenol, norethindrone, norethindrone acetate, ethynodiol diacetate, and norgestrel.[80]

Studies to evaluate the effect of progestins on ovarian morphology have led to different conclusions. Progesterone and 17α-hydroxyprogesterone caproate did not seem to have any effect on corpus luteum (CL) function despite the additive effect of progesterone as demonstrated by elevated serum levels.[81] Ovarian morphology was reported to be normal in women receiving injections of 250 to 300 mg of MPA every 6 months.[82] The histologic evaluation included germinal epithelium, tunica albuginea, ovarian cortical stroma, hilar cells, oocytes, and follicles from primordial to Graafian stage.[82] However, follicular cysts, sometimes involving the entire ovary, were found in 7 of 14 women receiving microdose progestins (mini-pills) for 6 to 18 months.[83] The cysts were lined by two to three layers of atrophic granulosa cells in which patchy luteinization and/or degeneration were apparent. Despite follicular cysts in 50% of the women, 71% ovulated, compared with 75% in the control group. No lesions were present in the corpora lutea except for one hematoma.[83] Ovarian blood vessels in women receiving oral progestins have a much higher incidence of degeneration than is found in other women.[84] The degenerative changes in these blood vessels remained after discontinuation of therapy. Gonads characteristically atrophy in both sexes when high levels of progesterone is administered either orally or subcutaneously.[85]

Cystic atrophy of large ovarian follicles together with an absence of corpora lutea were found when the baboon was treated with progesterone and several synthetic progestins which interrupted the estrus cycle.[74]

C. Uterus

In 1910, Bouin and Ancel first described the histologic changes in rabbit endometrium following ovulation and produced experimental evidence that these changes were dependent on corpus luteum function.[86] These observations later became the basis for a bioassay of progesterone. In 1971, a comprehensive review of the literature appeared concerning the histologic effects of progesterone on the vagina and uterus in several species.[87]

Most of the research concerning the effects produced by progesterone has been conducted using uterine tisues from various species in vivo and in vitro. The relationship between progesterone and estrogen has also been examined using this target organ. It was observed as early as 1938 that the progestational effect on the endometrium and myometrium of a rabbit's uterus could be antagonized by both natural and synthetic estrogens.[88]

Progesterone promotes uterine hypertrophy in the castrate rabbit uterus and stimulates labeled thymidine incorporation only in epithelial nuclei, both glandular and luminal, commencing 24 to 30 hr after hormone administration and reaching a peak at about 2 days.[89] Progesterone stimulates nuclear synthesis in the epithelium more vigorously than estradiol, causing formation of multinuclear cells or multilobed nuclei with extensive invagination of the epithelium.[89] Priming the rabbit uterus with low dosages of estrogen lowers the threshold of the epithelial response to progesterone,[90] a situation which is reversed from that in the mouse,[91,92] the rat,[93] and the guinea pig (Mehrota and Finn, personal communication cited by Lee and Dukelow)[90] where epithelial mitosis is induced by estrogen and suppressed by progesterone. One or two daily injections of 0.5 mg progesterone after estrogen priming produced maximal DNA synthesis and mitosis similar to that seen on the 4th day of pregnancy, and subsequent progesterone administration resulted in decreased cell proliferation.[90]

In the mouse uterus, estrogen is primarily responsible for controlling division and proliferation of glandular and luminal epithelial cells while progesterone inhibits both glandular mitoses (which begins 72 hr after estrogen administration) and luminal mitoses (which are maximal 24 hr after estrogen treatment).[94] Progesterone not only reverses the pattern of estradiol stimulation in the epithelium but also stimulates mitoses in the stroma.[95] When progesterone was administered simultaneously with 17α-estradiol to ovariectomized mice, 40% of the uterine luminal epithelial cells were prevented from entering DNA synthesis, but the G_1, S, or G_2 phases were not prolonged in the remainder of the cells.[96] However, the hormones do block the entry of these cells into a second round of DNA synthesis, which suggested that the uterine luminal epithelial cells were only sensitive to progesterone for a limited period during G_1.[96] Progesterone suppressed DNA synthesis in the uterine glandular epithelium in ovariectomized mice whether estrogen was administered or not, altered the nuclear morphology of the stromal cells, and increased the number of stromal cells synthesizing DNA.[97] The investigators concluded that progesterone stimulated stromal cells in the resting phase to enter the cell cycle and that estrogen then accelerated their passage through a single round of replication and division by shortening the interval between mitosis and DNA synthesis, following which the cells withdrew from the cycle.[97] Progesterone alone has no effect on the amount or rate of incorporation of ^{14}C lysine into mouse uterine stromal nuclear proteins, whereas in the epithelium, progesterone depressed incorporation into histone and acidic nuclear proteins, but did not abolish the subsequent response to 17β-estradiol.[98] Estradiol administered after progesterone produced mitoses only in the stroma and not in the epithelium.[98]

In the rat uterus, epithelial proliferation continues during the first two days of progestational influence and then ceases, while stromal mitoses begin about 70 hr after ovulation, reaching a maximal intensity during the 4th day of pregnancy or pseudopregnancy and subsiding gradually thereafter.[99] Myometrial proliferation also occurs during the progestational influence on days 4 and 5.[99] Treatment of ovariectomized Sprague-Dawley rats with progesterone (2.0 mg/day) reproduced in part the pattern of oxygen consumption by the uterus recorded in intact animals but prolonged the duration of uterine sensitivity to decidualization.[100] Addition of estrone to the progesterone resulted in a 24- to 48-hr advance in the pattern of oxidative metabolism in comparison with the progesterone controls and a decrease in both magnitude and duration of uterine sensitivity.[100] Progesterone (5 mg) administered concurrently with 17β-estradiol (1 μg) to ovariectomized Holtzman rats significantly reduced the uterine wet weight.[101] Some levels of progesterone also reduced the percent of water and glycogen concentration in the uterus.[101] These data illustrated that the estrogen to progesterone ratio and the time of progesterone administration relative to estrogen stimulation are important points to consider when studying the interrelationship between estrogen and progesterone on different parameters.[101]

In both ovariectomized and adrenalectomized rats, progesterone (5 mg/day) administered for at least 12 hr abolished the response of the uterine luminal epithelium to 17β-estradiol (0.2 mg) with respect to mitotic activity, nucleolar enlargement, and ^{3}H-uridine uptake.[102] The uptake of ^{3}H-17β-estradiol by epithelial cells was also suppressed. If progesterone pretreatment was extended for periods longer than 36 hr the mitogenic action of estradiol was redirected from the epithelium to the subepithelial stromal cells.[102] Progesterone prevented the induction of mitotic activity in glandular epithelium, but did not inhibit stimulation of ^{3}H-uridine uptake by these cells when stimulated by estradiol.[102]

When progesterone is administered to ovariectomized-adrenalectomized rats for 7 days, the solitary cilia are lost from the luminal cells of the uterus.[103] In addition, there is a threefold increase in the distance between the two centrioles and a distortion of the normal diplosome configuration, so that the centriolar axes are no longer in normal relationship to one another.[103] The nucleoli of the stromal cells are also enlarged due to massive accumulation of granular components, attended by augmentation of the rough endoplasmic reticulum and of the free ribosomal clusters in the cytoplasm.[104]

In the subhuman primate, estrogens stimulate the growth of both glands and stroma in preparation for maturation when stimulated by progesterone.[105] Progesterone produced increased secretion of glycogens and glycoproteins with resulting dilatation of the glands and also produced a direct effect on the stroma consisting of edema, increased vascular complexity, and predecidual cell formation.[105] Excessive amounts of either hormone inhibit the effects of the other.[105] The absolute amounts of both estrogen and progesterone administered were of greater importance than the ratio between the two.[105]

Progesterone stimulated both the synthesis and release of glycoproteins by estrogen-primed rabbit endometrium and regulated qualitatively and quantitatively the synthesis and secretion of total proteins[106] Uteroglobin, a progesterone-inducible protein, is produced by the uterus in ovariectomized rabbits by daily treatment for 5 days with progesterone but disappears when estradiol is added to the progesterone during the next 5 days.[107] These findings are consistent with uteroglobin levels found during early pregnancy which decreases when estradiol levels increase.[107] Progesterone produces histochemical and biochemical changes in the uterus consistent with secretory changes when the levels diminish. Acid phosphatase activity is elevated during metestrus in mice,[108] dogs,[109] pigs,[110] and humans.[111] In human endometrium during the secretory phase, there are three strongly active isoenzymes of acid phosphatase, whereas during the proliferative phase only one major band is evident.[111] One particular isoenzyme was found exclusively in secretory phase endometrium which might be of value in assessing progestin effects in both normal and pathologic conditions.[111] In addition to the increased acid phosphatase in pigs, a large increase in lysozyme and leucine aminopeptidase activity are stimulated by progesterone.[110] In contrast to the finding in the above-mentioned species, progesterone reduces acid and alkaline phosphatase activity in the uterus of Rhesus monkeys.[112] The pattern of acid phosphatase activity in the epithelia in all layers of the endometrium closely parallels that of alkaline phosphatase under the various hormonal treatments.[112]

Uterine glucose-6-phosphate dehydrogenase activity is controlled by both estradiol and progesterone. Estradiol (5 μg/day) produces an eightfold increase in G6PD when administered to ovariectomized rats for 3 days.[113] When progesterone (2 mg/day) is injected simultaneously with estradiol, the early increase in G6PD activity occurs, but further increase after 36 hr is blocked, with the resulting maximal level being 50% that reached with estradiol alone.[113] When progesterone was administered to ovariectomized pseudopregnant rats, the G6PD activity in the deciduoma increased whereas myometrial G6PD activity only increased after estrogen treatment.[114] Estrogen potentiated the effect of progesterone on the G6PD activity in the deciduoma, but progesterone suppressed the effect of estrogen on the myometrium.[114] G6PD activity in the nondecidualizing endometrium of the ovariectomized rat uterus did not respond to progesterone treatment, and progesterone suppressed the effects of estrone on endometrial G6PD activity.[114] Apparently, the cellular differentiation of the endometrium which occurs during decidualization alters the sensitivity of the G6PD activity in the tissue to progesterone.[114] In addition to the blocking effect of progesterone on G6PD activity, estrogen-induced increases in DNA and insoluble protein synthesis were suppressed by progesterone, while RNA and soluble protein synthesis were not affected.[115]

The induction of pseudopregnancy or administration of progesterone to rabbits stimulates succinate dehydrogenase and G6PD activity and decreases amylase and LDH activity.[116] In ovariectomized rabbits, glutamic-oxalacetic transaminase activity is increased following progesterone administration.[116] Clark and Yochim[117] found LDH activity to be reduced in rat uterus under all progestational conditions. Following decidualization or implantation on day 4 of the estrous cycle, the LDH activity showed an initial transient decline followed by a prolonged rise.[117] In contrast to changes in enzyme activity measured in the endometrium, LDH in the myometrium was more stable.

Carbonic anhydrase activity in the uterus is influenced by progesterone in the rabbit,[118-120] and has been suggested as a possible bioassay for progesterone.[120] However, the same enzyme is not stimulated by progesterone in the rat[119,121] or hamster[121] and is influenced primarily by estrogen in the guinea pig.[118] Progesterone decreases endometrial carbonic anhydrase in women.[122]

Other histochemical changes induced during progestation in the uterus include changes in lipid and glycogen. Glycogen granules were obvious in the mouse uterus during the major secretory periods of diestrus and proestrus, as well as during the catabolic phases of metestrus,[98] but in the canine uterus, large PAS-positive plugs occur during the estrogenic phase of the cycle.[123,124] Abundant lipid was present in the mouse uterus during diestrus and proestrus and especially during metestrus,[98] whereas two groups of investigators were unable to demonstrate lipid in either the dog or cat uterus during the estrous cycle.[123,125] The high concentration of uterine epithelial lipid found during late diestrus and proestrus in the rat reflect increased plasma progesterone levels of early diestrus acting in a low plasma estrogen environment.[126]

The influence of progesterone on various morphologic, biochemical, and histochemical parameters in the uterus has been the basis of several bioassays for progestins, namely proliferation of rabbit endometrium, endometrial carbonic anhydrase stimulation, Hooker-Forbes assay for nuclear appearance (the most sensitive of the assays), decidual reaction in the rat, pregnancy maintenance, and gonadotropin inhibition.[53] These have largely been replaced by radioimmunoassays and competitive protein-binding assays for progestins.

Progesterone possesses many biological actions which are not accurately mirrored by synthetic progestins.[127] Five different progestins were compared with progesterone using three different biological assays involving the chick, rat, mouse, and rabbit.[128] The biological assays used were the inhibition of oviduct growth, stimulation of decidual growth (Hooker-Forbes assay) and the proliferation of the rabbit endometrium (Clauberg assay) and the progestins tested included two 17 OH-progestins, two 19-nortestosterone derivatives, and 11-dehydroprogesterone.[128] Only 11-dehydroprogesterone mirrored all of the activity of progesterone and was consistently superior.[128] The other four progestins were less active in one or more of the assays. There are also marked species differences in their response to various synthetic progestins as well as to progesterone. Chlormadinone acetate possesses 62 to 225 times as much progestational activity as norethisterone in the beagle bitch, whereas the potency of chlormadinone acetate in man is only 5 times as great as norethisterone, illustrating the marked interspecies differences with respect to this progestin.[129] The progestational activity of progesterone and several other progestins was evaluated in the beagle bitch using the Clauberg assay, which was determined to be of only limited value for testing relative potency because of its insensitivity.[130] It was discovered, however, that in contrast to the hydroxyprogesterone derivative chlormadinone acetate, which has a wide range of potency in various species, the 19-nortestosterone derivatives failed to show this enormous discrepancy between man, rabbits, and dogs.[130]

The response of any one target organ to the synthetic progestins may be completely different. Biochemical changes were evaluated in the oviducts and uteri of Rhesus monkeys receiving megestrol acetate, norethynodrel, and ethynodiol diacetate, and it was determined that enzyme levels were evaluated in response to some of these steroids and depressed by others.[131]

The same synthetic progestin may have quite different effects on a given target organ, depending on dosage. For instance, low doses of norethynodrel stimulates estrogen uptake by the mouse uterus, but higher doses decrease estradiol uptake.[132] Chlormadinone acetate has a similar effect.[132] Norethindrone acetate increases uridine incorporation into RNA in the rat uterus when 100 μg are administered, but 10 mg significantly inhibit RNA synthesis.[132] Protein synthesis in the uterus is maximal with 100 μg of norethindrone acetate and inhibited with doses higher than 1 mg.[132]

Synthetic progestins alone, or combined with estrogen in contraceptive regimens, produce major changes in the uterus. Uterine endometrial histology was compared with the uterine weight after administration of 14 progestational steroids to immature New Zealand white rabbits, and excellent correlation was found between the appearance of significant secretory development in the endometrium and the occurrence of a sudden rise in uterine weight.[133] Ten oral contraceptives, nine of which were estrogen combined with progestin, were added to the culture medium of human endometrial explants, and the histologic, histochemical and biochemical changes indicated the hormones had a direct effect on the endometrium.[134] The effects in culture included proliferative and secretory changes similar to those caused by natural ovarian hormones, increased glycogen deposition in the glandular epithelium and stromal cells, and histologic changes in the stroma around glands and blood vessels.[134] However, high doses of MPA in women (330 mg) depress proliferative activity of the endometrium, and pseudostratification of the glandular epithelium is lost, but a decidual reaction develops in the endometrial stroma, indicating a definite dissocation between epithelial and stromal response.[135] This contrasts with the hyperplastic changes that occur in both glandular and stromal portions of the endometrium when MPA is administered for long periods to the beagle bitch.[109] The 19-nor-steroids, in either continuous or cyclic combinations with estrogens, also produced hyperinvoluted glands of the endometrium and a prominent predecidual reaction.[136] It was concluded that progestins produced a secretion indirectly and a decidual-like change directly.[136]

D. Cervix and Vagina

In the monkey cervix, progesterone prevents the squamous metaplasia of the cervical glands commonly found after treatment with estrogens.[137]

In the vagina of guinea pigs, estradiol benzoate alone will not produce complete cornification of the mucosa, but progesterone, when added to the estrogen, produces a normal smear (in that leukocytes tended to disappear and cornification became complete), which then progressed to a metestrus smear.[138] The amount of estrogen needed to induce these characteristic vaginal changes was greatly reduced by the presence of progesterone, illustrating the syngeristic action between these two steroid hormones.[138] In contrast to its effect in the guinea pig, progesterone had no consistent or significant stimulating effect on vaginal cornification in ovariectomized rats when given in conjunction with estrogen.[139] However, when progesterone (5 mg/day for 5 days) was administered subcutaneously to intact rats, mucification of the vagina occurred, but if the vagina was distended with glass beads and the vulvar orifices sutured closed, the same regimen of progesterone caused marked stratification and cornification of the vagina.[140]

E. Testicle

A number of synthetic progestins including chlormadinone acetate, MPA, and norgestrel have been found to inhibit spermatogenesis in several species.[141] Chlormadinone acetate was found to produce infertility in male rats without marked impairment of sexual activity.[142] The weight of the testicles and accessory sex glands was significantly depressed after 6 weeks of treatment (10 mg/day subcutaneously). This change, which included tubular atrophy of the testes, was completely reversible in 8 to 10 weeks after treatment was discontinued.[142] A single i.m. injection of MPA (1 gm) produced virtual azospermia in men by 79 days with significant impairment of spermatogenesis lasting as long as 6 months.[143] The prolonged action was thought to be due to the slow metabolic turnover of MPA. MPA influences testosterone metabolism by cultured human fibroblasts by inhibiting 3β-hydroxysteroid dehydrogenase activity resulting in a decrease in androstanediol and an increase in dihydrotestosterone.[144]

F. Mammary Gland

The role of progesterone in mammary gland development was reviewed as recently as 1971.[145] Progesterone administered to castrated male mice and rats stimulated only ductal development in mouse mammary glands after a total dose of 30 to 120 mg had been given over 10 to 70 days, whereas in rats both ductal and lobuloalveolar development occurred after 20 to 300 mg had been given over a 10- to 20-day period, indicating that rats are more sensitive to progesterone than mice.[146] This species variation with respect to how progesterone influences mammary gland structure, development, and function can be observed with several different species.

Selye concluded that large doses of progesterone would cause full development of the mammary gland in intact and castrated rats, but that sensitization by estrone was necessary.[147] Progesterone alone is sufficient to stimulate full ductal and lobuloalveolar development in guinea pigs if the daily dose is sufficiently high (2.4 mg).[148]

Marked lobular hyperplasia occurred in the mammary glands of dogs given high doses of progesterone subcutaneously over a period of 74 weeks.[149] When gonadectomized dogs were given progesterone alone, lobuloalveolar growth, similar to that produced by estrogen and progesterone together, occurred in the mammary glands.[150] Estrogen alone in moderate doses caused little or no growth of the mammary gland, whereas estrogen plus progesterone resulted in extensive growth of the gland. The rate and extent of mammary gland development with the combined hormone treatment closely resembled that approached during pregnancy, whereas progesterone alone caused similar alveolar development, but to a lesser and more variable extent.[150] The dose of progesterone required to produce complete alveolar development in the mammary gland of dogs was relatively much less than that required in rats.[150]

Crystalline progesterone was administered to three ovariectomized monkeys at the rate of 5 to 20 mg/day for 32 days.[151] Biopsies obtained before and after treatment revealed a dose-and-time-related response, with lobules increasing in size as their constituent alveoli dilated and multiplied. Individual alveolar cells grew larger, and mitotic figures appeared among the alveoli.[151]

Synthetic progestins affect mammary gland development much the same way that natural progesterone does. Norethynodrel alone, or combined with mestranol, caused marked lobuloalveolar development and secretory activity and pronounced growth of the nipples in the mammary gland of intact virgin female rats.[152] Nine cases of mammary gland hypertrophy were reported in cats, four of which were associated with pregnancy in young or aged queens, while the remaining five were in neutered animals that had been treated with megestrol acetate for periods ranging between 14 months and 5 years.[153] Prolonged administration of chlormadinone acetate to dogs, which is 63 times more potent in dogs than man or monkeys when measured by the Clauberg test, resulted in marked mammary gland hyperplasia together with other changes reminiscent of hypersecretion of growth hormone.[154]

Progesterone is generally believed to have a depressant effect on mammary gland function. When progesterone is injected simultaneously with prolactin into pseudopregnant rabbits, secretion is suppressed by depressing lactose synthetic activity and hence decreasing lactose synthetase.[155] Progesterone also suppressed the increased RNA content normally induced in the mammary gland by prolactin.[155] Progesterone (6 mg/day) prevented the appearance of casein in the mammary gland of ovariectomized pregnant rats and greatly diminished the incorporation of $^{32}PO_4^=$ into RNA of mammary tissue.[156] When progesterone is administered simultaneously with prolactin to pseudopregnant rabbits, the increase in prolactin receptors in the mammary tissue is completely prevented.[157] When progesterone is administered to pregnant rabbits, it reduces mammary secretion measured on the 24th day even though the number of mammary cells and RNA content is not decreased.[158] Progesterone administered alone to ovariectomized pregnant rabbits did not allow normal mammary gland growth, despite the fact that pregnancy was maintained.[158]

In contrast to the preceding studies, Bruce found that progesterone did not disturb the milk yield of lactating rats, growth of pups, or action of oxytocin on intramammary pressure.[159] Norethindrone, one of the 19-nortestosterone derivatives with progestational activity, also has weak estrogenic activity and showed some inhibitory action on lactation.[159]

In women, low-dose progestins do not have the same inhibiting effect on lactogenesis that estrogens do and in fact may be stimulatory. High dose progestins, on the other hand, cause some inhibition of lactation.[160] Women receiving 150 mg or 300 mg MPA at 3- or 6-month intervals were found to have a significant increase in prolonged lactation, compared with controls.[161] Protein content of the milk was also significantly increased in women receiving 150 mg MPA at intervals of 3 months, whereas it was significantly decreased in women receiving 300 mg every 6 months.[162] There was a significant decrease in the quantity of fat and calcium in the higher dosage group, indicating that the same progestin may have quite different effects on the mammary gland, depending on dosage.[162]

VI. INFLUENCE OF OTHER DRUGS AND HORMONES

A. Production

Progesterone production by the ovary is stimulated by LH.[163] Both FSH and LH stimulated increased progesterone levels when administered to Rhesus monkeys during the luteal phase of the cycle.[164] The effect of LH was dose related and linear, while that of FSH was not. Prolactin administration had no effect on progesterone level in Rhesus monkeys.[164] When corpora lutea from prolactin-treated rats were incubated in vitro, progesterone synthesis was increased fourfold over controls, but at the expense of 20α-hydroxypregn-4-en-3-one, so that total progestin level was not altered.[165] Prolactin depressed progesterone synthesis by the interstitial element of the ovary.[165] When LH was added to the medium in which corpora lutea from prolactin-treated rats were incubated, a 50% increase in total progestin accumulation was seen, most of which was due to the seven- to ninefold increase in progesterone synthesis.[165]

Luteinization of granulosa cells in vivo and in vitro is quite similar in monkeys, pigs, humans, and horses and requires stimulation by LH and FSH, resulting in elevated cyclic adenosine 5′-monophosphate (AMP) levels prior to luteinization.[166] The elevated cyclic AMP is thought to act on a receptor bringing about morphological luteinization and increased progestin synthesis.[166] Aminophylline, a substance known to alter cyclic AMP levels in tissue, is capable of stimulating progesterone synthesis, but not secretion.[167]

Other substances known to alter progesterone production and/or secretion rates include oxytocin and vasopressin, which increase adrenal but not ovarian secretion in dogs;[168] perphenazine, which increases progesterone levels 17-fold in the rat;[169] prostaglandin PGF$_{2\alpha}$, which increases progesterone biosynthesis by ovarian slices from immature rats hormonally primed to stimulate pseudopregnancy, but does not alter progesterone biosynthesis by slices of rabbit corpora lutea, rabbit ovarian interstitial tissue, or rat corpora luteal tissue[170] and methylcholanthrene, a polycyclic hydrocarbon causing mammary neoplasms in rodents, which produces elevated serum progesterone levels in both mice and rats.[171,172]

B. Metabolism and Binding

The influence of estrogen on metabolic enzymes of the uterus has been described earlier. Other hormones and drugs influencing progesterone metabolism include: human chorionic gonadotropin, FSH, and LH, which increase progesterone metabolism by the ovary;[173] chlormadinone acetate, which not only suppressed progesterone production, but also decreases progesterone metabolism;[62] thyroxin and thyroidectomy, which markedly diminish progesterone hydroxylation by the liver microsomes of male rats[174] and anesthetic agents, which create striking differences in the progesterone metabolite distribution in the adrenal gland.[32]

Progesterone receptors are under dual hormonal control, estrogen increasing the concentration through a mechanism that depends on synthesis of both RNA and protein, and progesterone decreasing the concentration of its own receptor probably by enhancing its own inactivation rate.[175] As stated earlier, progesterone administered simultaneously with estrogen will block receptor synthesis, actinomycin D and cycloheximide will prevent receptor formation,[176] and pronase, protamine sulfate, and p-hydroxymercuribenzoate will all abolish progesterone binding, which implies that the binding component(s) is (are) an acidic protein containing sulfhydryl groups necessary for binding.[41]

Progesterone binding is potentiated in the mammary gland and uterine cytosols of Sprague-Dawley rats by 7,12-dimethylbenz[a] anthracene (DMBA), another polycyclic hydrocarbon used to induce tumor formation in rodents.[177] The potentiation is greatest at weaning and declines gradually thereafter. Similar potentiation of progesterone binding was found in mammary gland and uterine cytosols from Wistar rats and guinea pigs.[177]

C. Activity

Progesterone and estrogen have long been known to be synergistic in some circumstances and antagonistic in others. The response of two target organs, the uterus and vagina, has primarily been used to evaluate the relationship between these two steroids. Progesterone and androgens both reduce the degree of vaginal cornification produced by natural and synthetic estrogens in ovariectomized mice.[178,179] When estradiol benzoate is administered to ovariectomized sheep before or during progesterone treatment, the vaginal response is partially suppressed.[180]

In the mouse uterine bioassay, the action of progesterone was completely inhibited, partially inhibited, not inhibited, or was stimulated by estrone or 17β-estradiol, depending on the proportion of the mixtures.[181] If progesterone and estradiol were mixed, there was partial or complete antagonism. The investigator concluded that the amount of estrogen in the circulation may exercise significant control on the action of progesterone.[181] Progesterone has been found to augment the response of the mouse uterus to low levels of estradiol, determined by the incorporation of ^{3}H-uridine, but 48 hr after progesterone administration, the vaginal response to estradiol is completely eliminated.[182]

In ovariectomized cats, a period of estradiol-induced differentiation is necessary before progesterone can antagonize the effect of estradiol on the oviduct epithelium.[183] Ciliated and secretory epithelial cells are restored in the oviduct by the estrogen treatment, and subsequent progesterone treatment results in atrophy of the epithelium equivalent to withdrawing estradiol.[184] The rate at which progesterone antagonism develops differs from one region of the oviduct to another.[183] In the uterus, progesterone treatment following estradiol priming will not lead to estradiol withdrawal symptoms but rather to a new stage of differentiation by altered and increased secretory activity.[184]

Estrone acts synergistically with progesterone in stimulating mammary gland growth and if progesterone is administered alone, six times as much is required for the same degree of stimulation.[185] If estrone is administered in large amounts, the stimulatory activity of the combination or of progesterone alone is decreased to a point where no alveolar growth can be demonstrated.[185]

An autoradiographic study of rat mammary gland revealed that DMBA combined with progesterone significantly increased DNA synthesis over that seen in the controls or with either compound alone, even though there appeared to be no interaction between DMBA and progesterone.[186]

VII. INFLUENCE ON TUMORIGENESIS

Nearly all of the published work regarding the role of progestins in tumorigenesis have implicated these steroid hormones in a promotional or at most cocarcinogenic role rather than as a carcinogen per se. As might be expected, tumors associated with these hormones are generally found in sites where progestins are produced or metabolized or have some effect. The majority of references reviewed for this chapter concerned the role of progestins in mammary neoplasia, perhaps in part reflecting the interests of the author, but also illustrating the importance of understanding the genesis of this very prevalent form of neoplasia which occurs in several different species.

A. General

There have been a number of cautions published regarding the widespread use of progestins, particularly as contraceptives. Some of the comments advising caution were published before many of the recent studies were reported, and for the most part, the advice would be regarded as correct. Almost 10 years ago (1968), the World Health Organization described the current knowledge concerning hormonal steroids in contraception and suggested additional research be done to determine how these steroids might affect the incidence of neoplasia.[187] Several years prior to the World Health Organization report, Muhlbock and Boot claimed that when growth-stimulating hormones act chronically on particular target organs tumors would be induced within their receptive sites.[188]

Definite differences of opinion exist concerning the value of animal studies in predicting the outcome of using these hormones in women, particularly when there are such great species differences in sensitivity to the progestins.[189-191] At least one investigator feels that the animal studies should be evaluated carefully and may in fact provide some indication of the hormonal effects and influence of cancer risks in women.[192] One of the arguments used against the predictability of rodents (and dogs) is the dissimilarity of metabolic disposition and feedback mechanisms controlling ovulation in these species, and the two species most closely resembling man were subhuman primates and guinea pigs.[191] Rodent strains were recommended only if they have low spontaneous tumor incidence, are free of oncogenic viruses, and are fed standardized diets.[191]

In comparing the metabolism of chlormadinone acetate in man, subhuman primates, and dogs, Goldzieher and Kramer found excretion patterns similar between man and subhuman primates and significantly different from the dog and reported significant differences in the response of the mammary gland in the different species with an increased incidence of nodules developing in the dog and a lack of such nodules in monkeys.[193]

B. Liver

Progesterone (20 mg/100 gm body weight [bw]) implanted subcutaneously in A×C rats increased the incidence of liver cell carcinomas induced by N-2-fluorenyldiacetamide in male rats, castrated male rats, and ovariectomized female rats, but did not affect the incidence in intact female rats.[194] The neoplasms in the progesterone-treated animals tended to be less differentiated carcinomas. Progesterone also increased the incidence of cirrhosis in the gonadectomized male and female rats.[194] Hepatocellular carcinogenesis was also accelerated in castrated male Wistar rats that had received progesterone weekly for life after they had received another carcinogen, 4-dimethylaminoazobenzene (DAB).[195] No increase in liver tumors was seen in intact male, intact female, or ovariectomized female rats treated with progesterone after receiving the carcinogen.[195]

The long-term toxicologic and tumorigenic effect of a contraceptive containing 98% norethisterone acetate and 2% ethinylestradiol was tested in Sprague-Dawley rats.[196] The contraceptive was added to the diet at the level of 75 ppm. In addition to the increased numbers of mammary tumors, the investigators found both increased regenerative nodules and increased adenomas in the liver.[196]

In tests sponsored and reported by the Committee on the Safety of Medicine (HMSO), two of the 19-nortestosterone derivatives used in contraceptive regimens were implicated in increasing the number of liver cell tumors found in either CF-LP strain mice or Wistar rats.[197] These two progestins were norethynodrel, which increased the incidence of benign liver tumors in male rats by 21% and resulted in 8% malignant hepatomas in male rats receiving medium to high levels, and norethisterone and norethisterone acetate, which increased the incidence of benign hepatomas in male mice by 15% but did not alter the incidence in female mice, and increased the incidence of benign hepatomas in male rats by 8%, but not in female rats.[197] Other progestins tested which did not alter the incidence of liver tumors in rats or mice included norgestrel, chlormadinone acetate, and ethynodiol diacetate.[197]

Only one of the several dog studies in which different progestins have been tested at various dosage levels has reported an increase in the number of liver adenomas at the time of sacrifice.[198]

C. Pituitary

Progesterone has been shown to have a synergistic effect with estrogens on the development of tumors in several organs including the anterior pituitary.[199] The progestins used in some contraceptives result in a high incidence of pituitary tumors in mice and male rats, and a decreased incidence in female rats.[200] Norethynodrel increased the incidence of pituitary tumors in both male and female CF-LP strain mice,[197] in C57Bl strain mice,[201] and in male Wistar rats.[197] Norethynodrel alone did not induce an increase of pituitary tumors in female Wistar rats, whereas norethynodrel plus mestranol (25:1) increased the incidence by 12%.[197]

Norethisterone alone increased the incidence of pituitary tumors in female CF-LP mice 15 to 18%, and norethisterone acetate plus ethynylestradiol (50:1) increased the incidence in both male and female CF-LP mice by about 23%.[197] Norethisterone acetate caused no increase in pituitary tumors when used alone.[197] Mice of the C57Bl strain receiving norethisterone plus ethinylestradiol also had an increase in pituitary tumors.[201] Neither norethynodrel nor norethisterone altered the incidence of pituitary tumors in C3H mice.[202]

Chlormadinone acetate plus mestranol (25:1) resulted in a five- to tenfold increase in pituitary tumors in CF-LP mice, whereas chlormadinone acetate alone produced no such increase.[197] Ethynodiol diacetate plus mestranol also increased the incidence of pituitary tumors in CF-LP mice by 21 to 29%, whereas no increase was seen when this progestin was given alone.[197] When combined with ethinylestradiol, the ethynodiol diacetate increased pituitary tumors in these mice by 28 to 86%![197] These experiments further substantiate the synergistic or cocarcinogenic effect between progestins and estrogens. Subcutaneous administration of progesterone (1 mg six times weekly for 17 weeks) caused a fivefold increase in the number of pulmonary metastases of a transplantable mammotropic pituitary tumor in LAF-l mice and resulted in increased local spread to thoracic wall, diaphragm, mediastinal lymph nodes, and thoracic duct.[203]

D. Ovary

Almost 30 years ago (1949), it was discovered that if progesterone (1 mg in oil) was administered weekly for several weeks to castrated male mice bearing intrasplenic ovarian grafts, tumors developed in the ovarian grafts.[204] The tumors varied in point of origin, some being granulosa cell tumors, and some were mixed. Since that time, several synthetic progestins have been prepared and tested for their tumorigenic potential. It has been learned that 19-norprogesterone has a more powerful effect on ovarian tumorigenesis than does natural progesterone.[205] Removal of the methyl group (CH^3) from the C-19 progesterone increases the progestational action of the hormone tenfold.

Administration of 15 mg of 19-norprogesterone per day for a minimum of 13 months produced granulosa cell tumors in 8 of 33 mice, with most of the ovaries in the treated animals containing nodules of lutein cells larger than those seen in normal control mice.[205]

Administration of norethindrone and norethynodrel to mice for 18 months or longer results in many microtumors in the ovaries.[206] Ovarian cysts occur in the norethynodrel-treated mice, which probably arise from the rete.[206] Norethindrone (7.7 mg), implanted as a s.c. pellet containing 40% progestin and 60% cholesterol in female BALB/c mice, produced a 53% incidence of ovarian tumors in 25 mice.[207] The tumors originated either from granulosa cells or possibly from germinal epithelium. The same concentration of norethynodrel administered to another group of female BALB/c mice by s.c. implant resulted in two granulosa cell tumors developing in 24 mice.[208] These same investigators who conducted the experiments described above (Lipschutz et al.) also produced granulosa cell tumors in mice after prolonged and continuous administration of progesterone.[209]

Diethylstilbestrol administration to 13 bitches resulted in ovarian tumors developing in all 13 in 13 to 14 months.[210] Progesterone administered together with the stilbestrol did not influence either the macroscopic or microscopic appearance of the neoplasms, nor did it influence behavior.[210]

E. Uterus

Progesterone and norethindrone administered to mice for prolonged periods produced cystic endometrial glands, endometriosis, and sarcomas in the endometrial stroma.[211] Subcutaneous implants of progesterone, norethynodrel, or another synthetic progestin (3β-17α-diacetoxy-6α-methyl-pregn-4-en-20-one, BL141) in B6AF female mice that had a thread impregnated with 20-methylcholanthrene (20-MC) placed through the cervical canal increased the total number of uterine tumors.[212] The tumors produced in the uterus by 20-MC and promoted by the progestins were adenoacanthomas. The percent of uterine tumors was increased by mestranol alone or a combination of mestranol and norethynodrel. The uterine effect of mestranol was not inhibited by simultaneous administration of either progesterone or BL141.[212]

Endometrial sarcomas developed in female BALB/c mice that had absorbed between 18 and 900 mg of progesterone per day for an 18-month period.[213] Progesterone suppressed the induction of uterine adenocarcinomas in WLL and Strong A strains of mice that had been implanted with carcinogens, but there was a corresponding increase in the incidence of connective tissue tumors.[214]

Progesterone was administered to intact and castrated rats that had received a local application of 1% DMBA weekly into the cervicovaginal canal.[215] Progesterone retarded and slightly decreased the induction of sarcomas, but increased the number of epithelial tumors in intact animals. The effect on either type of tumor in castrates was insignificant.[215] High doses of MPA significantly enhance tumor growth of a transplantable uterine adenocarcinoma in the rat and increase the rate of metastasis of the tumor.[216]

F. Cervix

Cervical carcinomas have been reported in A/J mice receiving norethynodrel, but did not develop in C3H/Hej mice.[217] Subcutaneous implants of progesterone and two synthetic progestins, including norethynodrel, increased the total number of cervical tumors in B6AF₁ female mice that had a thread implanted with 20-methylcholanthrene placed in the cervical canal.[212]

Norethynodrel and mestranol were administered continuously to BALB/c mice. Six mice receiving this combination for 518 to 721 days and two mice born to hormone-treated females that were in turn treated for 599 days had lesions of the uterine cervix diagnosed as early cancer or infiltrating cancer.[218] The cervical changes were believed due to mestranol, since no similar changes were seen due to norethynodrel alone.

Progestins were believed to exert a protective effect against viral carcinogenesis in the mouse cervix.[219] When herpesvirus type 2 was inoculated into the vagina of BALB/c mice that were implanted with progesterone-cholesterol pellets, one precancerous lesion and one squamous cell carcinoma of the cervix was found in 39 mice.[219] When norethynodrel plus mestranol (10 to 12.5 mg/day) was fed to 20 female BALB/c mice, 3 of 16 mice surviving 10 months or more developed precancerous lesions and 2 developed squamous carcinomas of the cervix and/or vagina, compared with a similarly treated group that had been inoculated with herpesvirus type 2 in which 1 of 31 developed precancerous lesions and 6 of 31 developed squamous cell carcinomas.[219] In contrast to this study, progesterone was found to have a cocarcinogenic effect with 20-methylcholanthrene on induction of cervical carcinomas in C57BL6 mice.[220] A progesterone pellet (15 mg) was implanted subcutaneously every 3 weeks for 9 weeks, and the mice were treated locally with methylcholanthrene. Forty-five of 50 mice so treated developed cervical carcinoma compared with 6 of 50 mice treated with methylcholanthrene alone ($p < 0.01$). Progesterone also selectively influenced the maturation of induced invasive carcinoma of the endocervix and produced a mucoepidermoid type of neoplasm, whereas it had no effect on the maturation of carcinoma developing in the vagina or ectocervix.[220]

One study revealed no cervical carcinomas developing in either mice or rats treated with norethynodrel or ethynodiol diacetate,[221] and in another report, the same investigator made the statement that cervical cancer was not increased in Rhesus monkeys, rats, mice, or dogs that had received high doses of progestins.[222]

G. Vagina

Subcutaneous implants of progesterone and two synthetic progestins, including norethynodrel, increased the total number of vaginal tumors in B6AF$_1$ mice that had a thread impregnated with 20-MC placed in the cervical canal. The 20-MC-induced tumors of the vagina promoted by progestins were squamous cell carcinomas.[212]

Progesterone administered to castrated mice that had received local applications of chemical carcinogens developed significantly more mucoepidermoid tumors.[223] Progesterone appeared to increase the extent of the columnar component and had a mucifying effect on the cervical-vaginal epithelium of the mice. When castrated mice were treated with progesterone, there was an increased adenocarcinomatous component of these tumors, while stilbestrol treatment resulted in the induction of only squamous cell carcinomas.[223]

Vaginal lesions bearing many resemblances to those seen in young women born from diethylstilbestrol-treated mothers have been found in mice exposed to sex steroids in neonatal life.[224] The lesions were more severe at 12 months of age in those mice exposed to a combination of progesterone and estradiol.

Rabbits exposed to vaginal strings containing 3-MC did not have any greater incidence of vaginal tumors when 10 mg of progesterone was injected subcutaneously twice each week.[225]

H. Mammary Gland

More information has been written about the effects of progestins on tumorigenesis in the mammary gland than on any other target organ. This undoubtedly is because mammary neoplasia is of such great concern and relatively high frequency in women and progestins are being used widely as human contraceptive agents. In addition, mammary neoplasms are frequently encountered spontaneously in several experimental animals and progestins have been generally found to increase the incidence of these lesions.

Problems arise in extrapolating experimental animal data to man, in part because of the difference in species responses to these steroids. Norethisterone enanthate, which is mainly progestational in the human and several other species, turns out to be predominantly estrogenic in rats, causing both hypophyseal and mammary tumors.[226] Another synthetic progestin, 4,6-dichloro-17-acetoxy-16α-methyl-4,6-pregnediene-3,20-dione, which is considered similar to chlormadinone acetate or medroxyprogesterone acetate, induces no signs of estrogenicity in dogs, but causes mammary nodules in this species.[226] It was pointed out in this article that the dosage regimen used to treat dogs (2, 10, and 25 times the human dose) was senseless from the biological point of view because the dog normally comes into estrus only twice a year, in contrast to the regular cycling schedule in humans and subhuman primates.[226] These investigators were not alone in their criticism of extrapolating animal data to humans, as pointed out earlier in this section.

In order to adequately cover the influence of progestins on mammary tumorigenesis, this subsection will be further subdivided by species.

1. Mice

There is no consistent susceptibility between different strains of mice to the different progestins and combinations of estrogens and progestins administered in high dosages throughout the life span.[191] It was therefore concluded that mice could be of little or no predictive value to determine potential carcinogenicity of any of these compounds in women.[191]

Natural progesterone is itself a potent cocarcinogen for mammary tumor induction in certain strains of mice, although it lacks carcinogenic potency by itself.[202] In the C3H strain, which bears the endogenous mammary tumor virus, progesterone administered five times per week for 19 weeks resulted in mammary tumors in 44% of the animals, compared with 6% in the controls.[227,228] Progesterone also increases the number of mammary tumors developing in methylcholanthrene-treated C3H virgin female mice resulting in 100% incidence, compared with approximately 20% incidence in animals treated with MC alone or 7.5% incidence in mice receiving progesterone alone.[229]

Over 35 years ago (1941), it was discovered that virgin A strain mice developed a higher incidence of mammary tumors when they were pseudopregnant.[230] Shortly thereafter, it was learned that administration of exogenous progesterone to pregnant mice of a low mammary tumor strain resulted in 50% of those mice developing mammary tumors within 56 to 145 days, illustrating the additive effect of the progesterone.[231] Pseudopregnancy was subsequently found to increase the potency of two carcinogens, DMBA and MC, for the mammary gland in C57BL mice.[232] (The reader should be reminded that in an earlier section of this chapter both of these carcinogens were implicated in elevating either progesterone binding in the mammary gland (DMBA) or the progesterone level in serum, thereby adding to the progestational influence on the mammary gland.) Pseudopregnancy caused the earliest and most rapid appearance of mammary tumors in three different genetic strains of mice after treatment with 3-MC, compared with pregnancy and lactation.[233] Continual pregnancies were a little less effective, while lactation had an inhibitory effect in all three strains of mice.[233]

Several investigators have found progesterone to be inhibitory or to have no effect on mammary tumor development in certain strains of mice. Progesterone (8 mg) was administered subcutaneously to female Marsh mice as a crystalline suspension mixed with saline and pooled female mouse serum and continued for 20 months with no statistically significant tumorigenic response.[234] The same strain of mouse when ovariectomized failed to develop mammary tumors after receiving 10 mg progesterone subcutaneously for 6 months, and progesterone (3 mg) combined with estrone failed to effect development of the mammary gland.[235] When MPA was administered intramuscularly to female Marsh mice at the rate of 5 mg/month for 2 months, there was a statistically insignificant tumorigenic response 20 months later, compared to controls.[236]

Natural progesterone was found to be inhibitory to mammary carcinoma formation in RIII mice.[235] The incidence of spontaneous mammary adenocarcinoma was reduced from 54% to 16.6%.[237] It should be noted that the incidence of mammary neoplasia was very high in these mice, and the tumors normally occurred at an early age. Even with some strains of mice in which progesterone does increase the incidence of mammary neoplasia, in other investigators' hands, no effect is reported. For instance, progesterone (1 mg) administered subcutaneously to female C3H mice for 34 weeks failed to alter the incidence of mammary tumors.[238] However, the incidence of mammary tumors was very high in both treated and untreated mice, and tumors occurred at an early age, possibly masking the effect of progesterone. Ethynodiol (1.0 mg) and mestranol (0.1 mg) administered daily to C3H or (C3H × RIII) F_1 mice from puberty until their natural death also failed to significantly modify the incidence of spontaneous breast cancer,[239] and one investigator even reported an inhibitory effect of norethynodrel plus mestranol on spontaneous mammary carcinogenesis in C3H female mice.[240] Norgestrel administered over long periods to mice also did not alter the incidence of mammary tumors.[197,241]

Early workers claimed that progesterone had no effect on the expectancy of mammary tumors in mice,[242-244] and one of these workers subsequently claimed that progesterone was effective only in the presence of prolactin by acting synergistically with this mammotropic hormone.[245] This is further underscored in a more recent study where norethynodrel and mestranol were administered to nulliparous C3H/HeJ female mice beginning at 1 month and terminating at 22 months of age. A significant increase in the incidence of mammary tumors was found over solvent-treated controls. However, if the prolactin inhibitor (CB/154) was given at the same time to the steroid-treated mice, a significant reduction of mammary tumor incidence and hyperplastic nodule development occurred, with the final level of tumors being similar to those found in controls.[246] However, many more investigators have claimed that progesterone and synthetic progestins increase the frequency of neoplasia, either as cocarcinogenic agents or as promoters of mammary gland growth and subsequently promoters of spontaneous mammary tumor growth. Progesterone not only maintained transplanted hyperplastic alveolar nodules (HANs) in C3H/Crgl mice, but also significantly increased the frequency of tumor development.[247] Mammary tumors developed earlier and in much higher incidence in mammary tumor virus-positive (MTV) C3H × A mice that received implants of progesterone (14 mg) every 28 days for 104 weeks.[248]

The results obtained from testing progestins used in contraceptive formulations have generally indicated that some are promotional for mammary neoplasia, at least in certain mouse strains. Norethynodrel and ethynodiol acetate plus combinations of these progestins with estrogens were fed to CF-LP strain mice for 78 weeks, 40 males and 40 females in each group, with feeding initiated when the mice were 4.5 to 5 weeks old.[189,249] Despite the feeding of very high levels (100 to 200 times the human dose), there was no significant induction of benign or malignant mammary tumors in these mice. These same progestins fed to the identical mouse strain at dosages equivalent to twice the level fed in the previous study resulted in a fivefold increase in malignant mammary tumors with one of the progestins (norethynodrel), but not with the other.[197] In another study using three other mouse strains (C3H, RIII, and (C3H × RIII)F_1), norethynodrel did not increase the frequency of mammary carcinomas and actually decreased the high tumor incidence in female mice.[250] However, norethynodrel did produce a high incidence (100%) and decreased latency (from 82 to 37 weeks) of mammary carcinoma in castrated male (C3H × RIII)F₁ mice.[250] Norethynodrel and ethyno-diol diacetate also increased the frequency and shortened the latency of mammary tumors in ovariectomized female mice.[251] Ethynodiol diacetate plus mestranol in-creased the incidence of mammary tumors in male (C3H × RIII)F₁ mice from 0 to 56% and in castrated males of the same strain from 16 to 75%.[251] Norethynodrel (125 mg/20 g bw two times a week) was administered to A/J mice (106 weeks) and C3H/HeJ mice (88 weeks).[217] Eight A/J mice developed type B adenocarcinomas in the mam-mary gland compared to 0 in the controls, and 28 of the C3H/HeJ mice developed mammary carcinomas compared to 12 in the controls.[217]

Chlormadinone acetate produced no increase in mammary tumors in the CF-LP strain mice,[197] nor any increased frequency or decreased latency in C3H, RIII, or (C3H × RIII)F₁ mice, no matter what their endocrine status.[251] Chlormadinone acetate plus ethinylestradiol increased the incidence of mammary tumors in both intact males (0 to 31.2%) and castrated males (32.8 to 77.8%) of the (C3H × RIII)F₁ hybrid and de-creased the latency period.[251]

Progesterone (100 μg) adinistered daily to neonatal BALB/c.f. C3H mice resulted in an earlier age of onset and higher incidence of mammary tumors which could be completely abolished by ovariectomy on day 40.[252,253]

2. Rats

It has been known for several years that pregnancy and pseudopregnancy markedly decrease the latent period and increase the frequency of mammary cancer development in rats receiving 3-MC.[254] Pregnancy had to occur before rather than following carcin-ogen administration in order to be effective, and any tumors developing during preg-nancy rapidly regressed following parturition, indicating the importance of the endog-enous hormonal milieu in the genesis of mammary cancer.[254] It was also discovered that the interval between carcinogen administration and pregnancy was critical, with more tumors developing as the interval increased, whereas if mating occurred imme-diately after carcinogen treatment, no mammary tumors developed.[225] Pregnancy ac-celerated the appearance of DMBA-induced tumors in rats and stimulated them to grow at a faster rate.[256] All rats that had received DMBA developed tumors during pregnancy, and all tumors grew rapidly until parturition.[257] Exogenous progesterone (6 mg/day) increased the growth rate in nearly 50% of the DMBA-induced tumors during the post-partum period.[257]

A few investigators have reported that progestins either have no effect on mammary tumor growth or actually are inhibitory. Progesterone does inhibit the growth of the adenomatous portion of spontaneous rat mammary fibroadenomas and inhibits the growth of the glandular portion of fibroadenomas found in castrated male rats, but does not alter the growth rate of fibroadenomas in pregnant rats.[258] Increasing dosages of progesterone, when combined with a constant daily dose of estradiol benzoate, pro-duced a slight but significant stimulation of DMBA-induced mammary tumors in Spra-gue-Dawley rats.[259] Estradiol benzoate alone or in increasing dosages with constant progesterone had a depressing effect on tumor appearance.[259]

Norethynodrel plus mestranol given to Wistar rats six times a week for 50 weeks produced no mammary tumors and did not enhance or retard mammary carcinogenesis produced by 3-MC.[260] In Sprague-Dawley rats, high levels of the same hormone com-bination reduced the incidence of DMBA-induced mammary tumors and lowered the multiplicity of tumors.[261]

Most investigators conclude, however, that progestins have a promotional influence on spontaneous and carcinogen-induced mammary neoplasia in rats. Norethynodrel plus mestranol, discussed in the last paragraph, increases malignant mammary tumors in female rats.[197] Norethynodrel alone was effective in male rats, but only the combi-nation was effective in females. Both benign and malignant mammary tumors were increased in Charles River CD female rats that received norethynodrel alone for 90 weeks.[189,249] Sprague-Dawley rats treated with DMBA and given norethynodrel alone, or combined with mestranol, developed a greater number of discrete mammary tumors at an earlier time, but there appeared to be no effect on the total number of rats that eventually developed mammary tumors.[262]

Norethisterone acetate plus ethinylestradiol fed to Sprague-Dawley rats increased the proportion of adenomas:fibroadenomas compared with controls, but did not alter the total number of benign tumors, and increased slightly the number of adenocarcinomas.[196] The dosage of contraceptive effective in increasing the incidence of mammary neoplasms was 100 times the human dose where 10 times the human dose produced no ill effect. Male Wistar rats had an increase in both benign and malignant mammary tumors when fed norethisterone alone or norethisterone plus mestranol (20:1).[197] The combination increased the malignant mammary tumors in female rats from 5% in controls to 30% in the treated animal.[197] Norethisterone acetate plus ethinylestradiol (50:1) increased the benign mammary tumors in male rats from 2% in controls to 28% in treated animals.[197]

Based on previous studies, the general consensus would be that progesterone administered before carcinogen to rats is inhibitory, whereas if given following the carcinogen it is stimulatory, but discrepancies in the literature exist concerning even this point. Progesterone (1.18 mg/day) administered for 10 days preceeding DMBA (20 mg) treatment of 50-day-old female Sprague-Dawley rats retarded the time of appearance of mammary tumors, but otherwise was ineffective.[263] Another investigator found that progesterone administered just prior to DMBA treatment of S-D rats or within 15 days after DMBA significantly increased the incidence of mammary neoplasms, with the progesterone given just prior to DMBA being as effective as when given after DMBA.[264] Still another investigator found that progesterone administered 0.5 days before or 4.5 days after DMBA reduced the mammary cancer from 82% found in controls receiving carcinogen alone to 42% in the treated group.[265] When progesterone (1.25 mg) was administered subcutaneously to 5-day-old S-D rats that later received DMBA (20 mg) at 55 days of age, there was an increased mammary carcinogenic response at 190 days of age with no effect on the benign tumors.[266] When progesterone (4 mg/day) was started at 30 days of age and 40 days later DMBA (5 mg) was given intravenously, the number of rats with tumors and the average number of tumors per rat were significantly decreased.[267]

An attempt was made a few years ago to resolve the question regarding time and duration of progesterone treatment relative to DMBA administration to Sprague-Dawley rats.[268] Tumor yield was reduced when progesterone was begun 25 days before DMBA and enhanced when begun 2 days after DMBA. The effects were not obvious when hormonal administration was brief. Continuation of progesterone some time after DMBA caused progressive diminution of inhibitory effect with 135 days of continuous hormone treatment entirely abolishing the effects of 25 days of pretreatment.[268] One of the investigators studying the interrelationship between progesterone and DMBA treatment used very high hormone levels (180 mg) and suggested that the high hormone level possibly interfered with tumor production.[265] A similar apparent interference was found when two contraceptive mixtures were fed to S-D rats that had received DMBA. Norethisterone plus ethinylestradiol (50:1) administered in low doses (0.5 mg added to the diet) for 10 days prior to DMBA resulted in an increased incidence of breast tumors (from 45% to 81%), whereas 1 mg resulted in no significant increase.[269] The same essential findings occurred when norethynodrel plus mestranol were fed, where 0.25 mg increased the incidence of mammary tumors and 1.0 mg did not.[269]

The relationship between progestins and other carcinogens affecting the rat mammary gland have also been studied, although not as extensively as DMBA. Repeated i.m. injections of progesterone (4 mg/day) decreased the latency period in 3-MC-treated rats and increased the incidence, even when the rats were ovariectomized.[270] Intramuscular injections of progesterone (0.5 mg, three times a week for life) increased the incidence of mammary tumors in Sherman and Wistar rats fed a diet containing 0.3% 2-acetylaminofluorene (AAF) from 17 of 56 AAF-treated rats having tumors to 22 of 26 progesterone-plus-AAF-treated rats bearing tumors.[271] Estradiol administration did not alter the incidence of mammary tumors. When ovariectomized rats were given AAF, they developed no mammary tumors.[272] Estrogen administration brought a very slight increase in the incidence, and only when progesterone was administered together with the estrogen was a normal incidence of breast cancer observed.[272]

Progesterone increased the latent period for mammary tumor development from 37 to 50 weeks in female hooded rats that had been implanted with estrone pellets, but the incidence of mammary tumors was not changed.[273] The progesterone caused temporary regression of established tumors. Female A × C rats implanted with pellets of diethylstilbesterol and exposed to 800 R of gamma irradiation were protected against developing mammary carcinoma if progesterone pellets (20 mg) were implanted subcutaneously.[274] Only 1 of 13 rats receiving both hormones plus irradiation developed seven tumors, whereas 12 of the 15 rats receiving only DES plus irradiation developed 56 mammary tumors.[274]

Most of the discussion regarding the influence of synthetic progestins on mammary tumor development in rats, with or without carcinogen administration, has centered on the 19-nortestosterone derivatives. Other progestins that have been evaluated include norgestrel, which does not produce tumors in rats,[197,241] and ethynodiol diacetate, which increased the incidence of benign mammary tumors in male Wistar rats by 10% and which, when combined with ethinylestradiol, increased the incidence of malignant mammary tumors by 10% in both males and females.[197] Another investigator evaluating ethynodiol acetate in Charles River CD rats found no increase in malignant tumors, but did find an increase in fibroadenomas in the rats.[189] Some of the 17α-hydroxyprogesterone derivatives that have been tested include chlormadinone acetate, which does not produce an increase in mammary tumors in Wistar rats after 104 weeks,[197] and medroxyprogesterone acetate, which has been shown to have a promotional effect on carcinogen-induced mammary tumors of rats[275] and an inhibitory effect on a transplantable mammary fibroadenoma.[276] Megestrol acetate plus ethinylestradiol administered subcutaneously to Wistar rats resulted in a high rate of fibroadenomas developing in the mammary gland.[277]

3. Dogs

In contrast to the findings in mice and rats, where some of the 19-nortestosterone derivatives increase the incidence and decrease the latency of mammary tumors and the 17α-hydroxyprogesterone derivatives have little effect, the reverse is true in dogs. The 17α-hydroxyprogesterone derivatives, chlormadinone acetate, medroxyprogesterone acetate, and megestrol acetate all decrease the latency and increase the incidence of mammary tumors, whereas few of the 19-nortestosterone derivatives seem to create any problem. This either indicates a marked species difference in the action and metabolism of these progestins or a difference in the endogenous hormonal changes resulting from progestin administration which may affect the mammary gland and subgross mammary tumors differently. Whatever the mechanism whereby mammary tumors are stimulated in the dog, most investigators who have reported these lesions and discussed the problem are of the opinion that the dog is an inappropriate model to test hormones designed for use in women because of their unusual sensitivity, different physiology, and the different morphological characteristics of their mammary tumors. The following paragraphs will discuss these differences and the controversy in more detail.

Before discussing the effects of progestins on the mammary gland of dogs, it is necessary to review some of the natural history of mammary neoplasia in dogs, particularly beagle bitches. In a colony of beagles located in Davis, California, 50% of 354 bitches between 6 and 8 years of age developed mammary tumors, especially virgin or rarely bred bitches.[278] The mammary glands of eight of these bitches (aged 7.6 to 8.5 years) were thoroughly evaluated using a whole-mount staining and examination technique, and 654 atypical glandular nodules were found in 32 glands.[279] Of these nodules, 94 (14%) were neoplasms, while the remainder were either hyperplastic or inflammatory lesions. Additional whole-mount evaluation of bitches between 2 and 3 years revealed that 50% had dysplasias of the mammary gland with the posterior pairs of glands developing more lesions than the anterior pairs.[280] The investigator concluded that the gradients for early onset of lesions coincided with the gradient of tumor frequency previously reported and suggested that preneoplastic potential should be ascribed to some of these dysplasias.[280]

High doses of progesterone administered to beagle bitches for at least 74 weeks produced marked lobular hyperplasia of the mammary gland, mimicking pregnancy, with secretory activity proportional to the progesterone level used.[281] Mixed mammary tumors (tumors composed of both an adenomatous and myoepitheliomatous portion) were found in two of the five dogs so treated.[281] A more complete report of this work indicated that the dosage of progesterone increased from 0.08 mg to 22.5 mg daily over this 74-week period and that alterations occurred in several organs of the endocrine and genital system.[149] Another group of investigators have found a dose-related increase in hyperplastic and benign neoplastic lesions in the mammary gland of beagle bitches receiving weekly i.m. injections of progesterone.[282]

Megestrol acetate and chlormadinone acetate, derivatives of 17α-hydroxyprogesterone, both promote the early appearance of hyperplastic and neoplastic lesions in beagle mammary glands.[283,284] These hormones were administered over a 4-year period with the dosages being 1, 10, and 25 times the projected human dose.[284] Numerous palpable mammary nodules were found in bitches treated with middle and high doses. Most of the nodules were nodular hyperplasias while a few (5 of 38 in the megestrol-treated bitches) were benign mixed mammary tumors. In the high-dose chlormadinone-treated group, 4 of 22 nodules were benign mixed tumors and 1 was an adenocarcinoma.[284]

Three other progestins, ethynerone, WY-4355, and anagestone acetate were all found to increase the appearance of mammary gland nodules and neoplasms in beagle bitches in a dose-related fashion.[285] Nearly all of the tumors produced were benign mixed tumors or adenomas, with only a few of the tumors being diagnosed as malignant. In a final report of this project, it was learned that clinically malignant mammary tumors occurred only in dogs receiving 25 times the human dose of ethynerone plus mestranol and either 10 or 25 times the human dose of anagestone plus mestranol.[286] Dogs receiving mestranol alone had no more nodules than were found in control animals.[286]

Medroxyprogesterone acetate was found several years ago to be associated with severe "fibrocystic" disease in the mammary glands of dogs who had received the drug for estrus control.[275] These bitches were presented to the clinic because of severe mucometra and pyometra that developed after using this progestin.[275] Since that time, several studies have been conducted or are now in progress (including this author's) to determine how MPA affects the mammary gland of beagle bitches.[109,198,282,287] Fowler's study has involved using low levels of depo-MPA, representing one tenth, one half, and one times the recommended human dose for contraception and has revealed adverse changes developing in mammary glands and uteri from both dosage levels that interrupt the estrous cycle (1.5 and 3.0 mg/kg every 3 months).[109] In a recent progress report, the author included the number of atypical mammary gland nodules that were present in five glands examined from 13 bitches in each of the four groups as follows:

Control	− 45
0.3 mg/kg	− 58
1.5 mg/kg	−164
3.0 mg/kg	−342

While many of these nodules were hyperplastic or inflammatory, there were several benign neoplasms (complex adenomas and adenomas) found in each group, more so in the higher dosage groups. Only one or two neoplasms were questionable as malignant neoplasms, and these only as low-grade malignancies based solely on lack of definite organization and limited extension into surrounding tissue. Not all of the bitches in the highest dosage groups had an increased number of atypical lesions, while some had many, indicating an individual animal susceptibility to the progestin. Of the 13 bitches examined in the 3.0 mg/kg group, 7 had 0 to 10 lesions, 2 had 11 to 20 lesions, 1 had 31 to 40 lesions, and 3 had over 50 atypical nodules (59, 67 and 113, 56 of which appeared in one gland!). An earlier report of beagle bitches receiving i.m. injections of MPA at 2.5 mg/kg or 62.5 mg/kg body weight for 20 and 15 months, respectively, revealed that the number of dogs developing nodules in the treated groups was not significantly different from the controls, but that the number of nodules developing in each dog was ten times higher in the treated animals than in the control.[287] An astounding 75% of the bitches in the highest dosage group developed malignant mammary tumors with metastases! All dogs receiving the highest dose had died or had been killed by the end of the 4th year. No malignant tumors were found in any dogs that died or were killed prior to the 42nd month of treatment in any group.[287]

Another group of investigators using 1, 6.1, and 23.7 times the recommended human contraceptive dose of depo-MPA found a dose-related increase in the number of nodules that developed.[282] None of these animals had malignant neoplasms, although the report did not include evaluations made after the animals had been on the drug over 40 months.

The conclusion to be drawn from these studies is that beagle bitches are sensitive to progestins and the mammary gland development is accentuated in intact bitches receiving progestins alone. Mammary tumors are increased in frequency and decreased in latency in bitches receiving these hormones, and the exact mechanism whereby progestins influence this growth or induction rate remains to be elucidated. Several investigators have refuted the validity of the dog as a model in which to test contraceptive progestins because of the mammary neoplasms that develop.[189-191,193,200,283,284,288-290]

4. Monkeys

Nearly all of the reports concerning the use of Rhesus monkeys for testing progestins and contraceptive combinations have indicated that they do not develop mammary gland nodules or neoplasms.[193-286,289,291] This is probably related to the fact that spontaneous mammary nodules and neoplasms rarely develop in this species. In one study, 2 of 20 control monkeys developed multiple palpable breast nodules varying from 2 to 7 mm in diameter, which were firm and freely moving.[292] Only one of these nodules was biopsied and diagnosed as focal nodular hyperplasia.

In a preliminary report of a study, reference was made to implicate contraceptives in mammary tumorigenesis in monkeys.[293] An infiltrating duct carcinoma was found in the mammary gland of a Rhesus monkey that had received 1 mg of Enovid® (norethynodrel plus mestranol) daily for 18 months. This was one of six females receiving this dosage regimen. No follow-up report on this study has been found.

5. Other

Estrogen induces tumors of the kidney in Syrian hamsters and at the same time increases the progesterone binding capacity in both the kidneys and the early tumors.[294] The amount of progesterone binding activity increased to a plateau after 2.5 months of diethylstilbestrol treatment and remained 17 times higher than in untreated control kidneys. This marked increase in cytosol progesterone binding activity represented the earliest consistent change reported during the induction period of renal tumors in this species.[294] Progesterone administered simultaneously with DES prevents renal carcinogenesis, and if administered after the renal tumors develop, the growth rate is retarded.[295,296] One investigator reported that progesterone had a synergistic rather than an antagonistic effect with estrogen on renal tumor development.[199]

Estrogen implanted subcutaneously in male BALB/c mice results in interstitial cell tumors developing in the testes after 1 year.[297] When pellets of progesterone (15 mg) were implanted subcutaneously in mice that were 2 to 3 months old, 1 week following DES implantation, and continued at intervals of 3 weeks until 12 progesterone implants had been given, the group showed a lower incidence of interstitial cell tumors and a higher average age of occurrence.[297] Another investigator had previously reported that progesterone retards estrogen-induced interstitial cell tumors in mice.[298]

Progesterone was found to be immunosuppressive in monkeys; physiological doses rendered a total of 30 (30 in the group) otherwise resistant juvenile and adult monkeys susceptible to the leukemogenic effect of the chicken sarcoma virus.[299] Further studies revealed that skin homografts were retained significantly longer in progesterone-treated monkeys compared with controls.[299] However, progesterone was found to have little effect on leukemogenesis in ovariectomized AKR female mice.[300]

VIII. CONCLUSION

Progesterone, a naturally occurring steroid hormone produced and secreted primarily by the corpus luteum as well as by granulosa and interstitial cells of the ovary and the adrenal cortex, is responsible for many biological effects, including maintenance of pregnancy and inhibition of estrus in both the pregnant and pseudopregnant animals. Synthetic progestins, produced from both naturally occurring progesterone and testerone generally have much greater progestational activity than progesterone, which varies not only with the progestin, but also with the species and assay in which the steroid is tested. There are few derivatives of progesterone or testosterone which mimic progesterone precisely, but several that inhibit estrus in certain species much more effectively than progesterone, a purpose for which they are primarily used, at least in women.

Because of their widespread use as contraceptive agents, many studies have been performed to evaluate the tumorigenic potential of these progestins, and the results have been of sufficient concern to stimulate the Food and Drug Administration (U.S.) to demand the removal of several products from the contraceptive market. Many of the 19-nortestosterone derivatives have estrogenic activity in rodents, including binding to estrogen receptors, and it is principally these species in which hepatic, pituitary, and ovarian tumors have been found using these progestins. Other progestins, such as the derivatives of 17α-hydroxyprogesterone, generally fail to stimulate such tumors unless combined with synthetic estrogens.

The mammary tumors that are stimulated by progestin administration present a more complex picture. Some of the 19-nortestosterone derivatives promote mammary tumors in rodents when used alone and in high dosage, as does progesterone, but these are generally seen in animals bearing the mammary tumor virus or which have received one of the chemical carcinogens, and the hormones appear to act as promoters or cocarcinogens. However, in the dog, derivatives of 17α-hydroxyprogesterone are the principal progestins implicated in mammary tumorigenesis; and tumors that appear are dose- and time-related and both benign and malignant. No known carcinogen or virus initiates these tumors, but it does appear that the hormones not only promote extensive mammary gland development but also early tumor growth, which normally occurs somewhat later and in high frequency in this species. The unusual sensitivity of the dog to these progestins, and the great variation in sensitivity not only of different species, but also of different strains within a species, has brought into serious question the validity of the animal studies for predicting tumorigenesis in women.

It should be evident from the information contained herein that synthetic progestins, as well as natural progesterone, are implicated as promoters or cocarcinogens of neoplasms in several species when administered in sufficient dosages and result in tumors developing in organs involved with production, metabolism, or response to these hormones.

Acknowledgments

The author wishes to thank his secretary, Ms. Mary C. Hawk, for her excellent assistance. This work was supported in part by contract number HD 73-2705 and Cancer Center Core Support Grant 5-P30-CA 11198-09, National Institutes of Health, Bethesda, Maryland.

REFERENCES

1. Allen, W. M., Physiology of the corpus luteum. V. The preparation and some chemical properties of progestin, a hormone of the corpus luteum which produces progestational proliferation, *Am. J. Physiol.*, 92, 174, 1930.
2. Allen, W. M., The preparation of purified progestin, *J. Biol. Chem.*, 98, 591, 1932.
3. Allen, W. M., Butenandt, A., Corner, G. W., and Slotta, K. H., Zur Nomenklatur des Corpus-luteum-Hormons, *Ber. Dtsch. Chem. Ges.*, 68, 1746, 1935.
4. Smith, M. S., Freeman, M. E., and Neill, J. D., The control of progesterone secretion during the estrous cycle and early pseudopregnancy in the rat: prolactin, gonadotropin and steroid levels associated with rescue of the corpus luteum of pseudopregnancy, *Endocrinology*, 96, 219, 1975.
5. Leavitt, W. W., Bosley, C. G., and Blaha, G. C., Source of ovarian preovulatory progesterone, *Nature (London)*, 234, 283, 1971.
6. Ryan, K. J. and Petro, Z., Steroid biosynthesis by human ovarian granulosa and thecal cells, *J. Clin. Endocrinol. Metab.*, 26, 46, 1966.
7. Fowler, R. E., Chan, S. T. H., Walters, D. E., Edwards, R. G., and Steptoe, P. C., Steroidogenesis in human follicles approaching ovulation as judged from assays of follicular fluid, *J. Endocrinol.*, 72, 259, 1977.
8. Friedrich, F., Breitenecker, G., Salzer, H., and Holzner, J. H., The progesterone content of the fluid and the activity of the steroid-3β OL-dehydrogenase within the wall of the ovarian follicles, *Acta Endocrinol. (Copenhagen)*, 76, 343, 1974.
9. Channing, C. P., Effects of stage of the menstrual cycle and gonadotropins of luteinization of Rhesus monkey granulosa cells in culture, *Endocrinology*, 87, 49, 1970.
10. Dorrington, J. H. and Kilpatrick, R., Effects of pituitary hormones on progestational hormone production by the rabbit ovary in vivo and in vitro, *J. Endocrinol.*, 35, 53, 1966.
11. McClellan, M. C., Diekman, M. A., Abel, J. H., Jr., and Niswender, G. D., Luteinizing hormone, progesterone and the morphological development of normal and superovulated corpora lutea in sheep, *Cell Tissue Res.*, 164, 291, 1975.
12. Shima, S., Urata, Y., and Pincus, G., Progestins biosynthesis in rats in vivo following infusion of cholesterol-7α-^{3}H and acetate-1-^{14}C into luteinized ovaries, *Proc. Soc. Exp. Biol. Med.*, 128, 673, 1968.

13. Shaikh, A. A. and Shaikh, S. A., Adrenal and ovarian steroid secretion in the rat estrous cycle temporally related to gonadotropins and steroid levels found in peripheral plasma, *Endocrinology,* 96, 37, 1975.

14. Resko, J. A., Sex steroids in adrenal effluent plasma of the ovariectomized Rhesus monkey, *J. Clin. Endocrinol. Metab.,* 33, 940, 1971.

15. Telegdy, G., Hergenroder, A., and Lissák, K., Effect of gonadal hormones on adrenal steroid production in the dog, *Acta Physiol. Acad. Sci. Hung.,* 31, 277, 1967.

16. Diczfalusy, E. and Troen, P., Endocrine functions of the human placenta. *Vitam. Horm. (N.Y.)* 19, 229, 1961.

17. Ainsworth, L. and Ryan, K. J., Steroid hormone transformations by endocrine organs from pregnant mammals. II. Formation and metabolism of progesterone by bovine and sheep placental perfusions in vitro, *Endocrinology,* 81, 1349, 1967.

18. Tait, J. F., Review: The use of isotopic steroids for the measurement of production rates in vivo, *J. Clin. Endocrinol. Metab.,* 23, 1285, 1963.

19. Taylor, W. and Wright, D. E., The distribution of metabolites or [7α-³H] progesterone in tissues of mice, *J. Endocrinol.,* 51, 727, 1971.

20. Little, B., Billiar, R. B., Rahman, S. S., Johnson, W. A., Takoaka, Y., and White, R. J., *In vivo* aspects of progesterone distribution and metabolism, *Am. J. Obstet. Gynecol.,* 123, 527, 1975.

21. Laumas, K. R. and Faroog, A., The uptake *in vivo* of [1,2-³H] progesterone by the brain and genital tract of the rat, *J. Endocrinol.,* 36, 95, 1966.

22. Tabei, T., Haga, H., Heinrichs, W., and Herrmann, W. L., Metabolism of progesterone by rat brain, pituitary gland and other tissues, *Steroids,* 23, 651, 1974.

23. Karavolas, H. J. and Nuti, K. M., Progesterone metabolism by neuroendocrine tissues, in *Subcellular Mechanisms in Reproductive Neuroendocrinology,* Naftolin, F., Ryan, K. J., and Davies, J., Eds., Elsevier, Amsterdam, 1976, 305.

24. DePaoli, J. and Eik-Nes, K. B., Metabolism *in vivo* of [7α-³H] pregnenolone by the dog ovary, *Biochim. Biophys. Acta,* 78, 457, 1963.

25. Ryan, K. J. and Smith, O. W., Biogenesis of steroid hormones in the human ovary, *Recent Prog. Horm. Res.,* 21, 367, 1965.

26. Huang, W. Y. and Pearlman, W. H., The corpus luteum and steroid hormone formation. II. Studies on the human corpus luteum *in vitro,* *J. Biol. Chem.,* 238, 1308, 1963.

27. Savard, K., Marsh, J. M., and Rice, B. F., Gonadotropins and ovarian steroidogenesis, *Recent Prog. Horm. Res.,* 21, 285, 1965.

28. Ryan, K. J., The conversion of pregnenolone-7-³H and progesterone-4-¹⁴C to oestradiol by a corpus luteum of pregnancy, *Acta Endocrinol. (Copenhagen),* 44, 81, 1963.

29. Saffran, J., Loeser, B. K., Haas, B. M., and Stavely, H. E., Metabolism of progesterone in rat uterus, *Steroids,* 23, 117, 1974.

30. Saffran, J., Loeser, B. K., Haas, B. M., and Stavely, H. E., Metabolism of progesterone in subcellular fractions of rat uterus, *Steroids,* 24, 839, 1974.

31. Francois, D., Johnson, D. F., and Wong, H. Y. C., *In vitro* metabolism of progesterone-4-¹⁴C by the adrenal gland of the Mongolian gerbil, *Steroids,* 7, 297, 1966.

32. Francois, D., Wong, H. Y. C., and Johnson, D. F., Effects of Nembutal® anesthesia on progesterone-4-¹⁴C metabolism in the adrenal gland of the Mongolian gerbil, *Steroids,* 8, 289, 1966.

33. Coffey, J. C., French, F. S., and Nayfeh, S. N., Metabolism of progesterone by testicular homogenates. IV. Further studies of testosterone formation in immature testis *in vitro,* *Endocrinology,* 89, 865, 1971.

34. Oh, R. and Tamaoki, B., *In vitro* steroidgenesis in feline testes, *Biochim. Biophys. Acta,* 316, 395, 1973.

35. Ficher, M. and Steinberger, E., *In vitro* progesterone metabolism by rat testicular tissue at different stages of development, *Acta Endocrinol. (Copenhagen),* 68, 285, 1971.

36. Frost, P., Gomez, E. C., Weinstein, G. D., Lamas, J., and Hsia, S. L., Metabolism of progesterone-4-¹⁴C *in vitro* in human skin and vaginal mucosa, *Biochemistry,* 8, 948, 1969.

37. Jensen, E. V. and DeSombre, E. R., Mechanism of action of the female sex hormones, *Annu. Rev. Biochem.,* 41, 203, 1972.

38. Falk, R. J. and Bardin, C. W., Uptake of tritiated progesterone by the uterus of the ovariectomized guinea pig, *Endocrinology,* 86, 1059, 1970.

39. Feil, P. D., Glasser, S. R., Toft, D. O., and O'Malley, B. W., Progesterone binding in the mouse and rat uterus, *Endocrinology,* 91, 738, 1972.

40. Philibert, D. and Raynaud, J.-P., Progesterone binding in the immature rabbit and guinea pig uterus, *Endocrinology,* 94, 627, 1974.

41. Reel, J. R. and Shih, Y., Oestrogen-inducible uterine progesterone receptors. Characteristics in the ovariectomized immature and adult hamster, *Acta Endocrinol. (Copenhagen),* 80, 344, 1975.

42. Rossier, G., Wilson, D. W., and Pierrepoint, C. G., Investigation of steroid-receptor interaction in pregnant sheep myometrium, *J. Endocrinol.,* 61, lix, 1974.
43. Flickinger, G. L., Elsner, C., Illingworth, D. V., Muechler, E. K., and Mikhail, G., Estrogen and progesterone receptors in the female genital tract of humans and monkeys, *Ann. N.Y. Acad. Sci.,* 286, 180, 1977.
44. Toft, D. O. and O'Malley, B. W., Target tissue receptors for progesterone: the influence of estrogen treatment, *Endocrinology,* 90, 1041, 1972.
45. Faber, L. E., Saffran, J., Chen, T. J., and Leavitt, W. W., Mammalian progesterone receptors: biosynthesis, structure and nuclear binding, in *Current Topics in Molecular Endocrinology,* Vol. 4, Menon, K. M. J. and Reel, J. R., Eds., Plenum Press, New York, 1976, 68.
46. Haukkamaa, M., The subcellular distribution of endogenous progesterone in pregnant rat myometrium, *J. Steroid Biochem.,* 5, 631, 1974.
47. Haukkamaa, M. and Luukkainen, T., Progesterone-binding properties of microsomes from pregnant rat uterus, *J. Steroid Biochem.,* 6, 1311, 1975.
48. Milgrom, E., Thi, M. L., and Baulieu, E. -E., Control Mechanisms of steroid hormone receptors in the reproductive tract, *Acta Endocrinol. (Copenhagen) Suppl.,* 180, 380, 1973.
49. Milgrom, E., Atger, M., Perrot, M., and Baulieu, E. -E., Progesterone in uterus and plasma. VI. Uterine progesterone receptors during the estrous cycle and implantation in the guinea pig, *Endocrinology,* 90, 1071, 1972.
50. Terenius, L., Affinities of progestogen and estrogen receptors in rabbit uterus for synthetic progesterone, *Steroids,* 23, 909, 1974.
51. Feil, P. D., Miljkovic, M. and Bardin, C. W., Medroxyprogesterone acetate: a steroid with potent progestational activity but low receptor affinity in the guinea pig uterus, *Endocrinology,* 98, 1508, 1976.
52. Goldman, B. D. and Zarrow, M. X., The physiology of progestins, in *Handbook of Physiology,* Section 7, Vol. 2, Part 1, Greep, R. O., Ed., American Physiological Society, Washington, D.C., 1973, 547.
53. Zarrow, M. X., The biological profile of progesterone and a consideration of the bioassay of progestogens, in *Hormonal Steroids, Biochemistry, Pharmacology, and Therapeutics,* Proc. 1st Intl. Congr. Hormonal Steroids, Milan 1962, Vol. 2, Martini, L. and Pecile, A., Eds., Academic Press, New York, 1965, 239.
54. Resko, J. A., Norman, R. L., Niswender, G. D., and Spies, H. G., The relationship between progestins and gonadotropins during the late luteal phase of the menstrual cycle in Rhesus monkeys, *Endocrinology,* 94, 128, 1974.
55. Frith, D. A. and Hooper, K. C., The action of progestational agents on oxytocinase activity in the female rabbit hypothalamus, *Acta Endocrinol. (Copenhagen),* 70, 429, 1972.
56. Aono, T., Miyake, A., Kinugasa, T., and Kurachi, K., Progesterone advancement of oestrogen-induced luteinizing hormone release during the midfollicular phase in normal cyclic women, *J. Endocrinol.,* 71, 451, 1976.
57. Knobil, E., Hormonal control of the menstrual cycle and ovulation in the Rhesus monkey, *Acta. Endocrinol. Suppl.,* (Copenhagen), 166, 137, 1972.
58. Ying, S.-Y. and Greep, R. O., Effect of age of rat and dose of a single injection of estradiol benzoate (EB) on ovulation and the facilitation of ovulation by progesterone (P), *Endocrinology,* 89, 785, 1971.
59. Uchida, K., Kadowaki, T. M., and Wakabayashi, K., Effects of exogenous progesterone on the ovarian progestin secretion and plasma LH and prolactin levels in cyclic rats, *Endocrinol. Jpn.,* 19, 323, 1972.
60. Greenwald, G. S., Exogenous progesterone: influence on ovulation and hormone levels in the cyclic hamster, *J. Endocrinol.,* 73, 151, 1977.
61. Spies, H. G. and Niswender, G. D., Blockade of the surge of preovulatory serum luteinizing hormone and ovulation with exogenous progesterone in cycling Rhesus (*Macaca mulatta*) monkeys, *J. Clin. Endocrinol. Metab.,* 32, 309, 1971.
62. Collins, W. P., Koullapis, E. N., and Sommerville, I. F., The effect of chlormadinone acetate on progesterone secretion and metabolism, *Acta Endocrinol. (Copenhagen)* 68, 271, 1971.
63. Saunders, D. M., Marcus, S. L., Saxena, B. B., Beling, C. G., and Connell, E. B., Effect of daily administration of 0.5 mg of chlormadinone acetate on plasma levels of follicle-stimulating hormone, luteinizing hormone, and progesterone during the menstrual cycle, *Fertil. Steril.,* 22, 332, 1971.
64. Larsson-Cohn, U., Johansson, D. B., Wide, L., and Gemzell, C., Effects of continuous daily administration of 0.1 mg of norethindrone on the plasma levels of progesterone and on the urinary excretion of luteinizing hormone and total oestrogens, *Acta Endocrinol. (Copenhagen),* 71, 551, 1972.
65. Aiyer, M. S., and Fink, G., The role of sex steroid hormones in modulating the responsiveness of the anterior pituitary gland to luteinizing hormone releasing factor in the female rat, *J. Endocrinol.,* 62, 553, 1974.

66. Taleisnik, S., Caligaris, L., and Astrada, J. J., Positive feed-back effect of progesterone on the release of FSH and the influence of sex in rats, *J. Reprod. Fertil.*, 22, 89, 1970.
67. Bhatia, S. K., Moore, D., and Kalkhoff, R. K., Progesterone suppression of the plasma growth hormone response, *J. Clin. Endocrinol. Metab.*, 35, 364, 1972.
68. Lawrence, A. M., and Kirsteins, L., Progestins in the medical management of active acromegaly, *J. Clin. Endocrinol. Metab.*, 30, 646, 1970.
69. Owen, L. N., Effects on the mammary glands of dogs dosed with the human contraceptive pill, *Clin. Oncol.*, 2, 305, 1976.
70. Mathews, J. H., Abrams, C. A. L., and Morishima, A., Pituitary-adrenal function in ten patients receiving medroxyprogesterone acetate for true precocious puberty, *J. Clin. Endocrinol. Metab.*, 30, 653, 1970.
71. Sadeghi-Nejad, A., Kaplan, S. L., Grumback, M. M., The effect of medroxyprogesterone acetate on adrenocortical function in children with precocious puberty, *J. Pediatr.*, 78, 616, 1971.
72. Haug, E. and Gantvik, K. M., Effects of sex steroids on prolactin secreting rat pituitary cells in culture, *Endocrinology*, 99, 1482, 1976.
73. Smollich, A., Voight, H. -J., Busch, W., Quantitativ-morphologische Untersuchungen zur Wirkung von Gestagenen auf das Hypothalamus-adenohypophysen-System des Rindes, *Endokrinologie*, 64, 39, 1974.
74. Mosca, L., Effects of progestational steroids on the cytology of the baboon pituitary gland, in *Hormonal Steroids, Biochemistry, Pharmacology, and Therapeutics*, Proc. 1st Intl. Congr. Hormonal Steroids, Milan, 1962, Vol. 2, Martini, L. and Pecile, A., Eds., Academic Press, New York, 1965, 301.
75. Baker, B. L., Eskin, T. A., and August, L. N., Direct action of synthetic progestins on the hypophysis, *Endocrinology*, 92, 965, 1973.
76. Baker, B. L., Eskin, T. A., and Clapp, H. W., The effect of medroxyprogesterone on cells of the pituitary pars distalis, *Proc. Soc. Exp. Biol. Med.*, 140, 357, 1972.
77. Wordinger, R., Dickey, J. F., and Hill, R., Jr., Influence of a progestogen on the cytophysiologic character of the bovine adenohypophysis, *Am. J. Vet. Res.*, 38, 449, 1977.
78. Buffler, G. and Roser, S., New data concerning the role played by progesterone in the control of follicular growth in the rat, *Acta Endocrinol. (Copenhagen)*, 75, 569, 1974.
79. Bland, K. P. and Donovan, B. T., Oestrogen and progesterone and the function of the corpora lutea in the guinea pig, *J. Endocrinol.*, 47, 225, 1970.
80. Boris, A., Trmal, T., and Nelson, E. W., Jr., The effect of some progestational steroids on pubertal ovulation in the rat, *Contraception* 5, 57, 1972.
81. Aksel, S. and Jones, G. S., Effect of progesterone and 17-hydroxyprogesterone caproate on normal corpus luteum function, *Am. J. Obstet. Gynecol.*, 118, 466, 1974.
82. Zanartu, J., Pupkin, M., Rosenberg, D., Davansens, A., Guerrero, R., Rodriguez-Bravo, R., Garcia-Huidobro, M., Long term effect of medroxyprogesterone acetate in human morphophysiology and sperm transport, *Fertil. Steril.*, 21, 525, 1970.
83. Aref, I., Hefnawi, F., and Kandil, O., Changes in human ovaries after long term administration of microdose progestogens, *Contraception*, 7, 503, 1973.
84. ten Berge, B. S., Histological changes in ovarian and uterine blood vessels after the use of oral contraceptive agents (estrogengestagen combinations) and Gestagens, *Intl. J. Fertil.*, 18, 57, 1973.
85. Rudel, H. W. and Kincl, F. A., The toxicity of progesterone, in *Pharmacology of the Endocrine System and Related Drugs: Progesterone, Progestational Drugs and Antifertility Agents*, Vol. 1, Tausk, M., Ed., Pergamon Press, New York, 1971, 405.
86. Bouin, P., and Ancel, P., Sur les fonctions du corps jaune gestatif. I. Sur le determinisme de la preparation de luterus a la fixation de l'oeuf, *J. Physiol. Pathol. Gen.*, 12, 1, 1910.
87. Madjerek, Z. S., Histological effects of progesterone on the vagina and the uterus, in *Pharmacology of the Endocrine System and Related Drugs: Progesterone, Progestational Drugs and Antifertility Agents*, Vol. 1, Tausk, M., Ed., Pergamon Press, New York, 1971, 65.
88. Robson, J. M., Antagonism between progesterone and the synthetic oestrogenic substance, triphenyl ethylene, *J. Physiol.*, 92, 401, 1938.
89. Koseki, Y. and Fujimoto, G. I., Progesterone effects contrasted with 17β-estradiol on DNA synthesis and epithelial nuclear proliferation in the castrate rabbit uterus, *Biol. Reprod.*, 10, 596, 1974.
90. Lee, A. E. and Dukelow, W. R., Synthesis of DNA and mitosis in rabbit uteri after oestrogen and progesterone injections, and during early pregnancy, *J. Reprod. Fertil.*, 31, 473, 1972.
91. Martin, L. and Finn, C. A., Hormonal regulation of cell division in epithelial and connective tissue of the mouse uterus, *J. Endocrinol.*, 41, 363, 1968.
92. Lee, A. E., The effect of continuous oestrogen on mitosis and [^{3}H] thymidine incorporation in the mouse uterus, in *Basic Actions of Sex Steroids on Target Organs*, Hubinont, P. O., Leroy, F., and Galand, P., Eds., Karger, Basel, 1971, 243.
93. Clark, B. F., The effect of oestrogen and progesterone on uterine cell division and epithelial morphology in spayed, adrenalectomized rats, *J. Endocrinol.*, 50, 527, 1971.

94. Finn, C. A. and Martin, L., Endocrine control of gland proliferation in the mouse uterus, *Biol. Reprod.*, 8, 585, 1973.
95. Martin, L. and Finn, C. A., Duration of progesterone treatment required for a stromal response to oestradiol-17β in the uterus of the mouse, *J. Endocrinol.*, 44, 279, 1969.
96. Martin, L., Das, R. M., and Finn, C. A., The inhibition by progesterone of uterine epithelial proliferation in the mouse, *J. Endocrinol.*, 57, 549, 1973.
97. Martin, L., Finn, C. A., and Trinder, G., DNA synthesis in the endometrium of progesterone-treated mice, *J. Endocrinol.*, 56, 303, 1973.
98. Smith, J. A., Martin, L., King, R. J. B., and Vertes, M., Effect of oestradiol-17β and progesterone on total and nuclear-protein synthesis in epithelial and stromal tissues of the mouse uterus, and progesterone on the ability of these tissues to bind oestradiol-17β, *Biochem. J.*, 119, 773, 1970.
99. Marcus, G. J., Mitosis in the rat uterus during the estrous cycle, early pregnancy and early pseudopregnancy, *Biol. Reprod.*, 10, 447, 1974.
100. Saldarini, R. J. and Yochim, J. M., Metabolism of the uterus of the rat during early pseudopregnancy and its regulation by estrogen and progestogen, *Endocrinology*, 80, 453, 1967.
101. Bo, W. J., Poteat, W. L., Krueger, W. A., and McAlister, F., The effect of progesterone on estradiol-17β dipropionate-induced wet weight, percent water, and glycogen of the rat uterus, *Steroids*, 18, 389, 1971.
102. Tachi, C., Tachi, S., and Lindner, H. R., Modification by progesterone of oestradiol-induced cell proliferation, RNA synthesis and oestradiol distribution in the rat uterus, *J. Reprod. Fertil.*, 31, 59, 1972.
103. Tachi, S., Tachi, C., and Lindner, H. R., Influence of ovarian hormones on formation of solitary cilia and behavior of the centrioles in uterine epithelial cells of the rat, *Biol. Reprod.*, 10, 391, 1974.
104. Tachi, C., Tachi, S., and Lindner, H. R., Effects of ovarian hormones upon nucleolar ultrastructure in endometrial stromal cells of the rat, *Biol. Reprod.*, 10, 404, 1974.
105. Good, R. G. and Moyer, D. L., Estrogen-progesterone relationship in the development of secretory endometrium, *Fertil. Steril.*, 19, 37, 1968.
106. Joshi, S. G. and Ebert, K. M., Effects of progesterone on labelling of soluble proteins and glycoproteins in rabbit endometrium, *Fertil. Steril.*, 27, 730, 1976.
107. Bullock, D. W., Progesterone induction of messenger RNA and protein synthesis in rabbit uterus, *Ann. N.Y. Acad. Sci.*, 286, 260, 1977.
108. Smith, M. S. R., Histochemical observations on the mouse uterus during the oestrus cycle, *J. Reprod. Fertil.*, 22, 461, 1970.
109. Fowler, E. H., Vaughan, T., Gotcsik, F., Reichhart, P., and Reed, C., Pathologic changes in mammary glands and uteri from beagle bitches receiving low levels of medroxyprogesterone acetate: an overview of research in progress, in *Pharmacology of Steroid Contraceptive Drugs*, Garantini, S. and Berendes, H. W., Eds., Raven Press, New York, 1977, 185.
110. Roberts, R. M., Bazer, F. W., Baldwin, N., and Pollard, W. E., Progesterone induction of lysozyme and pepidase activities in the porcine uterus, *Arch. Biochem. Biophys.*, 177, 499, 1976.
111. Sumner, N. A. and Brush, M. G., Acid phosphatase isoenzymes in normal human endometrium and pathological tissues, *J. Endocrinol.*, 57, xxxii, 1973.
112. Manning, J. P., Hisaw, F. L., Steinetz, B. G., and Kroc, R. L., The effects of ovarian hormones on uterine phosphatase of the Rhesus monkey (*Macaca mulatta*), *Anat. Rec.*, 157, 457, 1967.
113. Moulton, B. C. and Barker, K. L., A delayed antagonistic effect of progesterone on estradiol-induced increases in uterine glucose-6-phosphate dehydrogenase, *Endocrinology*, 92, 636, 1973.
114. Moulten, B. C., Progesterone and estrogen control of uterine glucose-6-phosphate dehydrogenase activity during deciduomal growth, *Biol. Reprod.*, 10, 526, 1974.
115. Yochim, J. M. and Pepe, G. J., Effect of ovarian steroids on nucleic acids, protein, and glucose-6-phosphate dehydrogenase activity in endometrium of the rat: a metabolic role for progesterone in "progestational differentiation," *Biol. Reprod.*, 5, 172, 1971.
116. Murdoch, R. N. and White, I. G., The activity of enzymes in the rabbit uterus and effect of progesterone and oestradiol, *J. Endocrinol.*, 43, 167, 1969.
117. Clark, S. W. and Yochim, J. M., Lactic dehydrogenase in the rat uterus during progestation, its relation to intrauterine oxygen tension and the regulation of glycolysis, *Biol. Reprod.*, 5, 152, 1971.
118. Hodgen, G. D. and Falk, R. J., Estrogen and progesterone regulation of carbonic anhydrase isoenzymes in guinea pig and rabbit uterus, *Endocrinology*, 89, 859, 1971.
119. Miyake, T. and Pincus, G., Hormonal influences on the carbonic anhydrase concentration in the accessory reproductive tracts of the rat, *Endocrinology*, 65, 64, 1959.
120. Pincus, G., Miyake, T., Merrill, A. P., and Longo, P., The bioassay of progesterone, *Endocrinology*, 61, 528, 1957.
121. Lutwak-Mann, C., Carbonic anhydrase in the female reproductive tract. Occurrence, distribution and hormonal dependence, *J. Endocrinol.*, 13, 26, 1955.
122. Morris, J. M., Mechanisms involved in progesterone contraception and estrogen interception, *Am. J. Obstet. Gynecol.*, 117, 167, 1973.

123. Erichson, S., Histochemical changes in the endometrium of the dog during the oestrus cycle, *Acta Pathol. Microbiol. Scand.*, 33, 263, 1953.
124. Fitch, K. L., A study of uterine glycogen during the oestrus cycle of the dog, *J. Morphol.*, 113, 331, 1963.
125. Dawson, A. B. and Kosters, B. A., Preimplantation changes in the uterine mucosa of the cat, *Am. J. Anat.*, 75, 1, 1944.
126. Boshier, D. P. and Holloway, H., Effects of ovarian steroid hormones on histochemically demonstrable lipids in the rat uterine epithelium, *J. Endocrinol.*, 56, 59, 1973.
127. Swyer, G. I., Potency and selectivity of action of progestogens, in *2nd Intl. Norgestrel Symp.*, Int. Congr. Ser. No. 344, Fairweather, D. V. I., Ed., American Elsevier, New York, 1974, 42.
128. Zarrow, M. X., Peters, L. E., and Caldwell, A. L., Jr., Comparative potency of several progestogenic compounds in a battery of different biological tests, *Ann. N.Y. Acad. Sci.*, 71, 532, 1958.
129. Hill, R., Averkin, E., Brown, W., Gagne, W. E., and Segre, E., Progestational potency of chlormadinone acetate in the immature beagle bitch: preliminary report, *Contraception*, 2, 381, 1970.
130. Graf, K. -J., El Etreby, M. F. A., Richter, K.-D., Gunzel, P., and Neumann, F., The progestogenic potencies of different progestogens in the beagle bitch, *Contraception*, 12, 529, 1975.
131. Iman, S. K., Sriastava, K., Dasgupta, P. R., and Kar, A. B., Biochemical changes in the fallopian tube and uterus of the Rhesus monkey (*Macaca mulatta*) under the influence of progestational contraceptive steroids, *Communications*, 11, 297, 1975.
132. Laumas, K. R. and Kasid, A., Low and high dose effects of progestogens at the molecular level in the uterus, in *Regulation of Growth and Differentiated Function in Eukaryote Cells*, Talwar, G. P., Ed., Raven Press, New York, 1975, 379.
133. Boris, A. and DeMartino, L., The utilization of uterine weight as an adjunct to histology in the evaluation of progestational steroids, *Steroidologia*, 2, 57, 1971.
134. Csermely, T., Hughes, E. C., and Demers, L. M., Effect of oral contraceptives on human endometrium in culture, *Am. J. Obstet. Gynecol.*, 109, 1066, 1971.
135. Khoo, S. K., MacKay, E. V., and Adam, P. R., Contraception with a six-monthly injection of progestogen. III. Effects on the endometrium, *Aust. N.Z. J. Obstet. Gynaecol.*, 11, 226, 1971.
136. Ober, W. B., Synthetic progestagen-oestrogen preparations and endometrial morphology, *J. Clin. Pathol.*, 19, 138, 1966.
137. Hisaw, F. L., Greep, R. O., and Fevold, H. L., The effects of oestrin-progestin combinations on the endometrium, vagina and sexual skin of monkeys, *Am. J. Anat.*, 61, 483, 1937.
138. Ford, D. H. and Young, W. C., The role of progesterone in the production of cyclic vaginal changes in the female guinea pig, *Endocrinology*, 49, 795, 1951.
139. Ford, D. H., The role of progesterone in the production of vaginal changes in ovariectomized female rats, *Endocrinology*, 55, 230, 1954.
140. Clarke, E. and Selye, H., The action of steroid compounds on the vaginal epithelium of the rat, *Am. J. Med. Sci.*, 204, 401, 1942.
141. Prasad, M. R. N. and Rajalakshmi, M., Recent advances in the control of male reproductive functions, *Intl. Rev. Physiol.*, 13, 153, 1977.
142. Dorner, G., Gotz, F., and Mainz, K., Infertility and maintained sexual behaviour in male rats treated with chlormadinone acetate, *J. Endocrinol.*, 52, 197, 1972.
143. Simon, S., Schiffer, M., Glick, S. M., and Schwartz, E., Effect of medroxyprogesterone acetate upon stimulated release of growth hormone in men, *J. Clin. Endocrinol. Metab.*, 27, 1633, 1967.
144. Saenger, P., Shanies, D. D., and New, M. I., Influence of medroxyprogesterone acetate on testosterone metabolism by cultured human fibroblasts: a model for drug-steroid interaction, *J. Clin. Endocrinol. Metab.*, 37, 760, 1973.
145. Hilgers, J., Progesterone and mammary gland development, in *Pharmacology of the Endocrine System and Related Drugs. Progesterone, Progestational Drugs and Antifertility Agents* Vol. 1, Tausk, M., Ed., Pergamon Press, New York, 1971, 83.
146. Chamorro, A., Action de la progesterone seule sur la glande mammaire, *C.R. Soc. Biol.*, 138, 453, 1944.
147. Selye, H., Activity of progesterone in spayed females not pretreated with estrin, *Proc. Soc. Exp. Biol. Med.*, 43, 343, 1940.
148. Benson, G. K., Cowie, A. T., Cox, C. P., and Goldzveig, S. A., Effects of estrone and progesterone on mammary development in the guinea pig, *J. Endocrinol.*, 15, 126, 1957.
149. Capel-Edwards, K., Hall, D. E., Fellowes, K. P., Vallance, D. K., Davies, M. J., Lamb, D., and Robertson, W. B., Long-term administration of progesterone to the female beagle dog, *Toxicol. Appl. Pharmacol.*, 24, 474, 1973.
150. Trentin, J. J., DeVita, J., and Gardner, W. U., Effect of moderate doses of estrogen and progesterone on mammary growth and hair growth in dogs, *Anat. Rec.*, 113, 163, 1952.
151. Speert, H., The normal and experimental development of the mammary gland of the Rhesus monkey, with some pathological correlations, *Carnegie Contrib. Embryol.*, 32, 9, 1948.

152. Kahn, R. H. and Baker, B. L., Effect of norethynodrel alone or combined with mestranol on the mammary gland of the adult female rat, *Endocrinology*, 75, 818, 1964.

153. Hinton, M., and Gaskell, C. J., Non-neoplastic mammary hypertrophy in the cat associated either with pregnancy or with oral progestagen therapy, *Vet. Rec.*, 100, 277, 1977.

154. Tucker, M. J., Some effects of prolonged administration of a progestogen to dogs, in *Proc. Eur. Soc. Study of Drug Toxicity* Vol. 12, Int. Congr. Ser. No. 220, Excerpta Medica, Amsterdam, 1971, 228.

155. Assairi, L., DeLousi, C., Baye, P., Houdebine, L. -M., Ollivier-Bousquet, M., and Denamur, R., Inhibition by progesterone of the lactogenic effect of prolactin in the pseudopregnant rabbit, *Biochem. J.*, 144, 245, 1974.

156. Davis, J. W., Coffelt, J. W., Eddington, C. L., The effect of progesterone on biosynthetic pathways in mammary tissue, *Endocrinology.* 91, 1011, 1972.

157. Djiane, J. and Durand, P., Prolactin-progesterone antagonism in self regulation of prolactin receptors in the mammary gland, *Nature (London)*, 266, 641, 1977.

158. Denamur, R. and Delouis, C., Effects of progesterone and prolactin on the secretory activity and the nucleic acid content of the mammary gland of pregnant rabbits, *Acta Endocrinol. (Copenhagen)*, 70, 603, 1972.

159. Bruce, J. D., Cofre, X., and Ramirez, V. D., Lactation and intra-mammary pressure in rats bearing oestrogen, progesterone or norethindrone mammary implants; effects of oxytocin, *Acta Endocrinol. (Copenhagen)*, 73, 713, 1973.

160. Chopra, J. G., Effect of steroid contraceptive on lactation, *Am. J. Clin. Nutr.*, 25, 1202, 1972.

161. Zañartu, J., Aquilera, E., Muñoz, G., and Peliowsky, H., Effect of a long-acting contraceptive progestogen on lactation, *Obstet. Gynecol.*, 47, 174, 1976.

162. Toddywalla, V. A., Joshi, L., and Virkar, K., Effect of contraceptive steroids on human lactation, *Am. J. Obstet. Gynecol.*, 127, 245, 1977.

163. Hilliard, J., Endroczi, E., and Sawyer, C. H., Stimulation of progestin release from rabbit ovary *in vivo*, *Proc. Soc. Exp. Biol. Med.*, 108, 154, 1961.

164. MacDonald, G. J. and Greep, R. O., Ability of luteinizing hormone (LH) to acutely increase serum progesterone levels during the secretory phase of the Rhesus menstrual cycle, *Fertil. Steril.*, 23, 466, 1972.

165. Armstrong, D. T., Miller, L. S., and Knudsen, K. A., Regulation of lipid metabolism and progesterone production in rat corpora lutea and ovarian interstitial elements by prolactin and luteinizing hormone, *Endocrinology*, 85, 393, 1969.

166. Channing, C. P., Influences of the *in vivo* and *in vitro* hormonal environment upon luteinization of granulosa cells in tissue culture, *Recent Prog. Horm. Res.*, 26, 589, 1970.

167. Horrell, E., Kilpatrick, R., and Major, P. W., A comparison of the effects of pituitary hormones and aminophylline on progestational hormone production by the rabbit ovary *in vivo*, *J. Endocrinol.*, 55, 205, 1972.

168. Telegdy, G. and Fendler, K., The effect of posterior pituitary hormones on adrenocortical and ovarian progesterone secretion in dogs, *Acta Physiol. Acad. Sci. Hung.*, 25, 359, 1964.

169. Chatterton, R. T., Jr., Chien, J., and Ward, D. A., Effect of perphenazine treatment of rats on serum ovarian and adrenal steroids. *Proc. Soc. Exp. Biol. Med.*, 145, 874, 1974.

170. Wilks, J. W., Forbes, K. K., and Norland, J. F., Prostaglandins and *in vitro* ovarian progestin biosynthesis, *Prostaglandins*, 3, 427, 1973.

171. Medina, D., O'Bryan, S. B., Warner, M. R., Sinka, Y. N., Vanderlaan, W. P., McCormack, S., and Hohn, P., Mammary tumorigenesis in chemical carcinogen treated mice. VII. Prolactin and progesterone levels in BALB/c mice, *J. Natl. Cancer Inst.*, 59, 213, 1977.

172. Moon, R. C. and Young, S., Progestin secretion in 3-methylcholanthrene-treated rats, *Intl. J. Cancer*, 9, 402, 1972.

173. Nishizawa, E. E. and Eik-Nes, K. B., On the secretion of progesterone and Δ-4-androstene-3,17-dione by the canine ovary in animals stimulated with human chorionic gonadotropin, *Biochim. Biophys. Acta*, 86, 610, 1964.

174. Kato, R., Takahashi, A., and Omori, Y., Effects of thyroid hormone on the hydroxylation of progesterone in liver microsomes of male and female rats, *J. Biochem.*, (Toyoko), 68, 603, 1970.

175. Vu Hai, M. T., Logeat, F., Warembourg, M., and Milgrom, E., Hormonal control of progesterone receptors, *Ann. N.Y. Acad. Sci.*, 286, 199, 1977.

176. Milgrom, E., Thi, L., Atger, M., and Baulieu, E. -E., Mechanisms regulating the concentration and the conformation of progesterone receptor(s) in the uterus, *J. Biol. Chem.*, 248, 6366, 1973.

177. Barlow, J. and Funder, J. W., DMBA and progesterone binding in breast and uterus, *Clin. Exp. Pharmacol. Physiol.*, 3, 268, 1976.

178. Robson, J. M. and Sharaf, A. A., Antagonisms of vaginal actions of oestrogen by progesterone and other steroids, *J. Endocrinol.*, 7, 177, 1951.

179. Robson, J. M., Quantitative data on the inhibition of oestrus by testosterone, progesterone, and certain other compounds, *J. Physiol.*, 92, 371, 1938.

180. Moore, N. W. and Robinson, T. J., The behavioral and vaginal response of the spayed ewe to oestrogen injected at various times relative to the injection of progesterone, *J. Endocrinol.,* 15, 360, 1957.
181. Forbes, T. R., Synergisms and antagonisms of estrogens and progesterone in a mouse uterine bioassay, *Endocrinology,* 79, 420, 1966.
182. Miller, B. G. and Emmens, C. W., The effects of oestradiol and progesterone on the incorporation of tritiated uridine into the genital tract of the mouse, *J. Endocrinol.,* 43, 427, 1969.
183. Verhage, H. G. and Brenner, R. M., A delayed antagonistic effect of progesterone on the estradiol-induced differentiation of the oviductal epithelium in spayed cats, *Biol. Reprod.,* 15, 654, 1976.
184. West, N. B., Verhage, H. G., and Brenner, R. M., Suppression of estradiol receptor system by progesterone in oviduct and uterus of cat, *Endocrinology,* 99, 1010, 1976.
185. Mixner, J. P. and Turner, C. W., Role of estrogen in the stimulation of mammary lobule-alveolar growth by progesterone and by the mammogenic lobule-alveolar growth factor of the anterior pituitary, *Endocrinology,* 30, 591, 1942.
186. Jabara, A. G., Toyne, P. H., and Fisher, R. J., An autoradiographic study of the early effects of 7,12-dimethylbenz[a] anthracene and progesterone on DNA synthesis in rat mammary epithelial cells and subsequent tumour development, *Br. J. Cancer,* 26, 265, 1972.
187. Report of a WHO Scientific Group, Hormonal Steroids in contraception, W.H.O. Tech. Rep. Ser., No. 386, 1968.
188. Muhlbock, O. and Boot, L. M., The mechanism of hormonal carcinogenesis, *Ciba Found. Symp.,* on Carcinogenesis: Mechanisms of Action, Wolstenholme, E. W., and O'Connor, M., Eds., Little, Brown, Boston, 1959, 83.
189. Drill, V. A., Experimental and clinical studies on estrogens, progestins, oral contraceptives and benign breast lesions, in *Experimental Model Systems in Toxicology and Their Significance in Man,* Vol. 15, Proc. Eur. Soc. Study Drug Toxicity, Exerpta Medica, Amsterdam, 1974, 192.
190. Hill, R. and Dumas, K., The use of dogs for studies of toxicity of contraceptive hormones, *Acta Endocrinol. (Copenhagen),* 75, 74, 1974.
191. Leonard, B. J., The use of rodents for studies of toxicity in contraceptive research, *Acta Endocrinol., (Copenhagen),* 75, 34, 1974.
192. Roe, F., The interpretation of animal studies, *Proc. R. Soc. Med.,* 69, 349, 1976.
193. Goldzieher, J. W. and Kraemer, D. C., The metabolism and effects of contraceptive steroids in primates, *Acta Endocrinol. (Copenhagen),* 71, 389, 1972.
194. Reuber, M. D. and Firminger, H. I., Effect of progesterone and diethylstilbestrol on hepatic carcinogenesis and cirrhosis in A×C rats fed N-2-fluorenyldiacetamide, *J. Natl. Cancer Inst.,* 29, 933, 1962.
195. Lacassagne, A., Hurst, L., Zajdela, F. and Royer, R., Influence des hormones sexuelles sur la production du cancer du foie chez le rat, *Acta Physiol. Lat. Am.,* 3, 136, 1953.
196. Schardein, J. L., Kaump, D. H., Woosley, E. T., and Jellema, M. M., Long term toxicologic and tumorigenesis studies on an oral contraceptive agent in albino rats, *Toxicol. Appl. Pharmacol.,* 16, 10, 1970.
197. Committee on the Safety of Medicine, Carcinogenicity tests of oral contraceptives, Her Majesty's Stationery Office, London, 1972.
198. Hansel, W., Concannon, P. W., and McEntee, K., Plasma hormone profiles and pathological observations in medroxyprogesterone acetate-treated beagle bitches, in *Pharmacology of Steroid Contraceptive Drugs,* Grattini, S. and Berendes, H. W., Eds., Raven Press, New York, 1977, 145.
199. Mühlbock, O., Steroid-induced tumors in animals, in *Biological Activities of Steroids in Relation to Cancer,* Pincus, G., and Vollmer, E. P., Eds., Academic Press, New York, 1960, 331.
200. Edgren, R. A., Are oral contraceptives and diethylstilbestrol (DES) involved in sex-linked cancer? in *Steroid Hormone Action and Cancer,* Menon, K. M. J. and Reel, J. R., Eds., *Current Topics in Molecular Endocrinology,* Plenum Press, New York, 1976, 95.
201. Poel, W. E., Pituitary tumours in mice after prolonged feeding of synthetic progestins, *Science,* 154, 402, 1966.
202. Poel, W. E., Bioassays with inbred mice: their relevance for the random bred animal, *Prog. Exp. Tumor Res.,* 11, 444, 1969.
203. Poel, W. E. and Haran-Ghera, N., Progesterone and tumour metastasis, *Lancet,* 2, 970, 1963.
204. Li, M. H. and Gardner, W. U., Further studies on the pathogenesis of ovarian tumors in mice, *Cancer Res.,* 9, 35, 1949.
205. Lipschütz, A., Iglesias, R., and Salinas, S., Ovarian tumours induced by a sterilizing steroid, *Nature (London),* 196, 946, 1962.
206. Lipschütz, A., Iglesias, R., Panasevich, V. I., and Salinas, S., Ovarian tumours and other ovarian changes induced in mice by two 19-norcontraceptives, *Br. J. Cancer,* 21, 153, 1967.
207. Lipschütz, A., Iglesias, R., and Salinas, S., Further studies on the recovery of fertility in mice after protracted steroid induced fertility, *J. Reprod. Fertil.,* 6, 99, 1963.
208. Lipschütz, A., Iglesias, R., Salinas, S., and Panasevich, V. I., Experimental conditions under which contraceptive steroids may become toxic, *Nature (London),* 212, 686, 1966.

209. Lipschutz, A., Iglesias, R., Panasevich, V. I., and Salinas, S., Granulosa-cell tumours induced in mice by progesterone, *Br. J. Cancer*, 21, 144, 1967.
210. Jabara, A. G., Induction of canine ovarian tumours by diethylstilbestrol and progesterone, *Aust. J. Exp. Biol. Med. Sci.*, 40, 139, 1962.
211. Lipschutz, A., Iglesias, R., Panasevich, V. I., and Salinas, S., Pathological changes induced in the uterus of mice with the prolonged administration of progesterone and 19-nor-contraceptives, *Br. J. Cancer*, 21, 160, 1967.
212. Blanzat-Reboud, S. and Russfield, A. B., Effect of parenteral steroids on induction of genital tumours in mice by 20-methylcholanthrene, *Am. J. Obstet. Gynecol.*, 103, 96, 1969.
213. Bischoff, F., Carcinogenic effects of steroids, *Adv. Lipid Res.*, 7, 165, 1969.
214. Kaslaris, E. and Jull, J. W., The induction of tumours following the direct implantation of four chemical carcinogens into the uterus of mice and the effect of strain and hormone thereon, *Br. J. Cancer*, 16, 479, 1962.
215. Glucksmann, A. and Cherry, C. P., The effect of oestrogens, testosterone and progesterone on the induction of cervicovaginal tumours in intact and castrate rats, *Br. J. Cancer*, 22, 545, 1968.
216. Sekiya, S., Takeda, B., Kikuchi, Y., Sakaguchi, S., and Takamizawa, H., Morphologic and enzymecytochemical changes in uterine adenocarcinoma cells of a rat by direct application of progesterone *in vitro*, *Gynecol. Oncol.*, 5, 5, 1977.
217. Kahn, R. H. and Baker, B. L., Effect of long-term treatment with norethynodrel on A/J and C3H/HeJ mice, *Endocrinology*, 84, 661, 1969.
218. Dunn, T. B., Cancer of the uterine cervix in mice fed a liquid diet containing an antifertility drug, *J. Natl. Cancer Inst.*, 43, 671, 1969.
219. Munôz, N., Effect of herpesvirus type 2 and hormonal imbalance on the uterine cervix of the mouse, *Cancer Res.*, 33, 1504, 1973.
220. Reboud, S. and Pageant, G., Co-carcinogenic effect of progesterone on 20-methylcholanthrene-induced cervical carcinoma in mice, *Nature (London)*, 241, 398, 1973.
221. Drill, V. A., Oral contraceptives: relation to mammary cancer, benign breast lesions, and cervical cancer, *Annu. Rev. Pharmacol. Toxicol.*, 15, 367, 1975.
222. Drill, V. A., Effects of estrogens and progestins on the cervix uteri, *J. Toxicol. Environ. Health Suppl.*, 1, 193, 1976.
223. Glucksmann, A. and Cherry, C. P., The effect of castration and of additional hormonal treatments on the induction of cervical and vulval tumours in mice, *Br. J. Cancer*, 16, 634, 1962.
224. Bern, H. A., Jones, L. A., Mills, K. T., Kohrman, A., and Mori, T., Use of the neonatal mouse in studying long-term effects of early exposure to hormones and other agents, *J. Toxicol. Environ. Health Suppl.*, 1, 103, 1976.
225. Alvizouri, M. and Ramirez de Pita, V., Experimental carcinoma of the cervix, hormonal influences, *Am. J. Obstet. Gynecol.*, 89, 940, 1964.
226. Neumann, F., von Berswordt-Wallrabe, R., Elger, W., Graf, K.-J., Hasan, S. H., Mehring, M., Nishino, Y., and Steinbeck, H., Special problems in toxicity testing in long acting depot contraceptives, *Acta Endocrinol. (Copenhagen) Suppl.*, 185, 315, 1974.
227. Poel, W. E., The co-carcinogenic effect of exogenous progesterone in C3H female mice, *Proc. Am. Assoc. Cancer Res.*, 7, 56, 1966.
228. Poel, W. E., Co-carcinogenicity of exogenous progesterone in C3H female mice, *Proc. Am. Assoc. Cancer Res.*, 8, 54, 1967.
229. Poel, W. E., Progesterone and the prolonged progestational state, co-carcinogenic factors in mammary tumour induction, *Br. J. Cancer*, 19, 824, 1965.
230. Law, L. W., Effect of pseudopregnancy on mammary carcinoma incidence in mice of the A stock, *Proc. Soc. Exp. Biol. Med.*, 48, 486, 1941.
231. Symeonidis, A., Mammakrebserzeugung bei Mausen durch Progesterone Verabreicht wahrend des Graviditat, *Acta Unio Int. Contra Cancrum*, 6, 163, 1948.
232. Marchant, J., The influence of pseudopregnancy on breast tumour induction in C57B1 mice by various chemical carcinogens, *Br. J. Cancer*, 17, 119, 1963.
233. Marchant, J., The influence of pseudopregnancy, pregnancy and lactation on the induction of breast tumours in agent free mice by methylcholanthrene (MC), *Acta Unio Int. Contra Cancrum*, 20, 1443, 1964.
234. Bryson, G. and Bischoff, F., Exogenous progesterone in female Marsh mice, *Proc. Am. Assoc. Cancer Res.*, 17, 4, 1976.
235. Bischoff, F. and Rupp, J. J., The production of a carcinogenic agent in the degradation of cholesterol to progesterone, *Cancer Res.*, 6, 403, 1946.
236. Bischoff, F. and Bryson, G., Medroxyprogesterone administration in female Marsh mice, *Proc. Am. Assoc. Cancer Res.*, 18, 3, 1977.
237. Heiman, J., The effect of progesterone and testosterone propionate on the incidence of mammary cancer in mice, *Cancer Res.*, 5, 426, 1945.

238. Burrows, H. and Hoch-Ligeti, C., Effects of progesterone on the development of mammary cancer in C3H mice, *Cancer Res.,* 6, 608, 1946.
239. Coezy, E. and Rudali, G., Action d'un contraceptif (Ovulene) sur la carcinogenese mammaire de souris, *Rev. Eur. Etud. Clin. Biol.,* 25, 205, 1970.
240. Heston, W. E., Vlahakis, G., and Desmukes, B., Effects of the antifertility drug Enovid® in five strains of mice, with particular regard to carcinogenesis, *J. Natl. Cancer Inst.,* 51, 209, 1973.
241. Lancaster, M. C., Long-term results of toxicological studies with norgestrel combinations, in *Proc. 2nd Int. Norgestrel Symp.,* Fairweather, D. V. I., Ed., American Elsevier, New York, 1974, 16.
242. Lacassagne, A., Tentatives pour modifier, par la progesterone ou par la testosterone, l'apparition des adenocarcinomes mammaires provoques par l'oestrone chez la souris, *C. R. Soc. Biol.,* 126, 385, 1937.
243. Mühlbock, O., Over de genese der ovarium tumoren, *Belg. Tijdschr. Geneeskd.,* 24, 1, 1951.
244. Gardner, W. U., Estrogens in carcinogenesis, *Arch. Pathol.,* 27, 138, 1939.
245. Mühlbock, O. and Boot, L. M., The mode of action of ovarian hormones in the induction of mammary cancer in mice, *Biochem. Pharmacol.,* 16, 627, 1967.
246. Welsch, C. W., Adams, C., Lambrecht, L. K., Hassett, C. C., and Brooks, C. L., 17-beta-oestradiol and Enovid mammary tumorigenesis in C3H/HeJ female mice: counteraction by concurrent 2-bromo-alpha-ergocryptine, *Br. J. Cancer,* 35, 322, 1977.
247. Nandi, S. and Bern, H. A., Effect of hormones on mammary tumor development from transplanted hyperplastic alveolar nodules in ovariectomized-adrenalectomized C3H/Crgl mice, *J. Natl. Cancer Inst.,* 28, 1233, 1962.
248. Trentin, J. J., Effect of long-term treatment with high levels of progesterone on the incidence of mammary tumors in mice, *Proc. Am. Assoc. Cancer Res.,* 1, 50, 1954.
249. Drill, V. A., Experimental and clinical studes on relationship of estrogens and oral contraceptives to breast cancer, in *Experimental Model Systems in Toxicology and Their Significance in Man,* Vol. 15, Proc. Eur. Soc. Study Drug Toxicity, Excerpta Medica, Amsterdam, 1974, 200.
250. Rudali, G., Coezy, E., and Chemama, R., Mammary carcinogenesis in female and male mice receiving contraceptives or gestagens, *J. Natl. Cancer Inst.,* 49, 813, 1972.
251. Rudali, G., Induction of tumors in mice with synthetic sex hormones, *Gann Monogr.,* 17, 243, 1975.
252. Bern, H. A., Jones, L. A., Mori, T., and Young, P. N., Exposure of neonatal mice to steroids: long-term effects on the mammary gland and other reproductive structures, *J. Steroid Biochem.,* 6, 673, 1975.
253. Jones, L. A. and Bern, H. A., Long-term effects of neonatal treatment with progesterone, alone and in combination with estrogen, on the mammary gland and reproductive tract of female BALB/cfC3H mice, *Cancer Res.,* 37, 67, 1977.
254. Dao, T. L. and Sunderland, J., Mammary carcinogenesis by 3-methylcholanthrene. I. Hormonal aspects in tumor induction and growth, *J. Natl. Cancer Inst.,* 23, 567, 1959.
255. Dao, T. L., Bock, F. G., and Greiner, M. J., Mammary carcinogenesis by 3-methylcholanthrene. II. Inhibitory effect of pregnancy and lactation on tumor induction, *J. Natl. Cancer Inst.,* 25, 991, 1960.
256. McCormick, G. M. and Moon, R. C., Effect of pregnancy and lactation on growth of mammary tumours induced by 7,12-dimethylbenz[a]anthracene (DMBA), *Br. J. Cancer,* 19, 160, 1965.
257. McCormick, G. M. and Moon, R. C., Hormones influencing post-partum growth of 7,12-dimethylbenzanthracene-induced rat mammary tumors, *Cancer Res.,* 27, 626, 1967.
258. Heiman, J., Comparative effects of estrogen, testoterone, and progesterone on benign mammary tumors in the rat, *Cancer Res.,* 3, 65, 1943.
259. McCormick, G. M. and Moon, R. C., Effect of increasing doses of estrogen and progesterone on mammary carcinogenesis in the rat, *Eur. J. Cancer,* 9, 483, 1973.
260. Gruenstein, M., Shay, H., and Shimkin, M. B., Lack of effect of norethynodrel (Enovid®) on methylcholanthrene-induced mammary carcinogenesis in female rats, *Cancer Res.,* 24, 1656, 1964.
261. Weisburger, J. H., Weisburger, E. K., Griswold, D. P., Jr., and Casey, A. E., Reduction of carcinogen-induced breast cancer in rats by an antifertility drug, *Life Sci.,* 7, 259, 1968.
262. McSweeney, E. D., Jr., and Fletcher W. S., Synthetic estrogen-progestin combinations: effect on hormone-sensitive breast cancer in the rat, *Arch. Surg., (Chicago),* 99, 652, 1969.
263. Briziarelli, G., Effects of hormonal pre-treatment against the induction of mammary tumors by 7,12-dimethylbenz[a]anthracene in rats, *Z. Krebsforsch.,* 68, 217, 1966.
264. Jabara, A. G., Effects of progesterone on 9,10-dimethyl-1,2-benzanthracene-induced mammary tumours in Sprague-Dawley rats, *Br. J. Cancer,* 21, 418, 1967.
265. Jull, J. W., The effect of infection, hormonal environment and genetic constitution on mammary tumor induction in rats by 7,12-dimethylbenz[a]anthracene, *Cancer Res.,* 26, 2368, 1966.
266. Shellabarger, C. J. and Soo, V. A., Effects of neonatally administered sex steroids on 7,12-dimethylbenz[a]anthracene-induced mammary neoplasia in rats, *Cancer Res.,* 33, 1567, 1973.

267. Welsch, C. W., Clemens, J. A., and Meites, J., Effects of multiple pituitary homografts or progesterone on 7,12-dimethylbenz[a]anthracene-induced mammary tumors in rats, *J. Natl. Cancer Inst.*, 41, 465, 1968.

268. Jabara, A. G., Toyne, P. H., and Harcourt, A. G., Effects of time and duration of progesterone administration on mammary tumours induced by 7,12-dimethylbenz[a]anthracene in Sprague-Dawley rats, *Br. J. Cancer*, 27, 63, 1973.

269. McCarthy, J. D., Influence of two contraceptives on induction of mammary cancer in rats, *Am. J. Surg.*, 110, 720, 1965.

270. Huggins, C., Briziarelli, G., and Sutton, H., Jr., Rapid induction of mammary carcinoma in the rat and the influence of hormones on the tumors, *J. Exp. Med.*, 109, 25, 1959.

271. Cantarow, A., Stasney, J., and Paschkis, K. E., The influence of sex hormones on mammary tumors induced by 2-acetaminofluorene, *Cancer Res.*, 8, 412, 1948.

272. Paschkis, K. E., Discussion: Molecular structure of steroids and phenanthracene derivatives related to growth of transplanted tumors, *Recent Prog. Horm. Res.*, 14, 89, 1958.

273. Cutts, J. H., Estrone-induced mammary tumors in the rat. II. Effect of alterations in the hormonal environment on tumor induction, behavior and growth, *Cancer Res.*, 24, 1124, 1964.

274. Segaloff, A., Inhibition by progesterone of radiation-estrogen induced mammary cancer in the rat, *Cancer Res.*, 33, 1136, 1973.

275. Brodey, R. S. and Fidler, I. J., Clinical and pathologic findings in bitches treated with progestational compounds, *J. Am. Vet. Med. Assoc.*, 149, 1406, 1966.

276. Glenn, E. M., Richardson, S. L., Bowman, B. J., and Lyster, S. C., Steroids and experimental mammary cancer, in *Biological Activities of Steroids in Relation to Cancer*, Pincus, G. and Vollmer, E. P., Eds., Academic Press, New York, 1960, 257.

277. Hisamatsu, T., Mammary tumorigenesis by subcutaneous administration of the mixture of megestrol acetate and ethinylestradiol in Wistar rats, *Gann*, 63, 483, 1972.

278. Anderson, A. C., Parameters of mammary gland tumors in aging beagles, *J. Am. Vet. Med. Assoc.*, 147, 1653, 1965.

279. Cameron, A. M. and Faulkin, L. J., Jr., Hyperplastic and inflammatory nodules in the canine mammary gland, *J. Natl. Cancer Inst.*, 47, 1277, 1971.

280. Warner, M. R., Age incidence and site distribution of mammary dysplasias in young beagle bitches, *J. Natl. Cancer Inst.*, 57, 57, 1976.

281. Vallance, D. K. and Capel-Edwards, K., Chlormadione and mammary nodules, *Br. Med. J.*, 2, 221, 1971.

282. Coleman, M. E., Murchison, T. E., and Frank, D., Mammary nodules in dogs receiving depo-provera and progesterone. An interim progress report, *Toxicol Appl. Pharmacol.*, 37, 181, 1976.

283. Nelson, L. W., Carlton, W. W., and Weikel, J. H., Jr., Canine mammary neoplasms and progestogens, *JAMA*, 219, 1601, 1972.

284. Nelson, L. W., Weikel, J. H., Jr., and Reno, F. E., Mammary nodules in dogs during four years treatment with megestrol acetate or chlormadinone acetate, *J. Natl. Cancer Inst.*, 51, 1303, 1973.

285. Wazeter, F. X., Geil, R. G., Cookson, K. M., Berliner, V. R., and Lamar, J. K., Five-year progress report on long-term oral contraceptive studies in female dogs and monkeys, *Toxicol. Appl. Pharmacol.*, 29, 98, 1974.

286. Wazeter, F. X., Geil, R. G., Cookson, K. M., Berliner, V. R., Lamar, J. K., Seven-year progress report on long-term oral contraceptive studies in female dogs and monkeys, *Toxicol. Appl. Pharmacol.*, 37, 178, 1976.

287. Finkel, M. J. and Berliner, V. R., The extrapolation of experimental findings (animals to man): the dilemma of the systemically administered contraceptives, *Bull. Soc. Pharmacol. Environ. Pathol.*, 4, 13, 1973.

288. Daniel, G. R., Chlormadinone contraceptive withdrawn, *Br. Med. J.*, 1, 303, 1970.

289. Goldzieher, J. W., Joshi, S., and Kraemer, D. C., Non-human primates in contraceptive research, *Acta Endocrinol. (Copenhagen)*, 75, 90, 1974.

290. Owen, L. N. and Briggs, M. H., Contraceptive steroid toxicology in the beagle dog and its relevance to human carcinogenicity, *Curr. Med. Res. Opinion*, 4, 309, 1976.

291. Drill, V. A., Martin, D. P., Hart, E. R., and McConnell, R. G., Effect of oral contraceptives on the mammary glands of Rhesus monkeys: a preliminary report, *J. Natl. Cancer Inst.*, 52, 1655, 1974.

292. Nelson, L. W., and Shott, L. D., Mammary nodular hyperplasia in intact Rhesus monkeys, *Vet. Pathol.*, 10, 130, 1973.

293. Kirschstein, R. L., Rabson, A. S. and Rusten, G. W., Infiltrating duct carcinoma of the mammary gland of a Rhesus monkey after administration of an oral contraceptive: a preliminary report, *J. Natl. Cancer Inst.*, 48, 551, 1972.

294. Li, A. S., Li, J. J., and Villee, C. A., Significance of the progesterone receptor in the estrogen-induced and dependent renal tumor of the Syrian Golden Hamster, *Ann. N.Y. Acad. Sci.*, 286, 369, 1977.

295. Kirkman, H., Estrogen-induced tumors of the kidney in the Syrian hamster, *Natl. Cancer Inst. Monogr.*, 1, 1, 1959.
296. Bloom, H. J. G., Dukes, C. E., and Mitchley, B. C. V., Hormone-dependent tumours on the kidney. I. The estrogen-induced renal tumor of the Syrian hamster-hormone treatment and possible relationship to carcinoma of the kidney in man, *Br. J. Cancer*, 17, 611, 1963.
297. Andervont, H. B., Shimkin, M. B., and Canter, H. Y., Some factors involved in the induction or growth of testicular tumors in BALB/c mice, *J. Natl. Cancer Inst.*, 25, 1083, 1960.
298. Gardner, W. U., Pfeiffer, C. A., and Trentin, J. J., Hormonal factors in experimental carcinogenesis, in *The Physiopathology of Cancer*, 2nd ed., Homburger, F., Ed., Hoeber and Harper, New York, 1959, 152.
299. Munroe, J. S., Progesteroids as immunosuppressive agents, *J. Reticuloendothel. Soc.*, 9, 361, 1971.
300. Rudali, G., Jullien, P., and Juliard, L., Action des hormones sur la leucemogenese des souris, *Rev. Fr. Etud. Clin. Biol.*, 4, 607, 1959.

Chapter 4

GLUCOCORTICOIDS

J. Stevens, Y. W. Stevens, and V. P. Hollander

TABLE OF CONTENTS

This review is concerned with the mechanism of glucocorticoid-mediated lympho-cytolysis in experimental tumor systems and in acute (ALL) and chronic lymphatic leukemia (CLL) in man. Among the animal models, the use of mouse lymphoma P1798 has been emphasized because of the authors' experience with the corticoid-sensitive (P1798/S) and corticoid-resistant (P1798/R) strains of this tumor for studying gluco-corticoid action on malignant lymphocytes. ALL will be discussed since glucocorti-coids are included in practically every successful combined therapy protocol currently used for treatment of this disease. CLL has been selected because this disorder fre-quently responds to corticoid therapy, which (as will be pointed out later) may be the treatment of choice, but only under specific circumstances.

I. EXPERIMENTAL TUMOR SYSTEMS

A. Historical

The adrenal cortex plays a major role in controlling the growth and development of normal and malignant lymphoid tissue. The first reference linking adrenal function to a specific lymphoid organ appears to be the report by Star in 1895 describing thymic enlargement in a case of Addison's disease.[1] Addison himself had noted the presence of hyperplastic lymphoid tissue in cases of adrenal insufficiency nearly 50 years earlier. Starting from the mid-1920s, the relationship between lymphatic organs and adreno-cortical hormones became the subject of intense investigation.

The discovery of dramatic effects of ACTH and adrenal extracts on normal lymph-oid cells soon prompted comparable studies on lymphoid tumors. Heilman and Ken-dall[2] demonstrated that cortisone administration caused regression of a solid trans-plantable mouse lymphosarcoma. Rats with transplantable leukemia and mice with spontaneous lymphoid leukemia showed regression of disease when treated with adre-nal extracts or ACTH.[3,4] Cortisone administration can also prevent the development of spontaneous lymphatic leukemia. Adrenalectomy increases both spontaneous and radiation-induced tumorigenesis.[5] Kaplan et al.[6] also showed that cortisone inhibited and adrenalectomy enhanced the susceptibility of C57Bl mice to the development of lymphoid tumors after total body irradiation. In a later study, Kaplan and Nagareda[7] showed that treatment of C57Bl mice with massive doses of hydrocortisone 50 or 100 days after induction of thymic lymphosarcoma with X-radiation resulted in permanent cure of half or more of the animals.

In the past 20 years, several corticoid-sensitive leukemias, such as L5178Y, P1798, ML388, S49, and YALL, have become available. The transplantable murine lymphob-lastic neoplasm L5178Y is best maintained as either a solid or an ascites tumor in mice of homozygous DBA/2 genotype but also grows well in hybrid strains such as AKDF and BDF. This neoplasm descended from a single cell cloned from a culture of the original lymphoid tumor.[8,9]

The L5178Y cells grow in culture with a generation time of 8 to 14 hr, which is approximately the rate of division when they are present in the mouse as an ascitic tumor.[10] After many years in culture, the response of these cells to glucocorticoid appears to have been greatly affected. Thus, Story and Melnykovych[11] found that 100 times more prednisolone and triamcinolone and 1000 times more cortisol were required to inhibit cell growth than previously reported by Jaffe et al.[10] In contrast, Kondo et al.[12] reported glucocorticoid sensitivity comparable to that originally described by Jaffe et al.[10] Interestingly, in some cultures of L5178Y cells, glucocorticoids cause only inhibition of growth but not cytolysis,[11] whereas other variants of this lymphoma undergo lymphocytolysis when exposed to corticosteroids.[12]

The origin of mouse lymphoma P1798 has been described in detail by McCain-Lampkin and Potter.[13] The tumor arose in the thymus of a male BALB/c mouse which had been implanted s.c. with a 20% diethylstilbestrol-cholesterol (DES) pellet. It was found to be exquisitely sensitive to the growth inhibitory effects of cortisone and could be carried serially in the ascites form, or as a s.c. neoplasm either in BALB/c or in (BALB/c × DBA/a)F$_1$ hybrid mice. A glucocorticoid-resistant subline was developed by means of intermittent treatment of an established subcutaneous sensitive tumor with cortisone.

In the authors' Institute, P1798 is maintained by s.c. transplantation. Animals bearing P1798/R are injected with 25 mg/kg 9α-fluoroprednisolone 48 hr and 24 hr prior to being used as donors for the next transplant generation. This procedure has resulted in a strain of P1798/R which is completely refractory to steroid treatment both in vivo[14] and in vitro,[15] and is therefore unlikely to consist of a mixed population of S and R cells as appears to be the case for another strain of P1798/R.[16] Studies from the authors' laboratory demonstrating the utility of P1798 for studying corticosteroid-mediated lymphocytolysis will be discussed later in this chapter.

Gabourel and Aronow[17] reported that cortisol inhibited the growth of mouse lymphoma ML388 in culture. It was noted that the structure-activity relationships demonstrated by steroids inhibiting the growth of ML388 were very similar to the spectrum of activity of antiinflammatory steroids and to their ability to cause thymic involution. Obvious exceptions were the inactivity of cortisone, prednisone and 11-dihydrocorticosterone in vitro.

The murine lymphoma line S49 was first transplanted from a 16-month-old female BALB/c mouse injected with T$_2$, T$_5$, and C bacteriophages at 3 and 4 months and with mineral oil at 4, 6, and 8 months of age. Subcutaneous transplantation yielded tumor growth at the site of injection, with enlargement of regional lymph nodes and the spleen of the host. Continuous cultures were initiated from a tumor in the seventh transplant generation.[18] A single clone isolated from the original cultures and designated S49.1 showed structure-activity relationships for growth inhibition by corticosteroids very similar to those described for the L5178Y and ML388 lines. An exception was aldosterone, which was twice as effective as cortisol in the S49.1 system, but only one twentieth as potent as cortisol against ML388.[19]

Recently, Yancey and Bleyer[20] described a transplantable murine leukemia (YALL) morphologically and pathologically similar to human acute lymphocytic leukemia, which arose spontaneously in a BALB/c × DBA/2F$_1$ male mouse. Administration of prednisolone or prednisolone plus vincristine resulted in an 11 to 36% increase in survival time. Apparently, this tumor has not been tested for sensitivity to corticosteroids in vitro. Finally, Huggins and Uematsu[21] described the development of lymphatic leukemia in adult female mice of the non-inbred CF-1 strain after feeding DMBA. The leukemia could be transmitted by s.c. injection of allogeneic newborn mice with blood from leukemic animals. Lymphosarcoma occurred at the site of injection. These lymphosarcomas regressed rapidly after the administration of cortisone or dexamethasone but frequently recurred.

B. The Effect of Glucocorticoid Structure on Inhibition of Lymphoid Growth in Experimental Animals

Dougherty et al.[22] found that conversion of cortisol to cortisone by oxidation of the 11 position resulted in loss of lympholytic activity. Furthermore, these authors showed that cortisone did not affect lymphocytes which lacked the ability to reduce cortisone to cortisol. Other essential structural features of the active glucocorticoids were the presence of an unsaturated A ring, a ketone at C-3 and the characteristic ketol side chain at C-17.

An excellent study correlating inhibition of growth of L5178Y leukemic cells in vitro and structure was done by Jaffe and colleagues.[10] Structural modification of the basic corticosteroid molecule affected the therapeutic efficacy of the drugs. Enhanced growth-inhibitory activity both in culture and in vivo was effected by α- or β-methylation at C-16, formation of a 16α, 17α-O-isopropylidene derivative or α-halogenation at C-6 or C-9. Introduction of a Δ' double bond or α-methylation at C-6 did not enhance the anti-leukemic potency of the basic cortisol molecule. However, combination of various substitutions leading to substances such as dexamethasone and triamcinolone acetonide gave rise to the most potent antileukemic substances. This paper is worth revisiting in terms of recent encouraging events in the treatment of acute leukemia. The authors were unable to increase longevity of leukemic mice, because as they raised the dose or potency of the steroid, toxicity also increased.

C. Morphological Changes Caused by Corticosteroids

Jaffe studied the regeneration of the thymus in rats after adrenalectomy.[23] When it was learned that ACTH could produce thymic involution,[24] Dougherty and White began a series of histological studies of the effects of adrenal hormones on lymphoid tissue in general.[25] Within 1 hr after administration of ACTH or adrenal extracts, lymphoid tissues were edematous. Many damaged lymphocytes could be seen leaving the cortex of the thymus for the medulla. Cellular damage consisted of pyknosis or alteration in normal chromatin structure. Pyknotic nuclei were ingested by macrophages. Lymph nodes of mice and rabbits responded like the thymus. Thymic involution produced by administration of hydrocortisone to mice has also been studied by ultramicroscopy.[26] The cytoplasmic budding described by Frank and Dougherty[27] was not observed. The ultramicroscopic study was particularly helpful in establishing that the nuclear changes caused by cortisol treatment preceded cytoplasmic alteration.

Such clear morphological changes after cortisol administration suggested that the lympholytic process could be investigated in vitro. However, the high concentration of steroid used in some of the early studies[28-30] make it difficult to evaluate the specificity of lysis. Burton et al.[31] found that suspensions of mouse and rat thymus cells could be maintained in good condition for 24 hr at 38° under 95% air-5% CO_2 with little cytologic change, either in Fisher's medium or medium 199 if supplemented with 10% equine or fetal bovine serum or purified serum proteins. Addition of corticosteroids produced cytolytic effects which were highly specific for compounds with an 11β-hydroxyl group.

Maximum effects were seen with 0.27 μM cortisol or 0.02 μM dexamethasone. As early as 2 hr after addition of steroid, electron microscopy showed nuclear edema and disappearance of normal chromatin pattern. The changes progressed until, by 8 hr, there was disruption of nuclear and cell membranes. No changes were seen with steroids devoid of glucocorticoid activity. In order to demonstrate lympholytic responses, the cells had to be metabolically active; cells maintained at 30° remained in good morphologic condition but steroid-mediated changes were much less pronounced than at 38°. Exposure of thymus cells to steroid for even 1 hr, followed by removal of the hormone and continued incubation in fresh, cortisol-free medium for a total of 8 hr allowed extensive nuclear changes to occur. Sensitive and resistant P1798 tumor lymphocytes were then incubated for 4 hr in the presence and absence of cortisol. Cortisol produced the expected nuclear changes in the sensitive cells but not in the resistant ones. However, it was noted that P1798 cells could not be incubated for more than 5 hr in control media without loss of morphologic integrity. Stevens and Stevens[15] recently described incubation conditions which allow the lympholytic effects of cortisol on P1798 lymphocytes to be studied in vitro, using trypan blue exclusion to measure loss of cell membrane integrity. This procedure has the advantage of being fast, inexpensive, easy to perform, and able to monitor large numbers of samples. As will be discussed later, lymphocytolysis was detected within 3 hr of exposure of P1798/S cells to cortisol.

D. Mechanism of Corticoid-induced Regression

1. Cell Cycle Dependence

In order to combine glucocorticoids with other chemotherapeutic agents for the treatment of lymphoid tumors, it is important to know whether the adrenal steroids act in a cell cycle-specific manner. Harris[19] reasoned that if the lethal action of steroids were cycle stage-specific, this should be reflected in fluctuations in the frequency of mitosis amongst surviving cells in a culture undergoing treatment. No significant frequency variations were found in the time intervals studied. Similar results were obtained by Story and Melnykovych,[11] who studied an L5178Y mouse lymphoma culture which was sensitive to pharmacologic concentrations of prednisolone (8 μM was required for 50% inhibition of growth). They concluded that the depression in growth rate was due to an increase in generation time and not in cytolytic effects of the steroid. When synchronous cell populations obtained by successive treatment with thymidine and Colcemid® were used, it became apparent that prednisolone had to be in contact with cells for longer than a complete cell cycle if cell multiplication was to be inhibited. However, no particular phase of the cycle was shown to be more sensitive than any other.

2. Requirement for P_i and Respiration for Loss of Nuclear Structure

Whitfield et al.[32] have been interested in the effects of radiation on loss of nuclear structure of lymphoid tissue. In previous work, they showed that pyknosis was caused indirectly by a respiration-linked and phosphate dependent reaction occurring during the first hour after radiation.[33-36]

A product of this reaction was found to sever the union between DNA and histones within nuclear protein granules. These authors were struck by similarities between the sensitivity of lymphoid tissue to radiation and adrenal hormone. During the first hour of continuous exposure to 0.27 μM cortisol, no pyknotic nuclei occurred in thymocytes suspended in medium containing inorganic phosphate. However, after 1 hr, the rate of pyknosis was a function of inorganic phosphate. Inorganic phosphate and cortisol exerted synergistic effects in the production of pyknosis; phosphate had no effect in the absence of cortisol. A linear relationship was found between the concentration of inorganic phosphate in the medium and the development of pyknosis in the presence of 0.27 μM cortisol. No effect of inorganic phosphate could be demonstrated if incubations were carried out anaerobically. Addition of 2,4-dinitrophenol also prevented the inorganic phosphate-respiration-linked increase in cortisol-induced pyknosis. Pyknosis apparently results when the large chromatin granules in normal lymphoid nuclei are disaggregated. These granules are formed by the combination of lysine-rich histones with DNA. Phosphate is transformed into an extremely powerful chromatin-dispersing agent when it combines with the hydroxyl groups of serine molecules in certain serine-rich nuclear proteins.[37-40] The authors suggested that cortisol might act by causing the formation of abnormal quantities of such a phosphate-rich, chromatin-dissociating phosphoprotein. Further studies in this area are clearly warranted.

3. Free Fatty Acids and Changes in Lipid Metabolism

Studies by Burton et al.[31] showed that free fatty acids with various chain lengths were quite toxic to rat thymocytes in vitro. Linoleic and azelaic acids produced 50% pyknosis at 3 μM. In subsequent work, Turnell et al.[41] and Turnell and Burton[42] found that incubation of P1798/S cells for 4 hr in Fischer's medium with 10% horse serum at 38° in the presence of 78 μM palmitate or 53 μM azelaic acid caused a significant increase in dead cells as determined by eosin exclusion. In contrast, P1798/R was only partially affected by concentrations of free fatty acid 10 times greater than those required to kill all S cells in 5.5 hr. This effect was temperature dependent.[43] Electron microscopy revealed that certain effects caused by free fatty acids in P1798/S cells, such as nuclear edema, focal dissolution, disintegration of the nuclear membrane, and ultimately karyolysis, were strikingly similar to those induced by corticosteroids. However, the biochemical changes caused by free fatty acids in P1798/S cells and thymocytes differed considerably from those observed after steroid treatment. Results of metabolic studies using radioactive palmitate suggested that P1798/R cells had a greater capacity for oxidizing free fatty acids. It was also found that thymocytes and P1798/S cells had a higher lipid content than P1798/R lymphocytes. Furthermore, in vivo treatment of mice with dexamethasone caused a 76% increase in free fatty acid content of thymus and a 14% increase in P1798/S, compared to a 22% decrease in P1798/R solid tumor. Inhibitors of fatty acid oxidation, either alone or in the presence of exogenous free fatty acid, caused resistant cells to undergo lysis. Based on these observations, Turnell et al. proposed that glucocorticoid-induced lymphocytolysis might result from accumulation of free fatty acids which damage primarily the nucleus. Resistance was attributed to the greater capacity for free fatty acid oxidation by corticoid-resistant cells.

Story and Melnykovych[11] investigated the influence of prednisolone on the uptake and incorporation of choline into logarithmically growing L5178Y lymphoblasts. They found that corticoid-sensitive cells showed 25% and 16% inhibition of total uptake of ^{14}C-choline 13 hr and 18.5 hr after addition of hormone, respectively. Similar inhibition of choline incorporation into the total lipid fraction of synchronized corticoid-sensitive lymphoblasts was detected 1.5 hr after exposure of these cultures to 10 μg/ml prednisolone. Story et al.[44] in a related study, reported a dose-dependent inhibition of ^{14}C-choline incorporation into purified plasma membranes of L5178Y lymphoblasts after only 6 min incubation of the cells with prednisolone. In order to demonstrate this very rapid effect, the cultures had to be starved of choline for 8 to 16 hr. This effect, together with the inhibition of ^{14}C-palmitate oxidation to $^{14}CO_2$ observed 30 min after exposure of P1798/S lymphocytes to cortisol,[41] are the fastest glucocorticoid-induced metabolic changes described so far in malignant lymphocytes.

4. The "Glucose" Hypothesis and Role of Biochemical Alterations Caused by Steroid Treatment

Based on extensive and detailed work with rat thymocytes, Hallahan et al.,[45] Mosher et al.,[46] and Munck[47] proposed the attractive hypothesis that reduced uptake of glucose occurring within 15 to 30 min of exposure of thymocytes to cortisol resulted in a fall in intracellular ATP which, in turn, caused lower rates of energy-dependent processes such as DNA, RNA, and protein synthesis and ultimately cell lysis.

The finding that incubation of P1798/S lymphocytes with cortisol also resulted in pronounced suppression of 2-deoxy-D-glucose uptake prior to steroid inhibition of precursor incorporation into RNA, DNA, and protein prompted Rosen et al.[48,49] to suggest that decreased glucose transport may likewise be involved in glucocorticoid-induced dissolution of tumor lymphocytes. However, the inhibitory effect of cortisol on incorporation of ^{3}H-uridine into RNA and of ^{14}C-leucine into protein was only partially diminished but was by no means abolished when the cells were incubated with steroid in glucose-free medium. This result, together with earlier work of Gabourel and Aronow[17] showing that cortisol caused a significant reduction in protein, ninhydrin-positive acid-soluble material, and deoxyribose content of ML388 lymphoma cells without affecting glucose utilization or lactate production prompted Stevens et al.[14] to reexamine the role of reduced glucose transport in the catabolic action of glucocorticoids on tumor lymphocytes.

They found that exposure of P1798/S lymphocytes to cortisol in vivo or in vitro, resulted in a pronounced decrease of uridine uptake and incorporation in vitro, while 2-deoxy-D-glucose-^{14}C entry into the cells was not affected.

These studies provided direct evidence that cortisol suppression of uridine uptake and incorporation by P1798/S lymphocytes could not be attributed to prior effects on glucose transport, since equally pronounced inhibition was observed whether or not the cells were supplied with an external source of glucose. Indeed, the inhibitory action of cortisol was more marked in medium supplemented with amino acids but lacking glucose than in glucose- and/or pyruvate-containing medium without amino acids. Furthermore, neither exogenous glucose nor pyruvate were necessary for maintaining maximal rates of uridine utilization by P1798 lymphocytes. A possible explanation for the discrepancy between this result and the report by Rosen et al.[49] that glucose deprivation caused marked suppression of uridine incorporation by P1798 cells is that the same tumor, grown for many years in two different laboratories, may have diverged in some of its biological properties. The different tissue culture medium used by Stevens et al. (Dulbecco's modified Eagle's medium as opposed to Roswell Park Memorial Institute (RPMI) Medium 1640 used by Rosen et al.) may also be a contributing factor.

A logical extension of this work was to determine whether glucocorticoid-induced lymphocytolysis itself was dependent upon inhibition of glucose uptake. This does not appear to be the case since, as shown by Stevens and Stevens[15] incubation of P1798/S lymphocytes for 3 to 4 hr with 1 μM cortisol resulted in an identical degree of cell lysis (as measured with trypan blue exclusion test) whether the cells had been exposed to the hormone in complete medium or in medium lacking glucose and pyruvate. The specificity of this effect was demonstrated in two ways. Epicortisol, the biologically inactive 11α epimer of cortisol, was totally ineffective. Also, there was complete absence of any lympholytic effect of cortisol on cell suspensions derived from the corticoid-resistant tumor. The reliability of the dye exclusion assay for detecting loss of cell membrane integrity of P1798 lymphocytes was established in experiments which demonstrated that trypan blue readily penetrated into physically damaged tumor cells. Thus, less than 1% of P1798 lymphocytes incubated at 56° for 15 min and only 8% of cells subjected to rapid freeze-thaw were still able to exclude the dye. No difference in behavior was noted between S and R cells with either of these procedures.[120]

Kondo et al.[12] found that glucocorticoid-resistant L5178Y lymphoblasts displayed substantial inhibition of uridine incorporation when exposed to 0.2 or 2 μM dexamethasone, in spite of which the steroid-treated cells continued to divide as fast as, or even faster than, the controls. Further evidence that some of the biochemical actions of the glucocorticoids may be unrelated to their capacity for causing cell damage has been provided by Giddings and Young.[50] In addition to their inhibitory effect on glucose transport, corticosteroids inhibit the entry of a variety of other small molecules into both normal and malignant lymphocytes. Among the substances which have been studied are ribonucleosides, deoxyribonucleosides, amino acids, K$^+$ and Rb$^+$. These effects have recently been reviewed elsewhere[51] and will not be discussed here. Suffice it to say that their relationship to the lympholytic process remains unclear, as mentioned above.

5. Membrane and Cell Coat Changes

The sensitive and resistant strains of lymphoma P1798 are similar by light micros-copy but differ in ultrastructure, cell surface chemistry, and biological behavior. When glutaraldehyde-fixed cells from lymphoma P1798/S and P1798/R were stained with Alcian blue, a prominent cell coat could be demonstrated on the surface of P1798/S cells which was lacking in P1798/R cells.[52] The existence of cell surface differences between sensitive and resistant cells was confirmed by chromatographic study of plasma membrane glycopeptides.[53] Between 6 and 8 hr after steroid treatment of mice bearing P1798/S, the sensitive cells lost the Alcian blue-staining coat. The relationship of this change to tumor involution remains to be established. A further difference in cell surface characteristics was reported by Roldan et al.,[121] who found that corticoid-sensitive P1798 lymphocytes had a significantly higher number of insulin binding sites than cells from the resistant tumor. There was no difference in the apparent affinity of insulin binding between P1798/S and P1798/R cells.

6. Nuclear Fragility and Changes in Chromatin Structure

Giddings and Young[50] found that nuclei from glucocorticoid-treated thymocytes showed increased nuclear fragility (i.e., reduced ability to survive hypotonic shock) within 0.5 to 1 hr after exposure of the cells to steroid. The effect did not require exogenous carbohydrate and appeared to involve cycloheximide-sensitive steps. In sim-ilar studies with lymphoma P1798, Nicholson and Young[54] demonstrated an analogous corticosteroid-induced increase in nuclear fragility of P1798/S lymphocytes which had been incubated with cortisol or dexamethasone for 2 hr. Interestingly, nuclei from P1798/R cells also showed increased fragility, except that 6-hr treatment was required.

Using a cytochemical approach (nuclear microfluorometry of acridine orange- or Feulgen-stained cell preparations), Alvarez and Truitt[55] concluded that there was an increase in thermal stability of rat thymus chromatin 15 to 30 min after administration of doses as low as 2.5 μg dexamethasone per kilogram of body weight to adrenalectom-ized rats.

7. Apparent Requirement for RNA and Protein Synthesis

As already mentioned, glucocorticoid treatment of normal or malignant lympho-cytes results in a variety of catabolic changes in nucleic acid, protein, carbohydrate, and lipid metabolism and ultimately in cell lysis. These alterations appear only after a lag period whose duration varies according to cell type and the effect being studied. Work from several laboratories[45,46,56,57] suggests that the following events take place during the lag period in normal rat thymocytes:

1. Formation of cytoplasmic hormone-receptor complexes and their translocation to nuclear acceptor sites
2. Transcription of new classes of RNA, including mRNA
3. Synthesis of specific proteins necessary for phenotypic expression of the hormone effect.

Rosen et al.[49] reported that simultaneous incubation of P1798/S tumor lymphocytes with cortisol and actinomycin D or cycloheximide prevented the suppressive effect of the hormone on 2-deoxyglucose uptake, and Baran et al.[58] showed that cycloheximide prevented cortisol inhibition of α-aminoisobutyric acid transport by human chronic leukemic lymphocytes when added to the cells together with the steroid. Stevens and Stevens[59] examined the influence of the above-mentioned antibiotics on the time course of cortisol action on P1798/S lymphocytes. Inhibition of uridine uptake and incorpo-ration was used to evaluate the effectiveness of hormone treatment. When tumor cells were incubated with 1 μM cortisol for 15 min and then washed free of steroid and reincubated in the absence of hormone, the expected decrease of uridine uptake failed to appear 1.5 hr later. In contrast, removal of cortisol after 30 or 60 min did not prevent subsequent development of the steroid effect. Addition of actinomycin D together with cortisol, or 15 min after hormone treatment was started, blocked steroid action. However, when actinomycin D was added 30 or 60 min after the initial exposure to cortisol, hormone-induced depression of uridine uptake was no longer prevented. To study the role of protein synthesis, cycloheximide was added to the tumor cell suspensions at various times after cortisol treatment was started. Cortisol suppression of uridine utilization was blocked when cycloheximide was added with the hormone or 30 min after the start of hormone treatment. Cycloheximide added together with cortisol and washed out with the steroid after 30 min did not prevent subsequent appearance of decreased nucleoside uptake. Hydroxyurea, an inhibitor of DNA synthesis, did not prevent cortisol action, even when present throughout a 2-hr exposure to the steroid. Hormone removal or actinomycin D addition after 1.5 to 2 hr (when uridine uptake was already inhibited about 25%) did not prevent intensification of the steroid effect during a subsequent 1.5 to 2 hr incubation period, while addition of cycloheximide at this time completely prevented its progression. Both actinomycin D and cycloheximide inhibited uridine utilization by the tumor cells. However, appropriate control experiments showed that the failure of cortisol to exert its usual inhibitory effect when added to the tumor cells together with the antibiotics was not due to inability of the steroid to further diminish the depressed levels of nucleoside accumulation caused by the antibiotics. These results suggest that:

1. Cortisol inhibition of uridine uptake by P1798 lymphocytes involves an early irreversible step and appears to require continuing RNA but not protein synthesis during the first 15 to 30 min of hormone action.
2. Protein synthesis but not RNA synthesis is required after 30 min.
3. Continuing protein synthesis but not RNA synthesis or hormone presence is necessary for the preestablished cortisol effect to progress.

Stevens and Stevens[60] also examined the influence of inhibitors of RNA and protein synthesis on cortisol-induced lymphocytolysis. Cordycepin, an inhibitor of rRNA synthesis and mRNA processing, completely prevented the steroid-induced decrease of dye-excluding cells when added together with cortisol. However, the antibiotic no longer blocked hormone action when added after 30 min.

As mentioned earlier in this chapter, addition of cycloheximide to P1798 cell suspensions completely prevented the progression of preestablished cortisol inhibition of uridine utilization. In contrast, cycloheximide did not prevent further intensification of the cortisol-induced loss of cell membrane integrity when added after lymphocytolysis had become apparent (2.5 hr after the start of hormone treatment). On the other hand, when cycloheximide was added prior to emergence of the cortisol-induced decrease in the number of dye-excluding cells (i.e., 1.5 hr after cortisol) the hormone effect failed to develop. It is interesting to note that the sensitivity of cortisol action to cycloheximide persisted far beyond the period of sensitivity to cordycepin, strongly suggesting that these two antibiotics influence hormone action via different mechanisms. Hydroxyurea, an inhibitor of DNA synthesis, had no effect on the cortisol-induced loss of cell membrane integrity.

To the best of the authors' knowledge, these results are the first demonstration that glucocorticoid-induced lymphocytolysis is mediated by specific cordycepin-sensitive, cycloheximide-sensitive steps. While the data suggest that a search for the key intermediary species of RNA and protein may be a fruitful area for future investigation, the authors caution, as have others,[51] against overinterpreting results obtained with the use of antibiotics which inhibit RNA and protein synthesis. While the data are consistent with a model involving sequential transcriptional and posttranscriptional events in the mechanism of action of glucocorticoids on tumor lymphocytes, this conclusion must be considered purely speculative until direct evidence for such steps has been obtained.

8. The Calcium Hypothesis

Kaiser and Edelman[61] found that A23187, a divalent cation ionophore, mimicked two of the characteristic actions of glucocorticoids on thymocytes: inhibition of uridine utilization and cytolysis. Removal of Ca^{2+} from the medium substantially diminished the lympholytic action of triamcinolone acetonide (as measured by the trypan blue exclusion test) and practically abolished that of A23187. Time course studies showed that triamcinolone acetonide and the ionophore caused a proportionate increase in ^{45}Ca uptake and in cell dissolution. These results suggest participation of enhanced Ca^{2+} uptake in the lympholytic process. However, as the authors point out, steroid-induced lysis was not abolished even in the virtual absence of Ca^{2+}. Furthermore, the possibility that increased ^{45}Ca uptake was simply a consequence and not a cause of the steroid-induced increase in membrane permeability could not be ruled out.

E. Degradative Enzymes

An important, yet still unanswered, question concerning glucocorticoid-induced regression of lymphoid tumors is whether the striking decrease in tumor mass results from the inhibition of synthetic processes without a concomitant reduction in the rate of normal intracellular breakdown reactions, or whether steroid treatment causes an actual increase in degradative processes (RNAse, DNAse, proteases).

1. RNase

When glucocorticoids were administered to animals bearing P1798/S, tumor cytosol acid ribonuclease was increased 18 hr after treatment. No such increase occurred in P1798/R when hosts were treated in a similar manner.[62] Incubation of P1798/S cells with glucocorticoid also increased the activity of this enzyme. However, treatment with other chemotherapeutic agents which cause regression of P1798 also resulted in an increase in acid ribonuclease. Therefore, the enzymic change appeared to be a consequence of cell damage, rather than a specific hormonal effect.[63]

2. DNase

Wiernik and MacLeod[64] reported that treatment of rats with 9α-fluoroprednisolone for 4 hr produced a 100% increase in the DNAse activity of thymic homogenates. Somewhat smaller increases have been described by Nakagawa and White[65] and by Sands and Haynes.[66]

3. Proteases

Stevens et al.[67] found that 3 hr after injection of 25mg/kg 9α-fluoroprednisolone (9FP) to mice bearing P1798/S, in vivo incorporation of basic amino acids into total tumor protein was decreased by 35%. In contrast, reduced incorporation of neutral amino acids only became apparent after 6 hr. These effects could not be attributed to inhibition of transport. Glucocorticoid treatment did not inhibit utilization of leucine, phenyalanine, and valine by P1798/R tumors, but caused a slight and nonprogressive decrease of arginine and lysine incorporation. Administration of 9FP had no differential effect on the incorporation of ^3H-arginine and ^3H-lysine into cytoplasmic and nuclear protein fractions of the tumor at either 3 or 6 hr. A similar lack of selectivity was observed with the neutral amino acids. Further fractionation of histones showed that the magnitude of steroid inhibition of lysine incorporation into F1 (lysine-rich) histone was no greater than in the remaining histones or whole homogenate protein. There was a sharp rise in the level of basic and most neutral amino acids in the corticoid-sensitive tumor 3 to 6 hr after injection of 9FP. All the amino acids that increased in the tumor were also elevated in host plasma. In marked contrast, steroid administration had no effect on free amino acid levels in the corticoid-resistant tumor, except for tyrosine which was decreased. However, treatment with 9FP did cause an increase in plasma levels of several neutral and basic amino acids in animals bearing P1798/R, perhaps due to systemic effect of the hormone. Whether the increased levels of amino acid in P1798/S were due to steroid-induced breakdown of tumor protein or to inhibition of protein synthesis was not clear. However, the earliest steroid effect on protein synthesis in a P1798 cell-free system was observed only 18 hr after administration of 9FP.[68]

These results suggest that accelerated degradation of tumor protein may be an important step in glucocorticoid-induced lymphocytolysis. Possibly, proteases are responsible for corticoid-induced changes in histones and nuclear acidic proteins. It has been shown that physiological concentrations of cortisol can elicit alterations in the circular dichroism spectrum of calf thymus nuclei. These changes have been interpreted as evidence for a key role of histones in the mechanism of corticoid-induced karyorrhexis.[69] It is tempting to speculate that the early inhibition of basic amino acid incorporation into P1798/S proteins after treatment with 9FP may reflect a steroid-mediated change in histone structure. Wong and Aronow[70] have shown that glucocorticoid treatment of mouse fibroblasts decreased labeled amino acid incorporation into a specific fraction of the lysine-rich histones. In view of the demonstration that histones play an essential role in maintaining the normal structure of chromatin,[71] the steroid-induced changes in acetylation of P1798/S histones mentioned by Libby may have profound structural and functional implications.[72]

F. Changes in Nucleic Acid Synthesis

Inhibition of one or more species of DNA-dependent RNA polymerase has been established as a late effect of glucocorticoid treatment in normal rat thymocytes.[73,74] Meulen et al.[75] found that cortisol may initially stimulate nucleoplasmic RNA polymerase in thymus, while simultaneously depressing the nucleolar enzyme. In a recent study, Bell and Borthwick[76] found that exposure of thymocytes to dexamethasone caused a rapid rise in RNA polymerase B activity within 10 min of steroid addition, followed by inhibition of both RNA polymerase A and B, 60 to 90 min after the start of hormone treatment. Dexamethasone effects on RNA polymerase A were prevented if cycloheximide was added to the cells 15 min prior to the steroid. However, the early stimulation and subsequent suppression of RNA polymerase B activity was not prevented by this inhibitor of protein synthesis. Gomez et al.[77] found that nuclei from mouse lymphoma ML388 cells which had been exposed to the synthetic glucocorticoid fluorocinolone acetonide for 24 hr, showed a 20 to 30% reduction in their ability to incorporate ^{3}H-ATP into RNA. Incorporation of ^{3}H-dATP into DNA was not diminished. Rosen et al.[78] found no change in DNA polymerase activity of high-speed supernatants prepared from lymphoma P1798/S homogenates 2 to 16 hr after injecting the tumor-bearing animals with 75 to 150 mg/kg cortisol.

G. Receptor Studies

1. Cytoplasmic Receptors

The binding of cortisol by subcellular fractions of liver, muscle, and thymus reported by several investigators prompted study of the binding of this hormone to cytosol from lymphosarcoma P1798.[79-83] Hollander and Chiu[84] obtained evidence for specific cortisol binding to a protein substance in P1798 by incubating radioactive cortisol with tumor cytosol and separating free from bound steroid by Sephadex® G-25 chromatography. In this early work, it was shown that the binding substance could be easily separated from corticosteroid binding globulin, and the possibility that specific cortisol binding might have physiological importance was pointed out. A significant advance in working with glucocorticoid receptor in tumor systems was made by Kirkpatrick and associates,[85] who demonstrated that when ^{3}H-triamcinolone acetonide (^{3}H-TA) was present at the time of cell breakage for the preparation of cytosol, the tracer protected the binding component from spontaneous inactivation. The stabilization of glucocorticoid receptor in tumor material achieved by using this tracer was striking. The rate of inactivation of the steroid-binding protein in the presence of this potent synthetic glucocorticoid was about 1% of that seen in the absence of ligand.

Kaiser et al.[16] compared the properties of the glucocorticoid-binding component, henceforth designated receptor, in P1798/S and P1798/R lymphocytes. After incubation of cell suspensions with 0.02 to 0.03 μM ^{3}H-TA at 0° for 30 min, most of the bound radioactivity was associated with the 27,000 G (constant of gravitation) supernatant obtained by homogenization of the cells in a low-salt buffer. Under these conditions, the sedimentation coefficient of the steroid-receptor complex was 7.10 ± 0.06S for P1798/S and 7.40 ± 0.04S for P1798/R. This difference was significant at the 0.01 level. When extracted at 0° with high-salt buffer (0.15 M KCl), hormone-receptor complexes from P1798/S sedimented at 4.60 ± 0.08S and those from P1798/R at 4.70 ± 0.10S. The relevance of these small differences to the mechanism of resistance of P1798/R to steroid therapy remains to be established. The total binding capacity and dissociation constant of binding for ^{3}H-TA by cytoplasmic preparations were then investigated. Saturation was achieved with 0.1 μM steroid. Scatchard analysis indicated that P1798/S cytoplasm bound somewhat more steroid than the resistant strain, confirming the original observations of Hollander and Chiu.[84] K_d varied from 0.7 to 1.9 × $10^{-8}M$ for both strains of tumor. The 25% decrease in binding sites observed in P1798/R is not of sufficient magnitude to explain resistance of this strain to glucocorticoid therapy. However, pretreatment in vivo with 75mg/kg cortisol acetate for 2 days, followed by a 3-day period without treatment to allow for elimination of exogenous steroid, reduced the number of binding sites in P1798/R to about 20% of those observed in the sensitive strain. Two possible explanations were offered by Kaiser et al.:

1. The solid P1798/R used in these experiments was composed of a mixture of S and R cells, and the latter are really characterized by a significantly lower number of glucocorticoid receptors.
2. Treatment with corticoids may impair synthesis and/or enhance degradation of receptor in P1798/R but not in P1798/S.

Reduced steroid transport or increased catabolism as a basis for resistance appear to be ruled out by the studies of Hollander and Chiu[86] and Kirkpatrick et al.[87]

Rosenau et al.[88] have investigated the binding of ^{3}H-dexamethasone by cytosol preparations of corticoid-sensitive and corticoid-resistant S49.1 lymphoma cells. The capacity of cytosol from steroid-resistant cells to bind ^{3}H-dexamethasone at equilibrium was about 10% of that from sensitive cells. Kondo et al.[12] obtained similar results with corticoid-sensitive and corticoid-resistant strains of L5178Y cells.

2. Nuclear Binding

Hormone binding by cytoplasmic receptors and translocation of the resulting hormone-receptor complexes to the nucleus appear to be essential steps in glucocorticoid action on lymphoid tissue.[51,89,90] Hence, nuclear binding of glucocorticoids by malignant lymphocytes has been investigated in several laboratories. Baxter et al.[91] incubated intact corticoid-sensitive and corticoid-resistant S49 lymphoma cells with ^{3}H-cortisol at 37°, after which cytosol and a crude nuclear fraction were obtained. The specific binding of steroid by both cell fractions was about 60% less in the resistant lines than in the parent sensitive cells. Uptake by the nucleus reached a maximum in about 45 min. Cytosol binding attained equilibrium by 5 min. Nuclear bound steroid represented 30 to 50% of total intracellular bound ^{3}H-cortisol in both sensitive and resistant cells. Subsequently, Rosenau et al.[88] examined nuclear binding by S49.1 cells in a cell-free system. When cytosol from sensitive or resistant cells was incubated with 0.08 μM ^{3}H-dexamethasone for 90 to 120 min at 0 to 4° with or without nonradioactive dexamethasone as competitor, the charged cytosols transferred hormone to nuclei when incubated at 20°. The transfer process did not occur if cytosol was omitted from the incubation mixture. Nuclei from both sensitive and resistant tumors incubated with charged cytosol from sensitive tumor gave a similar high transfer of hormone. When a similar experiment was performed with charged cytosol from resistant tumor, little nuclear transfer took place. Apparently, in S49.1, the capacity for nuclear transfer is limited by the amount of cytosol receptor available in a charged state. The presence of an inhibitor of nuclear transfer in resistant cells was ruled out in appropriate cross-mixing experiments. Similar results were obtained by Kondo et al.[12] using L5178Y lymphoblasts. These authors also showed that the transfer process was temperature dependent and did not proceed at 0°C, confirming the observation of Gehring and Tomkins[92] that an "activation" step was required for nuclear transfer.

Nuclear binding has also been investigated in the lymphoma P1798 system. Kaiser et al.[16] incubated intact P1798/S and P1798/R cells for 30 min with 0.02 μM ^{3}H-TA at either 0° or 37° and extracted crude chromatin pellets (27,000 G) from these cells with either low- or high-salt (0.15 M KCl) buffer. Sucrose density gradient analysis showed that the 27,000 G pellet from cells incubated with steroid at 0° contained little or no salt-extractable, macromolecular bound ^{3}H-TA. When the 27,000 G pellet from cells labeled at 37° was extracted with high-salt, ^{3}H-TA-receptor complexes which sedimented at 4.10 ± 0.11S for P1798/S and 3.70 ± 0.03S for P1798/R were obtained. This difference was significant at the 0.01 level. Further differences in nuclear glucocorticoid binding between P1798/S and P1798/R lymphocytes were found by Stevens et al.[93,123] Triton®-purified nuclei were isolated from cells which had been labeled with 0.01 μM ^{3}H-TA for 1 hr at 37° and extracted with increasing concentrations of KCl in the presence of 10 mM CBZ-L-phenylalanine (a chymotrypsin inhibitor) to prevent degradation of hormone-receptor complexes. Figure 1a shows that nuclei from sensitive cells released significantly more total ^{3}H-TA (bound and free) than nuclei from resistant cells when extracted with 0 to 0.1 M KCl. Figure 1b shows that with increasing salt concentrations there was a progressive rise in the fraction of bound steroid extracted. This fraction was significantly larger for resistant nuclei at each of the KCl concentrations used and reached a maximum of 84% bound for resistant, and 71% bound for sensitive nuclei in the 0.6 M KCl extract, with no further increase at higher salt concentrations. These levels of steroid correspond to 4585 ± 202 molecules of ^{3}H-TA/nucleus in sensitive cells and 2776 ± 160 molecules of ^{3}H-TA/nucleus in resistant cells (p < 0.001). If CBZ-L-phenylalanine was omitted from the extraction buffer, only 15 to 20% of ^{3}H-TA extracted with 0.6 M KCl was in the bound form. Over 90% of nuclear associated ^{3}H-TA was released from both sensitive and resistant nuclei with 0.6 M KCl. Purified sensitive nuclei behaved very differently from resistant nuclei when incubated at 4° with 4.5 mM MgCl$_2$ in the absence of KCl and CBZ-L-phenylalanine. As shown in Figure 2, 60% of the ^{3}H-TA associated with P1798/S nuclei was released within 7.5 min of exposure to divalent cation, compared to only a 10 to 20%

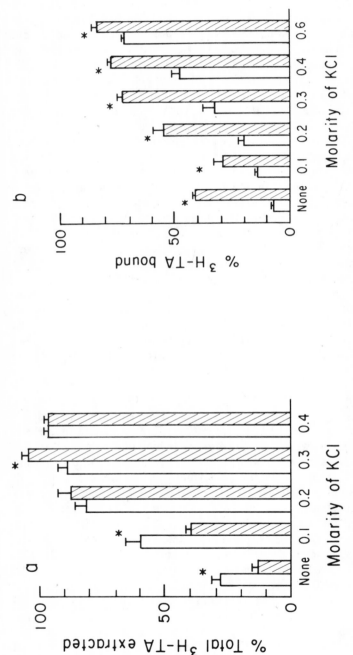

FIGURE 1.   KCl extractability of ³H-triamcinolone acetonide (³H-TA) from P1798/S and P1798/R nuclei. Open bars represent sensitive nuclei and shaded bars, resistant nuclei. Each bar depicts the mean ± S.E. of four experiments, except for the extractions with 0.6 M KCl in (b) which represent 8 to 10 experiments for each strain of tumor. (a) Percent of total nuclear ³H-TA (bound and free) extracted with increasing concentrations of KCl in 10 mM N-*tris*(hydroxymethyl)methyl-2-aminoethane sulfonic acid, 4 mM EDTA, 20 mM dithiothreitol, pH 7.5 at 4°C, containing 10 mM CBZ-L-phenylalanine. The amount of ³H-TA extracted with 0.6 mM KCl was arbitrarily set at 100%. (b) Influence of salt concentration on the fraction of bound steroid in the KCl extract. Asterisks denote statistically significant differences (p = 0.025 or less) between S and R nuclei. (Adapted from Stevens, J., Stevens, Y. W., Rhodes, J., and Steiner, G., *J. Natl. Cancer Inst.*, 61, 1477, 1978.)

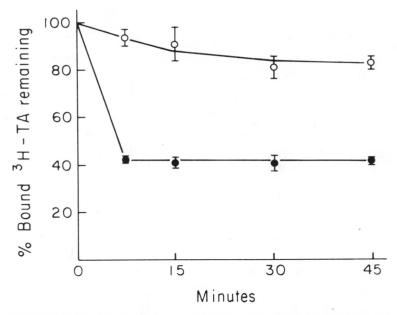

FIGURE 2. MgCl₂-induced release of ³H-TA from S and R nuclei. Purified nuclei were incubated at 4°C for the indicated periods of time in 10 mM N-tris(hydroxymethyl)-methyl-2-aminoethane sulfonic acid, 4.5 mM MgCl₂, 20 mM dithiothreitol (pH 7.5) with gentle shaking, then centrifuged 3 min at 27,000 G and the nuclear pellet extracted with 0.6 M KCl as described in Figure 1. Each point represents the mean ± S.E. of two to three experiments. Closed circles: nuclei from P1798/S lymphocytes. Open circles: nuclei from P1798/R lymphocytes. (From Stevens, J., Stevens, Y. W., Rhodes, J., and Steiner, G., *J. Natl. Cancer Inst.*, 61, 1477, 1978.)

loss of steroid from P1798/R nuclei under similar conditions. Further investigation of these differences may shed light on the mechanism of resistance to glucocorticoid therapy.

H. Genetic Approaches to Glucocorticoid Action

Sibley and Tomkins[94] studied the development of resistance to dexamethasone by S49 cells in culture. The rate of occurrence of resistant cells was similar in the presence and absence of the steroid, about 3.5×10^{-6} per cell per generation. This apparently random emergence of resistance could be increased by the addition of mutagenic agents to the cultures. These data are consistent with resistance as a trait explained by mutational events. Most resistant cells lacked cytosol receptor; others lacked the ability to translocate receptor to the nucleus, and some mutant cells with normal nuclear translocation still were unaffected by 0.05 μM dexamethasone. Further study of cytosol receptor showed that resistance was a property of receptor and not of nuclear binding. When cytosol from cells incapable of translocation was incubated with nuclei from dexamethasone-sensitive cells, no nuclear translocation occurred. Nuclei from cells incapable of translocation were able to accept cytosol hormone-receptor complex.[92] Although "absent" cytosol receptor cannot yet be studied, translocation-deficient receptors are known to differ in some respects from cytosol receptor derived from sensitive cells.

Sucrose gradient centrifugation revealed small differences between receptors from translocation deficient cells and receptors from dexamethasone-sensitive cells. Bio-Gel® A 0.5 M chromatography also revealed differences.[90]

Yamamoto et al.[90] showed that cytosol receptor from dexamethasone-sensitive cells bound to DNA cellulose after thermal activation. Cytosol from cells with a translocation deficiency also showed increased binding after activation at 20°; however, the total fraction bound was far less than that from sensitive cells. Hormone-receptor complex from resistant cells which had cytosol receptor and no translocation defect could bind to DNA cellulose after thermal activation similarly to hormone-receptor complexes from sensitive cells. Elution from DNA cellulose columns with a gradient of increasing ionic strength was able to distinguish different mutant types of defective cytosol receptor. Although these observations are consistent with defective or ineffective binding of cytosol receptor to DNA, they could also be explained by the presence of cytosol inhibitors of receptor interaction with DNA. Accordingly, Yamamoto and colleagues examined the binding of mixtures of cytosol from sensitive and resistant cells to DNA. No evidence for such inhibitors was found; the cytosols showed independent binding to DNA cellulose.

The negative complementation studies in vitro suggested that dexamethasone resistance resided in mutational changes in cytosol receptor. This concept was then examined by the powerful technique of somatic cell hybridization. Hybrids were produced with the aid of inactivated Sendai virus and cloned in appropriate selective media. Hybrid cells continued to make receptors characteristic of each parent. No intermediate or unique receptors were created by hybridization and one type of receptor did not extinguish expression of the other. Dominance of dexamethasone sensitivity was examined by measuring the relative cloning efficiency in soft agar, a technique more sensitive than measurement of cell survival in suspension cultures. Hybrids of sensitive and resistant cells showed sensitivity to dexamethasone to be codominant; (wild type × wild type) were very sensitive, (variant × variant) were completely resistant, and (wild type × variant) showed intermediate sensitivity. Additional studies are needed to understand the relationship between altered function of cytosol corticoid-receptor and lack of steroid-mediated lymphocytolysis in resistant cells with apparently "normal" nuclear binding.

II. HUMAN DISEASE

A. Chronic Lymphocytic Leukemia

Chronic lymphocytic leukemia (CLL) is characterized by an abnormally high content of morphologically normal but functionally abnormal small lymphocytes in blood accompanied by infiltration of many organs with this same cell. Etiology is unknown, but genetic and autoimmune factors play a prominent role. It is a disease of middle life and old age and is much more common in men than in women.

B. Clinical Features

Early CLL is asymptomatic and is discovered because a patient has a blood count for some other reason. Occasionally, vague symptoms appear of fatigue, fever, and loss of appetite and weight. Later, enlargement of the lymph nodes and spleen present a characteristic picture. An excellent description of the clinical features of this disease may be found in a recent review by Gunz.[95]

1. Light Microscopy of CLL Lymphocytes

Light microscopic examination shows that the characteristic cell in the peripheral blood of patients with CLL is a small, mature lymphocyte which cannot be distinguished from a normal blood cell. The CLL cell, however, is easily damaged, and blood smears of patients with CLL show an exceptionally large number of smudged white cells. This property is especially notable in view of the long life of the CLL cell.

2. Ultrastructure

Most CLL cells exhibit small mitochondria and smooth nuclei in contrast to normal lymphocytes.[96] Knospe et al.[97] have described different types of CLL cells based on EM criteria.

3. Metabolic and Functional Characteristics

The metabolic and immunological characteristics of CLL lymphocytes have been reviewed recently by Theml et al.[98] and will not be discussed here. While most CLL cells have the properties of B lymphocytes, they are deficient in many features of these cells. One metabolic deficit is the inability to secrete immunoglobulins. This defect may be the major reason why patients with CLL are immunologically crippled. The CLL cell has less surface Ig (immunoglobulin) and less receptor for aggregated Ig than normal lymphocytes; surface Ig tends to be monoclonal, and many cells react with antihuman T cell serum.[99] A localized concentration of surface Ig in one area of a normal lymphocyte, "cap formation" is not found in the CLL cell. CLL cells are less responsive to pokeweed mitogen than normal lymphocytes. Although blasts induced by PHA (phytohemagglutinin) from CLL lymphocytes appear normal, the overall response to this mitogen is blunted.

4. Proliferation Kinetics

Major proliferation defects are found in the disease. Autoradiographic analysis of ^{3}H-thymidine-labeled lymphocytes in patients indicated that separate short- and long-lived lymphocyte populations were present. About 15 times more lymphocytes were produced per day in CLL-afflicted than in normal individuals. The production rate of short-lived lymphocytes was increased 25-fold, but these cells had a normal life span. Long-lived lymphocytes showed a 12-fold increase in production rate and a fivefold increase in life span. Thus, increased production and delayed destruction result in exponential accumulation of lymphoid cells.[98]

C. Glucocorticoids

1. Role of Glucocorticoids as a Possible Physiological Control

It is not known whether CLL involves expansion of a small subpopulation of normal lymphoid cells over which the organism no longer exerts adequate control or if the CLL lymphocyte arises by malignant transformation of a hitherto normal precursor cell.

There is much to suggest that glucocorticoids play a role in regulating blood lymphocyte levels. While patients with Addison's disease may have a relative increase in lymphocyte count and those with Cushing's syndrome a relative decrease, such glucocorticoid control is only partial, since adenopathy is not a feature of Addison's disease. However, lymph follicle formation comparable to that observed in myasthenia gravis has been found in the thymus of patients with Addison's disease.[100] Although the human lymphocyte is not particularly sensitive to the lympholytic action of glucocorticoids, CLL lymphoid tissue regresses when pharmacologic doses of adrenal steroids are administered. For these reasons, it is believed that studies on the precise role of adrenal hormone in the control of human lymphoid cell populations could be very important.

D. The Role of Glucocorticoids in Treatment of CLL

Glucocorticoids are used in the treatment of CLL for two reasons. Administration of pharmacologic doses will decrease tumor mass and also alleviate complications of the disease such as hemolytic anemia and thrombocytopenia. Unfortunately, large doses of glucocorticoids produce undesirable effects in all patients, and especially in patients with CLL. The CLL patient has an already compromised immunologic defense mechanism and administration of steroid may further impair the system. Consequently, the reduction in tumor mass can best be achieved by other agents. The use of high-dose glucocorticoid treatment for the alleviation of hemolytic anemia or thrombocytopenic purpura may justify the undesirable side effects, since often there is no better agent to bring about the desired clinical improvement. When large doses of steroid are administered to CLL patients, there is usually a shrinking of large lymph nodes and diminution in the size of the enlarged spleen. The earliest response in peripheral blood is an increase in lymphocyte count. It is usually assumed that this rise in lymphocytes is due to an efflux of cells from the shrinking tumor tissue. Several weeks after treatment is started, the lymphocyte count begins to decrease and may fall to normal levels.[101]

1. In Vitro Effects of Glucocorticoids on CLL Cells

Schrek,[102] and more recently Knospe et al.,[97] found that incubation with 3 μM prednisolone for 7 days at 37° resulted in greater lysis of CLL cells than of normal human lymphocytes in 21 out of 37 patients. Werthamer and Amaral[103] exposed normal lymphocytes and 14 separate CLL preparations to 10 μM cortisol for 2 hr. Pronounced ultrastructural cytoplasmic alterations were observed in the normal cells but not in the malignant ones. These authors[104] have also demonstrated rapid inhibition of uridine and leucine utilization in CLL lymphocytes by cortisol. The suppression of leucine incorporation required plasma, and a possible role of transcortin in glucocorticoid action was suggested. Exposure of CLL cells to steroid appeared to result in enhanced degradation of prelabeled RNA. This effect was not abolished by actinomycin D. Baran et al.[58] and Frengley et al.[105] found that incubation of CLL cells with cortisol resulted in markedly decreased α-amino-isobutyric acid uptake and that this effect could be prevented by cycloheximide.

E. Glucocorticoid Binding by CLL Cells

There are conflicting reports concerning the presence of glucocorticoid receptors in CLL cells. Gailani et al.[106] reported a lack of specific binding of ^{3}H-triamcinolone acetonide in the cytoplasmic fraction of freshly isolated lymphocytes from eight patients with CLL. In contrast, Homo et al.[107] found that peripheral lymphocytes from 19 patients with CLL bound ^{3}H-dexamethasone to a greater or to a lesser degree than normal human lymphocytes, with identical affinity as determined by Scatchard analysis. These studies were performed with intact cells at 4°, and binding was measured in the cytoplasmic fraction only. Terenius et al.[108] also obtained evidence for the existence of glucocorticoid receptors in lymphocyte cytosol preparations from 17 out of 22 patients with CLL. Recent studies from the authors' laboratory[93,123] indicate the presence of specific glucocorticoid binding in Triton X-100-purified nuclei isolated from intact CLL cells previously incubated with ^{3}H-triamcinolone acetonide for 1 hr at 37° in tissue culture medium (RPMI 1640) without serum. As described earlier in this review for the corticoid-sensitive strain of mouse lymphoma P1798, exposure of the isolated CLL nuclei to dilute $MgCl_2$ resulted in rapid release of nuclear ^{3}H-TA-receptor complexes. In addition, the protease inhibitor CBZ-L-phenylalanine was required for preserving the integrity of nuclear hormone-receptor complexes during extraction with 0.6 M KCl. Further study of corticoid receptors in CLL cells may lead to understanding of a possible physiological role of corticoid in the control of lymphoid proliferation.

F. Acute Lymphocytic Leukemia

Acute lymphocytic leukemia (ALL) is a disease characterized by progressive malignant lymphoblastic infiltration of lymphatic organs and bone marrow. It is not the purpose of this general discussion of the biology of the disease to attempt differentiation from conditions which fulfill this definition but are also associated with considerable lymphoma development or aberrations in the peripheral white cell count. The disease arises because of faulty control of proliferation and differentiation. Diagnosis is made by demonstrating lymphoblastic infiltration of the marrow. Marrow examination will have been carried out for study of anemia, a bleeding disorder, unexplained fever, or an accidentally discovered abnormality in the peripheral blood. Although ALL may occur at any age, the incidence is highest in the first 5 years of life and only slightly favors males. The etiology is unknown; exposure to radiation does increase the incidence but is not a factor in the vast majority of patients. Although chromosomal abnormalities are common, no single one predominates. The increased incidence of ALL in Trisomy-21 (Down's syndrome) is totally unexplained.

G. Proliferation Kinetics

The doubling time of leukemic cells in patients with ALL in relapse is 4 to 6 days. However, generation times (Tg) of individual lymphoblasts are about 20 hr, with a smaller population of 60 hr.[109] The doubling times and Tg are different because most lymphoblasts are not actively dividing.

H. Glucocorticoid Therapy

Farber et al.[110] and Pearson and associates[111] were the first to demonstrate remission of ALL with ACTH and the corticosteroids. Prednisone alone causes 60% complete remissions in children and 35% complete remission in adults with ALL. Substantial improvement in the rate of remission-induction (80% or more in children, 50% in adults) is currently achievable with drug regimens that include prednisone, and values of 90 to 97% have been reported when three or four chemotherapeutic agents were combined.[112] Before such multiple-agent therapy was developed for the treatment of acute lymphoblastic leukemia, the major problem in curing the disease was the rapid development of drug resistance. Now that many lymphocytolytic substances are available for treatment and their combinations for optimal therapy are under active study, a new problem has emerged. The leukemic cell population before treatment is expanding because of the many stem cells present which are capable of sustaining the leukemic population. However, commitment to maturation clearly occurs in leukemic populations, and the committed cells eventually die. Unfortunately, there are also many dormant cells which can reenter the stem cell population long after the tumor burden has been materially reduced by administration of effective therapeutic agents. This reentry of the dormant cells is probably the key factor preventing cure in many patients today. Glucocorticoid therapy does not destroy normal hematopoietic tissue and is not cell cycle specific. Thus, further study may expand the role of hormonal treatment in acute leukemia, since it is not known whether the dormant cell is insensitive to glucocorticoid and what factors would make for sensitivity.[113]

Ernst and Killmann[114] reported that in vivo prednisone therapy destroyed quiescent lymphoblasts and affected proliferating leukemic cells to the same degree. In addition, prednisone appeared to reduce efflux from G_1 into S. It was not clear whether this was due to killing of cells in G_1 or to decreased progression from G_1 to S. There was no preferential killing of cells which were in S phase at the start of treatment. Further biochemical study of the precise effects of glucocorticoids on the very heterogeneous cell population in ALL may lead to improvement in therapy.

I. Glucocorticoid Receptors

Lippman and associates[115] studied the glucocorticoid-binding protein in human acute lymphatic leukemia cells. Although normal human lymphocytes are relatively resistant to steroid-mediated lysis,[102,116] ALL is often treated with glucocorticoids. Accordingly, it was reasonable to determine whether ALL cells contained corticoid-binding protein (CBP) and whether its presence correlated with clinical sensitivity. Specific binding was determined as the difference in binding of ^{3}H-dexamethasone to cell-free extracts in the presence or absence of a 1000-fold excess of nonradioactive cortisol or dexamethasone. Leukemic cell extracts were saturated at 2.5 μM ^{3}H-cortisol or 0.25 μM ^{3}H-dexamethasone. Saturation analysis was performed at 0.4 μM dexamethasone on lysate from 22 untreated patients with ALL. Although there was a wide variation about the mean of 0.3 pmol/mg cytosol protein, all patients tested had abundant binding protein. In contrast, lymphocytes from normal healthy volunteers and from ALL patients resistant to corticoid and other therapy showed little binding. Lymphocytes from patients who had been treated with corticoid and other agents but were still capable of responding demonstrated ample binding protein. ^{3}H-Thymidine uptake and CBP in sensitive and resistant ALL cells were then compared. The sensitive cells showed characteristic saturation with ^{3}H-dexamethasone and comparable inhibition of ^{3}H-thymidine incorporation with increasing dexamethasone concentration. In contrast, resistant cells showed no binding or inhibition of ^{3}H-thymidine incorporation over a wide concentration range of steroid. ALL cells resemble lymphoma cells in that the presence of cytosol receptor is no guarantee of lytic response.[117,118]

Further comparison of glucocorticoid binding to intact human lymphocytes and cytosol may be rewarding. As mentioned above, little or no receptor was found in cytosol preparations from normal, untransformed cells. However, about 2700 specific glucocorticoid binding sites could be demonstrated when glucocorticoid binding was measured by incubating purified intact human lymphocytes with ^{3}H-dexamethasone at 21°.[119] It is not yet clear whether the difference in these observations simply lies in a rapid transfer to the nucleus from a small pool of rapidly turning over cytosol receptor or whether the observed binding involves the plasma membrane in some way. Basal binding of the purified human lymphocytes was increased two- to threefold by incubation with PHA.

The achievement of long-term remissions in many, and apparent cure in some, children with ALL represents a dramatic improvement in therapy. Glucocorticoid therapy must get some of the credit. Further understanding of the mechanism of glucocorticoid sensitivity and resistance may allow hormonal agents to play an even wider role in extinguishing malignant lymphoid cells.

III. ADDENDUM

Since this review was completed in August 1977, Stevens et al. have published a detailed report on the differences in nuclear glucocorticoid binding between P1798/S and P1798/R tumor lymphocytes[122] and on nuclear binding of triamcinolone acetonide in lymphocytes from patients with chronic lymphatic leukemia.[123] McPartland et al.[124] have also described differences in nuclear glucocorticoid binding between the corticoid-sensitive and -resistant strains of mouse lymphoma P1798. Further details on the effect of glucocorticoids on nuclear fragility in P1798 lymphocytes can be found in the article by Nicholson and Young,[125] and Kaiser and Edelman[126] have presented data which suggest that increased calcium uptake may not be the basic cause of glucocorticoid-induced lymphocytolysis. Finally, several reports on glucocorticoid binding in normal and malignant lymphocytes were presented at the John E. Fogarty International Center Conference on Hormones and Cancer,[127-132] held at the National Cancer Institute, Bethesda, Md.

ACKNOWLEDGMENTS

Work performed in the authors' laboratories was supported by Grant CA 10064, P

30-14194 and CA 14987 from the National Cancer Institute, Department of Health, Education, and Welfare and by the Dworetz-Wolf Foundation for Leukemia Research. John Stevens is a Scholar of the Leukemia Society of America, Inc.

REFERENCES

1. Star, P., An unusual case of Addison's disease; sudden death; remarks, *Lancet,* 1, 284, 1895.
2. Heilman, F. R. and Kendall, E. C., The influence of 11-dihydro-17-hydroxy-corticosterone (compound E) on the growth of a malignant tumor in the mouse, *Endocrinology,* 34, 416, 1944.
3. Murphy, J. B. and Sturm, E., Effect of adrenal cortical extract on transplanted leukemia in rats, *Science,* 99, 313, 1944.
4. Law, L. W. and Spiers, R., Response of spontaneous lymphoid leukemias in mice to injection of adrenal cortical extracts, *Proc. Soc. Exp. Biol. Med.,* 66, 226, 1947.
5. Law, L. W., Effect of gonadectomy and adrenalectomy on the appearance and incidence of spontaneous lymphoid leukemia in C58 mice, *J. Natl. Cancer Inst.,* 8, 157, 1947.
6. Kaplan, H. S., Sumner, M. N., and Brown, M. B., Adrenal cortical function and radiation-induced lymphoid tumors of mice, *Cancer Res.,* 11, 629, 1951.
7. Kaplan, H. S. and Nagareda, C. S., On the possibility of cure of malignant lymphoid tumors. I. Treatment of autochthonous lymphoid tumors in C57BL mice with massive doses of lymphocytolytic agents, *Blood,* 18, 166, 1961.
8. Fischer, G. A. and Welch, A. D., Effect of citrovorum factor and peptones on mouse leukemic cells, L5178Y in tissue culture. *Science,* 126, 1018, 1957.
9. Fischer, G. A., Studies of the culture of leukemic cells *in vitro*, *Ann. N. Y. Acad. Sci.,* 76, 673, 1958.
10. Jaffe, J. A., Fischer, G. A., and Welch, A. D., Structure-action relationships of corticosteroid compounds as inhibitors of leukemic L5178Y cell reproduction *in vivo* and *in vitro*, *Biochem. Pharmacol.,* 12, 1081, 1963.
11. Story, M. T. and Melnykovych, G., Growth inhibition of mouse lymphoma cells, L5178Y, *in vitro*, by glucocorticoids, *Exp. Cell Res.,* 77, 437, 1973.
12. Kondo, H., Kikuta, A., and Noumura, T., Studies on glucocorticoid-induced cytolysis in cultured mouse lymphoma cells, L5178Y, *Exp. Cell Res.,* 90, 285, 1975.
13. McCain-Lampkin, J. and Potter, M., Response to cortisone and development of cortisone resistance in a cortisone-sensitive lymphosarcoma of the mouse, *J. Natl. Cancer Inst.,* 20, 1091, 1958.
14. Stevens, J., Stevens, Y. W., and Hollander, V. P., Substrate requirements and kinetic analysis of the cortisol effects on uridine uptake and incorporation by mouse lymphoma P1798 cells *in vitro*, *Cancer Res.,* 34, 2330, 1974.
15. Stevens, J. and Stevens, Y. W., Cortisol-induced lymphocytolysis of P1798 tumor cells in glucose-free, pyruvate-free medium, *J. Natl. Cancer Inst.,* 54, 1493, 1975.
16. Kaiser, N., Milholland, R. J., and Rosen, F., Corticoid receptors and mechanism of resistance in the cortisol-sensitive and -resistant lines of lymphosarcoma P1798, *Cancer Res.,* 34, 621, 1974.
17. Gabourel, J. D. and Aronow, L., Growth inhibition effects of hydrocortisone on mouse lymphoma ML-388 *in vitro*, *J. Pharmacol. Exp. Ther.,* 136, 213, 1962.
18. Horibata, K. and Harris, A. W., Mouse myelomas and lymphomas in culture, *Exp. Cell Res.,* 60, 61, 1970.
19. Harris, A. W., Differentiated functions expressed by cultured mouse lymphoma cells, *Exp. Cell Res.,* 60, 341, 1970.
20. Yancey, S. T. and Bleyer, W. A., Characteristics and response to certain cancer chemotherapeutic agents of an acute lymphocytic leukemia arising in a BALB/c × DBA/2 F_1 mouse, *Cancer Res.,* 34, 1866, 1974.
21. Huggins, C. B. and Uematsu, K., Induction of lymphatic leukemia in non-inbred mice and its control with glucocorticoids, *Cancer,* 37, 177, 1976.
22. Dougherty, T. F., Berliner, M. L., Schneebeli, G. L., and Berliner, D. L., Hormonal control of lymphatic structure and function, *Ann. N. Y. Acad. Sci.,* 113, 825, 1964.
23. Jaffe, H. L., The influence of the suprarenal gland on thymus. I. Regeneration of the thymus following double suprarenalectomy in the rat, *J. Exp. Med.,* 40, 325, 1924.

24. Crede, R. H. and Moon, H. D., Effect of adrenocorticotropic hormone on the thymus of rats, *Proc. Soc. Exp. Biol. Med.*, 43, 44, 1940.
25. Dougherty, T. F. and White, A., Functional alterations in lymphoid tissue induced by adrenal cortical secretion, *Am. J. Anat.*, 77, 81, 1945.
26. Cowan, W. K. and Sorenson, G. D., Electron microscopic observations of acute thymic involution produced by hydrocortisone, *Lab. Invest.*, 13, 353, 1964.
27. Frank, J. A. and Dougherty, T. F., Cytoplasmic budding of human lymphocytes produced by cortisone and hydrocortisone in *in vitro* preparations, *Proc. Soc. Exp. Biol. Med.*, 82, 17, 1953.
28. Trowell, O. A., The action of cortisone on lymphocytes *in vitro*, *J. Physiol.* (London), 119, 274, 1953.
29. Schreck, R., Cytotoxicity of adrenal cortex hormones on normal and malignant lymphocytes of man and rat, *Proc. Soc. Exp. Biol. Med.*, 108, 328, 1961.
30. Makman, M. H., Dvorkin, B., and White, A., Alterations in protein and nucleic acid metabolism of thymocytes produced by adrenal steroids *in vitro*, *J. Biol. Chem.*, 241, 1646, 1966.
31. Burton, A. F., Storr, J. M., and Dunn, W. L., Cytolytic action of corticosteroids on thymus and lymphoma cells *in vitro*, *Can. J. Biochem.*, 45, 289, 1967.
32. Whitfield, J. F., Perris, A. D., and Youdale, T., Destruction of the nuclear morphology of thymic lymphocytes by the corticosteroid cortisol, *Exp. Cell Res.*, 52, 349, 1968.
33. Perris, A. D. and Whitfield, J. F., The release of free deoxyribonucleic acid in rat thymocytes after whole-body irradiation, *Intl. J. Radiat. Biol.*, 11, 399, 1966.
34. Perris, A. D., Youdale, T., and Whitfield, J. F., The relation between nuclear structural changes and the appearance of free deoxyribonucleic acid in irradiated rat thymocytes, *Exp. Cell Res.*, 45, 48, 1966.
35. Whitfield, J. F., *EURATOM Bull.*, 4, 166, 1965.
36. Whitfield, J. F., Youdale, T., and Perris, A. D., Early postirradiation changes leading to the loss of nuclear structure in rat thymocytes, *Exp. Cell Res.*, 48, 461, 1967.
37. Allfrey, V. G., Meudt, R., Hopkins, J. W., and Mirsky, A. E., Sodium-dependent "transport" reactions in the cell nucleus and their role in protein and nucleic acid synthesis, *Proc. Natl. Acad. Sci. U.S.A.*, 47, 907, 1961.
38. Kleinsmith, L. J., Allfrey, V. G., and Mirsky, A. E., Phosphoprotein metabolism in isolated lymphocyte nuclei, *Proc. Natl. Acad. Sci. U.S.A.*, 55, 1182, 1966.
39. Kleinsmith, L. J., Allfrey, V. G., and Mirsky, A. E., Phosphorylation of nuclear protein early in the course of gene activation in lymphocytes, *Science*, 154, 780, 1966.
40. Whitfield, J. F. and Perris, A. D., Dissolution of the condensed chromatin structures of isolated thymocyte nuclei and the disruption of deoxyribonucleoprotein by inorganic phosphate and a phosphoprotein, *Exp. Cell Res.*, 49, 358, 1968.
41. Turnell, R. W., Clarke, L. H., and Burton, A. F., Studies on the mechanism of corticosteroid-induced lymphocytolysis, *Cancer Res.*, 33, 203, 1973.
42. Turnell, R. W. and Burton, A. F., Studies on the mechanism of resistance to lymphocytolysis induced by corticosteroid, *Cancer Res.*, 34, 39, 1974.
43. Turnell, R. W. and Burton, A. F., Glucocorticoid receptors and lymphocytolysis in normal and neoplastic lymphocytes, *Mol. Cell. Biochem.*, 9, 175, 1975.
44. Story, T. M., Standaert, M. M., and Melnykovych, G., Glucocorticoid-induced alterations in phosphatidylcholine metabolism in mouse lymphoma cells, L5178Y, *in vitro*, *Cancer Res.*, 33, 2872, 1973.
45. Hallahan, C., Young, D. A., and Munck, A., Time course of early events in the action of glucocorticoids on rat thymus cells *in vitro*. Synthesis and turnover of a hypothetical cortisol-induced protein inhibitor of glucose metabolism and of a presumed ribonucleic acid, *J. Biol. Chem.*, 248, 2922, 1973.
46. Mosher, K. M., Young, D. A., and Munck, A., Evidence for irreversible, actinomycin D-sensitive and temperature-sensitive steps following binding of cortisol to glucocorticoid receptors and preceding effects on glucose metabolism in rat thymus cells, *J. Biol. Chem.*, 246, 654, 1971.
47. Munck, A., Glucocorticoid inhibition of glucose uptake by peripheral tissues: old and new evidence, molecular mechanisms, and physiological significance, *Perspect. Biol. Med.*, 14, 265, 1971.
48. Rosen, J. M., Fina, J. J., Milholland, R. J., and Rosen, F., Inhibition of glucose uptake in lymphosarcoma P1798 by cortisol and its relationship to the biosynthesis of deoxyribonucleic acid, *J. Biol. Chem.*, 245, 2074, 1970.
49. Rosen, J. M., Fina, J. J., Milholland, R. J., and Rosen, F., Inhibitory effect of cortisol *in vitro* on 2-deoxyglucose uptake and RNA and protein metabolism in lymphosarcoma P1798, *Cancer Res.*, 32, 350, 1972.
50. Giddings, S. J. and Young, D. A., An *in vitro* effect of physiological levels of cortisol and related steroids on the structural integrity of the nucleus in rat thymic lymphocytes as measured by resistance to lysis, *J. Steroid Biochem.*, 5, 587, 1974.
51. Munck, A. and Leung, K., Glucocorticoid receptors and mechanism of action, in *Receptors and Mechanism of Action of Steroid Hormones*, Vol. 8, Pasqualini, J. R., Ed., Marcel Dekker, New York, 1977, 311.

52. Behrens, U. J., Mashburn, L. T., Stevens, J., Hollander, V. P., and Lampen, N., Differences in cell surface characteristics between glucocorticoid-sensitive and -resistant mouse lymphomas, *Cancer Res.*, 34, 2926, 1974.

53. Behrens, U. J. and Hollander, V. P., Cell membrane sialoglycopeptides of corticoid-sensitive and -resistant lymphosarcoma P1798, *Cancer Res.*, 36, 172, 1976.

54. Nicholson, M. L. and Young, D. A., An effect of glucocorticoid hormones *in vitro* on the structural integrity of nuclei in cortisol-sensitive and -resistant P1798 tumor cells as measured by resistance to lysis, 59th Annual Meeting of The Endocrine Society, Abstr. No. 382, Chicago, Ill., 1977.

55. Alvarez, M. R. and Truitt, A. J., Rapid nuclear cytochemical changes induced by dexamethasone in thymus lymphocytes of adrenalectomized rats, *Exp. Cell Res.*, 106, 105, 1977.

56. Makman, M. H., Nakagawa, S., Dvorkin, B., and White, A., Inhibitory effects of cortisol and antibiotics on substrate entry and ribonucleic acid synthesis in rat thymocytes *in vitro*, *J. Biol. Chem.*, 245, 2556, 1970.

57. Young, D. A., Barnard, T., Mendelsohn, S., and Giddings, S., An early cordycepin-sensitive event in the action of glucocorticoid hormones on rat thymus cells *in vitro*: evidence that synthesis of new mRNA initiates the earliest metabolic effects of steroid hormones, *Endocr. Res. Commun.*, 1, 63, 1974.

58. Baran, D. T., Lichtman, M. S., and Peck, W. A., Alpha-aminoisobutyric acid transport in human leukemic lymphocytes: *in vitro* characteristics and inhibition by cortisol and cycloheximide, *J. Clin. Invest.*, 51, 2181, 1972.

59. Stevens, J. and Stevens, Y. W., Sequential irreversible, actinomycin D-sensitive, and cycloheximide-sensitive steps prior to cortisol inhibition of uridine utilization by P1798 tumor lymphocytes, *Cancer Res.*, 35, 2145, 1975.

60. Stevens, J. and Stevens, Y. W., Cortisol (F)-induced loss of tumor lymphocyte cell membrane integrity, *Proc. Am. Assoc. Cancer Res.*, 18, 710, 1977.

61. Kaiser, N. and Edelman, I. S., Calcium dependence of glucocorticoid-induced lymphocytolysis, *Proc. Nat. Acad. Sci. U.S.A.*, 74, 638, 1977.

62. MacLeod, R. M., King, C. E., and Hollander, V. P., Effect of corticosteroids on ribonuclease and nucleic acid content in lymphosarcoma P1798, *Cancer Res.*, 23, 1045, 1963.

63. Ambellan, E. and Hollander, V. P., The role of ribonuclease in regression of lymphosarcoma P1798, *Cancer Res.*, 26, 903, 1966.

64. Wiernik, P. H. and MacLeod, R. H., The effect of a single large dose of 9-alpha-fluoroprednisolone on nucleodepolymerase activity and nucleic acid of rat thymus, *Acta Endocrinol.* (Copenhagen), 49, 138, 1965.

65. Nakagawa, S. and White, A., Response of rat thymic nuclear RNA polymerase to cortisol injection, *Endocrinology*, 81, 867, 1967.

66. Sands, H. and Haynes, R. C., Jr., Effect of glucocorticoids on the acid DNase of the thymus, *Endocrinology*, 86, 144, 1970.

67. Stevens, J., Stevens, Y. W., and Hollander, V. P., Early effects of glucocorticoid treatment on amino acid metabolism in lymphosarcoma P1798, *Cancer Res.*, 33, 370, 1973.

68. Hollander, V. P., Gordon, C., and Hollander, N., Effects of corticoid injection and of adrenalectomy on *in vitro* amino acid incorporation into microsomes of P1798 lymphosarcoma, *Nature* (London), 213, 1036, 1967.

69. Wagner, T. W., A trypsin-sensitive site for the action of hydrocortisone on calf thymus nuclei, *Biochem. Biophys. Res. Commun.*, 38, 890, 1970.

70. Wong, M. D. and Aronow, L., Identification of a glucocorticoid sensitive histone protein from mouse fibroblast nuclei, *Biochem. Biophys. Res. Commun.*, 71, 265, 1976.

71. McCarty, K. S. and McCarty, K. S., Jr., Hormonal induction of postsynthetic modifications of chromosomal proteins in mammary neoplasia, in *Control Mechanisms in Cancer*, Criss, W. E., Ono, T., and Sabine, J. R., Eds., Raven Press, New York, 1976, 37.

72. Libby, P. R., Histone acetylation and hormone action, *Biochem. J.*, 134, 907, 1973.

73. Fox, K. E. and Gabourel, J. D., Effect of cortisol on the RNA polymerase system of rat thymus, *Mol. Pharmacol.*, 3, 479, 1967.

74. Nakagawa, S. and White, A., Properties of an aggregate ribonucleic acid polymerase from rat thymus and its response to cortisol injection, *J. Biol. Chem.*, 245, 1448, 1970.

75. Meulen, N. V. D., Marx, R., Sekeris, C. E., and Abraham, A. D., Differential effects of cortisol on nucleolar and extranucleolar RNA synthesis of rat thymocytes, *Exp. Cell Res.*, 74, 606, 1972.

76. Bell, P. A. and Borthwick, N. M., Glucocorticoid effects on DNA-dependent RNA polymerase activity in rat thymus cells, *J. Steroid Biochem.*, 7, 1147, 1976.

77. Gomez, J., Kemper, B. W., Pratt, W. B., and Aronow, L., Effects of glucocorticoids on nucleic acid synthesis in mouse lymphoma cells growing *in vitro* and on nuclei isolated from these cells, *Biochem. Pharmacol.*, 19, 1471, 1970.

78. Rosen, J. M., Rosen, F., Milholland, R. J., and Nichol, C. A., Effects of cortisol on DNA metabolism in the sensitive and resistant lines of mouse lymphoma P1798, *Cancer Res.*, 30, 1129, 1970.

79. Brunkhorst, W. K. and Hess, E. L., Interactions of hormones with thymus-cell fractions, *Biochim. Biophys. Acta,* 82, 385, 1964.
80. Bellamy, D., Phillips, J. G., Chester Jones I., and Leonard, R. A., The uptake of cortisol by rat tissues, *Biochem. J.,* 85, 537, 1962.
81. Litwack, G., Fiala, E. S., and Filosa, R. J., Intracellular binding of ^{14}C-hydrocortisone prior to enzymatic induction, *Biochim. Biophys. Acta,* 111, 569, 1965.
82. DeVenuto, F. and Chader, G., Report # 639, U.S. Army, Medical Research Laboratory, 1965.
83. Morris, D. J. and Barnes, F. W., Jr., Intracellular distribution of 4-^{14}C-cortisol in rat liver, *Fed. Proc. Fed. Am. Soc. Exp. Biol.,* 25, 281, 1966.
84. Hollander, N. and Chiu, Y. W., *In vitro* binding of cortisol 1,2-^{3}H by a substance in the supernatant fraction of P1798 mouse lymphosarcoma, *Biochem. Biophys. Res. Commun.,* 25, 291, 1966.
85. Kirkpatrick, A. F., Kaiser, N., Milholland, R. J., and Rosen, F., Glucocorticoid-binding macromolecules in normal tissues and tumors, *J. Biol. Chem.,* 247, 70, 1972.
86. Hollander, N. and Chiu, Y. W., Relation between cortisol metabolism and its lympholytic effect in P1798 lymphosarcoma, *Endocrinology,* 79, 168, 1966.
87. Kirkpatrick, A. F., Milholland, R. J., and Rosen, F., Stereospecific glucocorticoid binding to subcellular fractions of the sensitive and resistant lymphosarcoma P1798, *Nature (London) New Biol.,* 232, 216, 1971.
88. Rosenau, W., Baxter, J. D., Rousseau, G. G., and Tomkins, G. M., Mechanism of resistance to steroids: glucocorticoid receptor defect in lymphoma cells, *Nature (London) New Biol.,* 237, 20, 1972.
89. Lippman, M., Steroid hormone receptors in human malignancy, *Life Sci.,* 18, 143, 1976.
90. Yamamoto, K. R., Gehring, U., Stampfer, M. R., and Sibley, C. H., Genetic approaches to steroid hormone action, *Rec. Prog. Horm. Res.,* 32, 3, 1976.
91. Baxter, J. D., Harris, A. W., and Cohn, M., Glucocorticoid receptors in lymphoma cells in culture: relationship to glucocorticoid killing activity, *Science,* 171, 189, 1971.
92. Gehring, U. and Tomkins, G. M., A new mechanism for steroid unresponsiveness: loss of nuclear binding activity of a steroid hormone receptor, *Cell,* 3, 301, 1974.
93. Stevens, J., Stevens, Y. W., Hollander, V. P., Rosenthal, R. L., and Sloan, E., Differences in Nuclear Glucocorticoid Binding between Corticoid-sensitive (S) and -resistant (R) Mouse Lymphoma P1798 and Human Chronic Lymphocytic Leukemia (CLL) Cells, presented at the Meeting of the American Chemical Society, Abstr. No. 143, Chicago, Ill., August 1977.
94. Sibley, C. H. and Tomkins, G. M., Isolation of lymphoma cell variants resistant to killing by glucocorticoids, *Cell,* 2, 213, 1974.
95. Gunz, F., Chronic lymphocytic leukemia, in *Cancer Medicine,* Holland, J. and Frei, E., III, Eds., Lea & Febinger, Philadelphia, 1974, 1256.
96. Schrek, R., Ultrastructure of blood lymphocytes from chronic lymphocytic and lymphosarcoma cell leukemia, *J. Natl. Cancer Inst.,* 48, 51, 1972.
97. Knospe, W. H., Gregory, S. A., Trobaugh, F. W., Jr., Stedronsky, J. A., and Schrek, R., Chronic lymphocytic leukemia: correlation of clinical course and therapeutic response with in vitro testing and morphology of lymphocytes, *Am. J. Hematol.,* 2, 73, 1977.
98. Theml, H., Love, R., and Begemann, H., Factors in the pathomechanism of chronic lymphocytic leukemia, *Annu. Rev. Med.,* 28, 131, 1977.
99. Whiteside, T. L., Winkelstein, A., and Rabin, B. S., Immunologic characterization of chronic lymphocytic leukemia cells, *Cancer,* 39, 1109, 1977.
100. Sloan, H. E., Jr., The thymus in myasthenia gravis, with observations on the normal anatomy and histology of the thymus, *Surgery,* 13, 154, 1943.
101. Shaw, R. K., Boggs, D. R., Silberman, H. R., and Frei, E., III, A study of prednisone therapy in chronic lymphocytic leukemia, *Blood,* 17, 182, 1961.
102. Schrek, R., Prednisolone sensitivity and cytology of viable lymphocytes as tests for chronic lymphocytic leukemia, *J. Natl. Cancer Inst.,* 33, 837, 1964.
103. Werthamer, S. and Amaral, L., Effect of cortisol on ultrastructure of normal, leukemic and cultured human lymphocytes, *In Vitro,* 11, 313, 1975.
104. Werthamer, S. and Amaral, A., The response of leukemic lymphocytes to cortisol: a suggested role of transcortin, *Blood,* 37, 463, 1971.
105. Frengley, P. A., Lichtman, M. S., and Peck, W. A., Specificity and sensitivity of cortisol-induced changes in alpha-aminoisobutyric acid transport in human leukemic small lymphocytes and leukemic myeloblasts, *J. Clin. Invest.,* 52, 1518, 1973.
106. Gailani, S., Minowada, J., Silvernail, P., Nussbaum, A., Kaiser, N., Rosen, F., and Shimaoka, K., Specific glucocorticoid binding in human hemopoietic cell lines and neoplastic tissue, *Cancer Res.,* 33, 2653, 1973.
107. Homo, F., Duval, D., and Meyer, P., Binding of dexamethasone in normal human lymphocytes and in leukemic patients, *C. R. Acad. Sci. Ser. D,* 280, 1923, 1975.

108. Terenius, L., Simonsson, B., and Nilsson, K., Glucocorticoid receptors, DNA synthesis, membrane antigens and their relation to disease activity in chronic lymphatic leukemia, *J. Steroid Biochem.*, 7, 905, 1976.

109. Killman, S. A., Acute leukemia: the kinetics of leukemic blast cells in man, *Series Haematol.*, 1, 38, 1968.

110. Farber, S., Schwachmann, H., Toch, R., Downing, V., Kennedy, B. H., and Hyde, J., The effect of ACTH in acute leukemia in childhood, in *Proc. First Clinical ACTH Conf.*, Mote, J. R., Ed., Blakston, Philadelphia, 1950.

111. Pearson, O. H., Eliel, L. P., and Rawson, R. W., Regression of lymphoid tumors in man induced by ACTH and cortisone, in *Proc. First Clinical ACTH Conf.*, Mote, J. R., Ed., Blakston, Philadelphia, 1950.

112. Henderson, E. S., Acute lymphoblastic leukemia, in *Cancer Medicine*, Holland, J. and Frei, E., III, Eds., Lea & Febinger, Philadelphia, 1974, 1173.

113. Clarkson, B. D., The survival value of the dormant state in neoplastic and normal cell populations, in *Control of Proliferation in Animal Cells*, Vol. 1, Clarkson, B. and Baserga, R., Eds., Cold Spring Harbor, N. Y., 1974, 945.

114. Ernst, P. and Killmann, S. A., Perturbation of generation cycle of human leukemic blast cells by cytostatic therapy *in vivo*: effect of corticosteroids, *Blood*, 36, 689, 1970.

115. Lippman, M. E., Halterman, R. H., Leventhal, B. G., Perry, S., and Thompson, E. B., Glucocorticoid-binding proteins in human acute lymphoblastic leukemic blast cells, *J. Clin. Invest.*, 52, 1715, 1973.

116. Claman, H. N., Moorhead, J. W., and Benner, W. H., Corticosteroids and lymphoid cells *in vitro*. I. Hydrocortisone lysis of human, guinea pig and mouse thymus cells, *J. Lab. Clin. Med.*, 78, 499, 1971.

117. Bird, C. C., Waddell, A. W., Robertson, A. M. G., Currie, A. R., Steel, C. M., and Evans, J., Cytoplasmic receptor levels and glucocorticoid response in human lymphoblastoid cell lines, *Br. J. Cancer*, 33, 700, 1976.

118. Lippman, M. E., Perry, S., and Thompson, E. B., Cytoplasmic glucocorticoid-binding proteins in glucocorticoid-unresponsive human and mouse leukemic cell lines, *Cancer Res.*, 34, 1572, 1974.

119. Neifeld, J. P., Lippman, M. E., and Tormey, D. C., Steroid hormone receptors in normal human lymphocytes, *J. Biol. Chem.*, 252, 2972, 1977.

120. Stevens, J. and Stevens, Y. W., unpublished results.

121. Roldan, A., Stevens, J., and Hollander, V. P., Difference in the number of insulin binding sites between cortisol-sensitive and cortisol-resistant lymphoma P1798 cells, *Proc. Soc. Exp. Biol. Med.*, 151, 711, 1976.

122. Stevens, J., Stevens, Y. W., Rhodes, J., and Steiner, G., Differences in nuclear glucocorticoid binding between corticoid sensitive and -resistant P1798 tumor lymphocytes and stabilization of nuclear hormone receptor complexes with carbobenzoxy-L-phenylalanine, *J. Natl. Cancer Inst.*, 61, 1477, 1978.

123. Stevens, J., Stevens, Y. W., Sloan, E., Rosenthal, R., and Rhodes, J., Nuclear glucocorticoid binding in chronic lymphatic leukemia lymphocytes, *Endocr. Res. Commun.*, 5, 91, 1978.

124. McPartland, R. P., Milholland, R. J., and Rosen, F., Nuclear binding of steroid-receptor complex to lymphosarcoma P1798 resistant and sensitive cells and effect of concanavalin A on receptor levels, *Cancer Res.*, 37, 4256, 1977.

125. Nicholson, M. L. and Young, D. A. Effect of glucocorticoid hormones in vitro on the structural integrity of nuclei in corticosteroid-sensitive and -resistant lines of lymphosarcoma P1798, *Cancer Res.*, 38, 3673, 1978.

126. Kaiser, N. and Edelman, I., Further studies on the role of calcium in glucocorticoid-induced lymphocytolysis, *Endocrinology*, 103, 936, 1978.

127. Lippman, M. E., Yarbro, G. K., and Leventhal, B. G., Clinical implications of glucocorticoid receptors in human leukemia, *Cancer Res.*, 38, 4251, 1978.

128. Iacobelli, S., Ranelletti, F. O., Longo, P., Riccardi, R., and Mastrangelo, R., Discrepancies between in vivo and in vitro effects of glucocorticoids in myelomonocytic leukemic cells with steroid receptors, *Cancer Res.*, 38, 4257, 1978.

129. Duval, D and Homo, F., Prognostic value of steroid receptor determination in leukemia, *Cancer Res.*, 38, 4263, 1978.

130. Crabtree, G. R., Smith, K. A., and Munck, A., Glucocorticoid receptors and sensitivity of isolated human leukemia and lymphoma cells, *Cancer Res.*, 38, 4268, 1978.

131. Norman, M. R., Harmon, J. M., and Thompson, E. B., Use of a human lymphoid cell line to evaluate interactions between prednisolone and other chemotherapeutic agents, *Cancer Res.*, 38, 4273, 1978.

132. Bourgeois, S., Newby, R. F., and Huet, M., Glucocorticoid resistance in murine lymphoma and thymoma lines, *Cancer Res.*, 38, 4279, 1978.

Chapter 5

INSULIN AND MAMMARY CANCER

J. T. Harmon and R. Hilf

TABLE OF CONTENTS

I. INTRODUCTION

When consideration is given to hormones that are involved in the etiology of breast cancer, those that are foremost in the literature are the steroids from the ovaries and the pituitary hormone, prolactin. The role of the ovary, as initially pointed out by the success that Beatson[1] reported in the treatment of women with breast cancer, has been amply demonstrated in both clinical and laboratory settings. As understanding of endocrinology has progressed, the hormones from the pituitary were implicated. Prolactin, because of its role in lactation, was considered as an important factor, and tumor regression following hypophysectomy was considered to be a response to removal of prolactin as well as to the reduction of steroidogenesis due to removal of ACTH and gonadotrophins. However, as progress was made to elucidate the exact role of these hormones alone and in various combinations, it has become apparent that other hormonal factors need to be considered as important in both neoplastic transformation and growth. One such hormone is insulin, and the purpose of this chapter will be to review the pertinent studies that implicate a role for insulin in breast cancer.

II. INSULIN IN THE NORMAL MAMMARY GLAND

The classic studies by Lyons et al.[2] in the rat clearly demonstrated the hormonal complement required by the mammary gland. Using triply operated (ovariectomized-adrenalectomized-hypophysectomized) rats, these investigators demonstrated that the animal required replacement of estrogen, progesterone, glucocorticoids, growth hormone, and prolactin to stimulate the lobulo-alveolar development attending the naturally occurring differentiation during pregnancy and lactation. After parturition, continued lactation required prolactin and adrenal glucocorticoids. Thus, in vivo, insulin may not play a critical role in mammary gland growth and differentiation. However, there are data that implicate a role for insulin in lactogenesis. For example, postpartum rats injected with 3 units of insulin daily showed increased total milk yield,[3] and Martin and Baldwin[4] clearly demonstrated that insulin insufficiency (alloxan-induced diabetes) resulted in an immediate depression of lactational performance, as reflected by decreased synthesis of lactose, casein, and lipids of mammary gland slices in vitro. In this latter study, insulin reversed these effects during the early stages of diabetes. On the basis of his earlier experiments,[5,6] Ahren[7] examined extensively the ability of insulin to augment the effects of estrogen and progesterone on mammary gland growth. In castrate rats, estrogen plus progesterone has synergistic actions to cause mammary gland development, but no effect was seen in castrate-hypophysectomized rats. Insulin given with estrone produced a slight development in the mammary duct system in castrate-hypophysectomized rats, a response that was less than that seen alone in animals with intact pituitaries; long-term injection of estrone, progesterone, and insulin did result in some alveolar development in the castrate-hypophysectomized rat. Thus, even in the absence of pituitary hormones, insulin did demonstrate some ability to stimulate development of the mammary gland.

The most extensive and convincing evidence of a role for insulin in mammary growth and development has come from the studies of Topper and colleagues, using the explanted gland in vitro. An excellent review of these studies has been published recently,[8] and a brief summary will be presented here. In this system, it has been shown that mammary gland proliferation arises after exposure to insulin and, in the presence of insulin, prolactin, and glucocorticoids, casein synthesis increased markedly along with the appearance of α-lactalbumin. It was also established that insulin-free serum can stimulate epithelial DNA synthesis in explants from pregnant mice, whereas it required a time in culture (24 hr) for the gland from virgin mice to acquire this sensitivity. Prolactin, while not mitogenic under these conditions in vitro, renders the mammary gland in vivo sensitive to the mitogenic effects of insulin in vitro. Thus, under the proper hormonal milieu, mammary gland epithelial cells respond to insulin as though insulin was a mitogen. If these experiments in vitro have their counterpart in vivo, consideration needs to be given to the potential role of insulin in growth of abnormal mammary cells.

III. EFFECT OF INSULIN ON NEOPLASTIC TISSUES

Although there are a number of reports in the literature in which insulin or its lack was examined for effects on tumor growth, no clear picture has emerged.[9] One reason for this is the variety of experimental tumors that were examined. For example, Goranson and Tilser[10] reported that growth of the Novikoff hepatoma or the Walker 256 carcinoma was reduced in alloxan-diabetic rats. Their data also indicated that the rate of tumor growth showed a relationship to the severity of the alloxan-induced diabetes. In contrast, Salter et al.[11] reported that insulin, either alone or with glucagon, inhibited growth of the Walker 256 carcinosarcoma, a finding that they stated was in keeping with other earlier reports. (see above). As will be seen later, such dichotomies of results are still present among more recent reports in different mammary tumors and it is this apparent conflict that should warrant further investigation in light of our increasing fund of knowledge. We will therefore limit the following discussion to experimental mammary tumors, which have been more thoroughly explored in the last decade.

A. Insulin-dependent Mammary Tumors

Dependence is defined here as a requirement of the tumor for insulin for its continued growth and metabolism. On the basis of the earlier reports by numerous investigators, it was astutely reasoned by Heuson that a role for insulin might be ascertained by studying tumors that were known to be hormonally dependent rather than those that were not influenced by the hormonal milieu in vivo. With this as a basis, Heuson and colleagues[12] examined the effects of insulin in vitro on rat mammary tumors that had been induced with 7,12-dimethylbenz(a)anthracene (DMBA); the majority of tumors produced by this technique are known to be dependent on ovarian and pituitary hormones.[13] Using an explant system, they found that 5/12 tumors demonstrated an insulin-induced stimulation of thymidine incorporation into DNA, an effect correlated with an increased labeling index and mitotic index. The fact that a large proportion of the tumors did not respond to insulin in vitro suggested to these investigators that some tumors were insulin independent. Heuson and Legros[14] then performed experiments directed towards elucidation of the role of insulin as a stimulator of DNA synthesis as related to carbohydrate metabolism. They found that stimulation of thymidine incorporation occurred with little or no effect on glucose consumption and that elevating the level of glucose in the medium did not increase cell proliferation. However, at low concentrations of glucose, thymidine incorporation was reduced, and it is curious that their results indicated that the lowest amount of thymidine incorporation relative to glucose consumption occurred in tumors exposed to 100 mg/100 mℓ of glucose, a level that approximates the physiological level of blood glucose. From these experiments, Heuson concluded that the effect of insulin to promote growth was not mediated through a stimulating effect on glucose uptake and utilization.

Having determined an effect of insulin in vitro, Heuson and Legros[15] then examined the effects of insulin and glucose on tumor growth in vivo. They found that increased glucose intake (in the drinking water) or injection of insulin (2.5 IU/100 g body weight per day except on Sundays) increased the average surface area of DMBA-induced tumors. Animals that received both glucose and insulin demonstrated an eightfold increase in total tumor surface per rat compared to intact control animals. When tumor-bearing animals were treated with alloxan to induce diabetes, approximately 90% of the tumors present at the time of administration of alloxan showed regression of growth. A more extensive investigation of the effects of insulin deprival on DMBA tumor growth was reported later by these investigators.[16] They observed that administration of estradiol benzoate failed to prevent tumor regression produced by alloxan diabetes. Because of the severe weight loss resulting from alloxan treatment, they examined the effect of food restriction on tumor growth and found that tumor regression did occur under these nutritional restrictions. It is possible that the effects of nutritional deprivation could have caused a decrease in tumor growth indirectly through a decreased insulin secretion, but no measurements of circulating insulin levels were made. Another interesting observation reported was that induction of diabetes 3 or 4 weeks after carcinogen feeding completely prevented mammary tumor formation, results that implicate insulin as having a role in the early stages of neoplastic transformation. To examine the interplay between insulin and other hormones, Heuson et al.[17] administered insulin together with glucose to tumor-bearing animals that had been ovariectomized; tumor regression was not prevented. However, treatment with insulin significantly reactivated tumor growth in hypophysectomized rats that also received daily injections of prolactin; prolactin alone did not activate tumor growth (it should be noted that body weight loss occurred as a result of hypophysectomy). Thus, a conclusion was reached that insulin does play a role in stimulating growth of DMBA-induced tumors and needs to be considered, along with estrogens and prolactin, as another hormonal factor in mammary tumor growth.

Studies in this laboratory were initiated to investigate the role of insulin in growth and metabolism of DMBA-induced tumors, particularly to elucidate metabolic (biochemical) similarities and differences in tumors designated as insulin dependent vs. insulin independent. To induce diabetes, we chose to use streptozotocin, which will produce hyperglycemia and decreased circulating insulin levels relative to the dose of drug administered. The authors' criteria[18,19] for diabetes were >250 mg/100 ml blood glucose, urinary glucose levels exceeding 0.5 g/ml, and serum insulin levels $\sim 10^{-10}$ M. Applying these conditions to animals with DMBA-induced mammary carcinomas, 56% (50/89) of the tumors regressed (>20% decrease in volume during at least a 10-day observation period) in diabetic rats, 21% remained static (±20% change), and 23% (20/89) continued to grow. The difference in results reported here with those of Heuson may be attributed, at least in part, to differences in body weight loss; diabetic animals in our laboratory showed less than a 5% difference in body weight from that of intact control animals. Administration of 2 IU insulin per day to diabetic rats reversed the effects of diabetes so that the distribution of tumor growth patterns was identical to that seen in intact animals. Analysis of cellular macromolecules in insulin-dependent and insulin-independent tumors revealed some differences. The RNA level in dependent (regressing) tumors was reduced below that in growing tumors from intact or diabetic rats; tumors from rats receiving insulin treatment had significantly elevated levels of RNA compared to all others. Regressing tumors demonstrated a modest increase in DNA levels, which were observed to be the same in tumors from intact animals, and in neoplasms classified as insulin independent. However, DNA levels were the highest in tumors of animals treated with insulin, a response in vivo compatible with the findings of Heuson and his colleagues in vitro. Cohen and Hilf[20] also reported that estrogen treatment of tumor-bearing diabetic rats resulted in regression of all tumors, an effect that was not observed with either hormonal manipulation alone.

In attempting to gain insight into the role of insulin in tumor growth, certain aspects of carbohydrate metabolism were examined in DMBA-induced tumors that were classified as either insulin dependent or independent. Tumors regressing in diabetic animals were found to have lowered activities of pyruvate kinase, phosphofructokinase, and glucose-6-phosphate dehydrogenase compared to those in insulin-independent tumors or to those in tumors growing in intact hosts.[18] Administration of 2 IU insulin per day to diabetic tumor-bearing rats caused an increase in glucose-6-phosphate dehydrogenase activity to levels observed in tumors from intact animals; this level of insulin treatment did not significantly alter the activities of the other enzymes measured. Glucose utilization in vitro was also examined by incubating tumor slices with radioactive-labeled glucose as a substrate, and both the $^{14}CO_2$ evolved and the ^{14}C incorporated into fatty acids by tumor tissue in the presence of C-1-labeled, C-6-labeled, or uniformly labeled glucose were determined. Tumors that were insulin dependent (regressing in diabetic hosts) showed a significant decrease in $^{14}CO_2$ evolved from either glucose-1-^{14}C or uniformly labeled glucose; addition of 1 IU of insulin in vitro returned glucose utilization to levels comparable to that demonstrated by growing tumors from intact animals. Glucose utilization was estimated on the basis of percent conversion of substrate per milligram of tumor DNA, an approach that would tend to normalize differences in cell number. These calculations also showed that regressing tumors from diabetic rats had lower glucose uptake (μmol/mg DNA) and the percent contribution of the pentose phosphate pathway was reduced (~40%) compared to that in growing tumors in intact rats. Thus, tumor regression arising from insulin deprivation was accompanied by decreased carbohydrate metabolism, results that suggest a role for insulin in influencing glucose utilization.

Measurement of glucose utilization and substrate throughput are valuable approaches to elucidate glucose metabolism, but a major role of insulin is in regulation of glucose transport, which is related to cellular metabolism.[21] It may, therefore, be more appropriate to examine the effects of insulin on transport of substrate, such as glucose and, by so doing, gain some insight into very early events in hormone action. The authors recently[22] had an opportunity to measure glucose transport on dissociated cells of three DMBA-induced tumors from the same diabetic rat; one tumor was regressing (insulin dependent), the second lesion was classified as static, and the third tumor was continuing its growth (insulin independent). Glucose transport was measured using labeled 3-O-methylglucose (discussed in greater detail below) at 15, 30, 45, and 60 sec in the absence or presence of added insulin ($10^{-10}M$). The initial velocity of transport (v_i^T) was lowest in the regressing tumor and highest in the growing tumor; addition of insulin significantly elevated glucose transport in the insulin-dependent lesion and caused an inhibition of transport in the insulin-independent tumor. No effect of insulin was seen in the cells from the static tumor. Since all three lesions were obtained from the same animal, differences in hormonal milieu can be ruled out as a cause of the divergence of response. These data indicate that transport of glucose into tumor cells may be regulated by insulin and that control of substrate entry may be directly related to growth behavior of the neoplasm under varied hormonal states.

B. Insulin-responsive Tumors

Response is defined as any alteration in growth or metabolism that can be attributed to the administration or exposure of tumors to insulin. It is to be distinguished from dependence as defined earlier, in that tumor growth may be equal or greater in the diabetic host when compared to the intact host; a dependent tumor would not demonstrate equal growth in the absence of endogenous insulin. The authors have defined the R3230AC tumor as an autonomous (not dependent), insulin-responsive tumor on the basis of their observation that this mammary adenocarcinoma grew as well, if not faster, in the diabetic host and that growth of the neoplasm was inhibited by daily administration of insulin to intact or diabetic tumor-bearing hosts.[23] It was also observed in these experiments that treatment with estrogen plus insulin was additive in causing inhibition of tumor growth, which implied that these two hormones might be altering tumor growth by different mechanisms. Although activities of several selected glycolytic enzymes (pyruvate kinase, phosphofructokinase, hexokinase, glucose-6-phosphate dehydrogenase, and 6-phosphogluconate dehydrogenase) were essentially unaltered in tumors from diabetic rats, there did appear to be a modest decrease in the utilization of labeled glucose (reduction in the ratio of utilization of glucose-1-C^{14} to glucose-6-C^{14}) in vitro by tumors from diabetic rats. A curious observation was the finding that tumor slices from diabetic rats demonstrated even lower utilization of glucose-1-C^{14} when insulin was added in vitro; this effect was seen in the amount of label evolved as $^{14}CO_2$ or as radioactivity incorporated into fatty acids. These results prompted the authors to examine in greater detail the role of insulin in the R3230AC carcinoma.

It is well accepted that the initial event in hormone action is the interaction of the ligand with its receptor, and considerable data have accumulated to demonstrate the presence of insulin receptors on the plasma membrane of a variety of cells.[24-27] Studies were initiated in the authors' laboratory to identify and characterize insulin binding to the R3230AC tumor. Tumor cell suspensions were prepared by enzymatic dissociation in order to establish an experimental system to examine insulin binding as well as substrate transport on the same preparation in vitro. Optimum conditions of time and temperature for binding, for separation of bound and free hormone, and for minimal degradation of labeled ligand were ascertained for tumor cell preparations. Specific insulin binding was defined as the difference between binding in the absence (total) or presence (nonspecific) of 1000-fold excess unlabeled insulin. Specificity of binding was examined by competition with insulin analogues. Proinsulin, guinea pig insulin, and desocatpeptide insulin were capable of competing for insulin binding in an order of potency related to their biological activity; prolactin and glucagon were unable to compete for insulin binding.[28] Scatchard analysis of binding data yielded a curvilinear plot, a result similar to that reported for other tissues.[27] Binding of labeled insulin was estimated over a concentration range from 10^{-11} to 10^{-10} M insulin; over this concentration range, the binding sites showed a high affinity for insulin (10^{10} M^{-1}) and the number of sites estimated was greater in tumors from diabetic animals than in tumors from either intact animals or intact animals given insulin prior to sacrifice. Reversibility of insulin binding was studied by dissociation experiments; dissociation of bound insulin was enhanced by the presence of unlabeled insulin. It was observed that the maximum dissociation of bound insulin occurred in the presence of 10^{-7} M unlabeled insulin, and less of an effect was observed with either lower or higher concentrations of unlabeled hormone. These data regarding saturability, reversibility, and specificity of insulin binding strongly support the existence in this tumor of an insulin receptor with properties similar to those found in other cells.

There are two of these properties that are worthy of additional comment. First, the apparent negative control of insulin receptor by circulating levels of insulin (diabetic vs. intact animals), or "down regulation,"[29] appears to operate in this adenocarcinoma and, as will be discussed below, regulation of insulin receptors may be under control of other hormones as well. The fact that such regulation occurs in the tumor implies the existence of an intact response system for regulation of the insulin receptor. The second property, namely, more rapid dissociation of bound insulin in the presence of unlabeled hormone than in the absence of added unlabeled ligand, has been interpreted as reflecting negative cooperative interactions for the insulin receptor.[30] The data obtained with the tumor are compatible with such an interpretation. However, other interpretations of the binding and dissociation data, as fitting with other proposed models such as a hormone-receptor-effector model, i. e., two-step model or a mobile-receptor model, are not ruled out by these results.[31,32]

A most critical aspect of hormone receptor interaction is the resultant translation of the initial step into an event that has physiological consequences. Since insulin is known to affect glucose and amino acid uptake in many normal tissues, the authors initiated experiments to examine glucose transport into dissociated R3230AC tumor cells.[19] Initial experiments dealt with the characterization of glucose transport systems. It was found that glucose entered these mammary tumor cells by a nonsaturable (diffusion) system and by a passive carrier system. The properties of the passive carrier were identified by specificity for glucose, by competition studies, by its temperature sensitivity, and by inhibition of transport with phloretin but not by phloridzin. Using labeled 3-O-methylglucose (3-O-MG) as the probe, it was determined that the passive carrier exhibited a K_m of 3 to 4 mM. The properties of the passive carrier in the tumor were similar to those reported for normal cells.[33,34] Having characterized how glucose entered these tumor cells, the authors then examined the effects of insulin in vitro on glucose entry.[35] Unexpectedly, a time- and dose-related decrease in the v_i for 3-O-MG entry into cells of this carcinoma was observed. The effect of insulin occurred with as little as 10^{-11} M, with the major effects observed between 10^{-10} to 10^{-8} M insulin in vitro; the effects were seen when glucose was present in the medium at 2 and 5 mM, but not at 20 mM glucose. Thus although the response observed was somewhat surprising, the authors also observed a similar effect for cells from DMBA-induced tumors that were insulin independent.[22] From these studies, it was concluded that the ability of insulin to inhibit growth of this tumor in vivo could be due in part to the hormone's ability to decrease glucose transport. These results, taken together with earlier findings of the lack of insulin to stimulate hexokinase activity and the decreased utilization of glucose labeled at C-1, appear to be compatible with decreased substrate entry and utilization leading to a retardation of growth of this carcinoma. Faster tumor growth in the diabetic rat might result from alleviation of this negative control by insulin. Thus, a role for insulin in mammary tumor growth may need to be considered either as an adjunct to therapy or as a facilitator of other hormonal agents.

The authors have now completed a series of experiments directed towards characterization of the transport process of neutral amino acids into cells of the R3230AC mammary carcinoma, and the effects of insulin thereon. Using proline as a probe for the "A" carrier system, the authors found that its entry was a concentrative process, was Na⁺-dependent, pH- sensitive and sensitive to metabolic inhibitors, and was completely inhibited by methyl α-aminoisobutyrate, an analogue that enters only by the "A" system; the Km for proline transport was in good agreement with that reported for other tissues.[36] When α-aminoisobutyrate (AIB) was used as another probe for the "A" system, the authors found both a Na⁺-dependent and Na⁺-independent carrier-mediated entry, the former demonstrating all of the characteristics of the "A" system, and the latter displaying characteristics quite similar to those of the "L" system.[36a] These findings with AIB resemble those reported by others for fetal rat calvaria[37] and chick embryo heart cells,[38] findings that support the recently suggested biochemical similarities between tumor and embryonic tissues. Tumor cells from diabetic rats demonstrate an enhanced entry of proline and AIB via the Na⁺-dependent carrier; entry of phenylalanine, leucine or AIB via the Na⁺-independent carrier, amino acids that utilize the "L" system, was unchanged in tumors from diabetic rats.[38a] Administration of insulin to diabetic tumor-bearing rats resulted in a time- and dose-related reduction in proline transport and incorporation, with no effect on phenylalanine transport.[38a] Thus, the biological behavior of the tumor to altered insulin milieu, i.e., more rapid tumor growth in the diabetic rat and inhibition of tumor growth by insulin therapy, was correlated with alterations in the transport capacity of the "A" system but not the "L" system. These results demonstrate the specificity of the insulin effects and provide an opportunity to explore a cause-effect relationship between entry of substrates and subsequent cell growth. An examination of the effects of other hormones on substrate transport and utilization and the interactions between insulin-mediated effects in the presence or absence of these other hormones would provide better insight into possible mechanisms of hormonal regulation of tumor growth; such an investigation is currently in progress.[38b]

C. Insulin, Hormone Receptors, and Regulation of Receptors

It is now accepted that hormone receptors, like other cellular proteins are dynamic components subject to regulation and, as such, the response of a cell to a hormone may be markedly influenced by the amount of receptor present. In the case of insulin, data have been presented to indicate that insulin receptors are influenced by insulin itself. Thus, it has been shown that the insulin binding capacity is inversely proportional to the circulating levels of insulin, a response referred to as "down-regulation," and it has been suggested that such type of regulation may be a widespread phenomenon among target cells exposed to chronic high levels of a hormone.[39] In the case of insulin, data were presented implicating that such a regulatory response could be demonstrated directly in cell culture systems.[29] Complete agreement among investigators that such a mechanism may explain insulin resistance, such as that seen in obesity, has not been reached, as exemplified by reports citing differences in insulin binding[40] and those showing no differences in insulin binding[41] to fat cells from obese humans. Data obtained with the R3230AC tumor indicate that insulin binding capacity was inversely related to endogenous insulin levels, since insulin binding capacity was increased in tumors from diabetic rats and decreased in tumors from intact animals administered insulin.[19,42] Furthermore, it has also been observed that the binding capacity for ¹²⁵I-insulin was increased in DMBA-induced tumors that regressed after animals were made diabetic, although insulin binding capacity was unchanged in lesions that remained static in diabetic rats; insulin binding was reduced in lesions that continued to grow in diabetic hosts.[43] Thus, a simple unifying mechanism for self-regulation of insulin receptors may not apply to all target cells.

A most interesting observation has been recently made by Shafie et al.[42] regarding a relationship between estrogen and insulin binding. The insulin binding capacity of R3230AC mammary carcinomas obtained from ovariectomized rats showed a marked increase, an increase that represented a two- to threefold elevation in specific ^{125}I-insulin binding above that seen in tumors from intact rats. Careful analysis of the saturation kinetics of binding revealed that this elevated binding capacity was not attributable to a change in receptor affinity, an alteration in degradation of ligand, or to changes in rates of dissociation, and it was concluded that the enhanced binding most probably resulted from an increase in the number of receptors. Additional data supporting a role for estrogen in regulation of insulin binding were obtained by the demonstration that injection of estradiol valerate caused a significant reduction in insulin binding to cells prepared from tumors of ovariectomized rats. A direct effect of estradiol in decreased insulin binding was also found in experiments employing short-term culture (3 to 6 days) of R3230AC tumor cells. Thus, it appears that insulin binding may be regulated by ovarian hormones. Such an estrogen-insulin axis may also be a component of the insulin resistance seen in obesity, pregnancy, or in women taking oral contraceptives; circulating levels of estrogen are increased in these clinical situations and may lead to a decrease in insulin binding capacity.

A second important role for insulin action on the mammary gland has been described as "permissive," a role that would allow or enhance the action of other hormones. An example of such a proposal is that reported by Mukherjee et al.,[44] in which insulin acted along with prolactin to enhance mitoses. A permissive role of insulin for other hormones could be manifest by effects on receptors, and data to support this suggestion have recently appeared. In a series of experiments with rodent mammary tumors, Smith et al.[45,46] reported that prolactin binding to tumor membrane preparations was significantly reduced in diabetic rats. It is also of interest that livers from diabetic tumor-bearing rats demonstrated a reduction in prolactin binding. In an earlier report, Gibson and Hilf[47] showed that estrogen binding capacity was reduced in DMBA-induced tumors, which regressed after induction of diabetes. Shafie et al.[42] reported a significant decrease in estrogen receptor content in R3230AC tumor cells from diabetic rats. Taken together, these data indicate that insulin may exert its permissive role by influencing receptor levels for prolactin and estrogen, and although this effect may not be an exclusive action of insulin, it does add insight regarding the role of insulin in mammary tumor growth. The observation that such a role may have useful therapeutic implications is alluded to in a later section.

IV. EFFECTS OF INSULIN IN VITRO

Although some success has been achieved with normal mammary glands in tissue culture, a great number of studies have been conducted with mammary gland explants in organ culture, a technique originally developed by Elias[48] and studied extensively by Topper.[49] Although most of these studies dealt with mouse and rat tissues, it is clear that insulin plays an essential role in preserving the morphology of these tissues and in causing an enhancement of DNA synthesis. It is to be noted, however, that the ability of insulin alone to maintain the integrity of the explant was found to be dependent on the stage of differentiation of the explant. The early prelactating glands retained to some extent their alveolar integrity in the presence of 5 μg/mℓ insulin, whereas nonpregnant gland explants were maintained by insulin alone at either 5 or 50 μg/mℓ.[50] Insulin is apparently required in the medium for the maximum expression of differentiated product formation resulting from the addition of prolactin. Insulin alone provoked a slight transitory increase in casein synthesis, but its major effect was to maintain the initial level of casein synthesis, which dropped off when explants were cultured in the absence of any added hormones.[51] Most investigators have used a final concentration of 5 μg/mℓ of insulin in the medium, a level that is approximately 10^{-6} M. This contrasts to the levels in vivo, which are 10^{-10} to 10^{-8} M, and it is necessary to consider that some of the effects reported for insulin in vitro may be attributed to the high concentrations required for maintenance of the cultured tissue.

The ability of insulin to simulate DNA synthesis in mammary gland tumor explants was reported for tumors of mice.[52,53] Some DMBA-induced tumors of rats were found to be responsive to insulin in vitro,[14] and in a study of 20 tumors in organ culture, Pasteels et al.[54] found that 17 neoplasms were dependent on insulin for DNA synthesis. Interestingly, in the presence of insulin, variable responses were observed after addition of prolactin, progesterone, and/or estradiol, with 9/12 insulin-dependent tumors showing enhanced DNA synthesis after addition of prolactin plus progesterone in vitro. Somewhat similar results were reported by Welsch et al,[55] in which both mouse tumors and DMBA-induced mammary tumors were examined simultaneously. In these experiments, the effects of insulin on labeled thymidine incorporated into DNA were more dramatic in mouse tumors (average of 375% increase) than in rodent tumors (average increase of 127%); addition of prolactin to insulin-containing media showed a further increase in thymidine incorporation into rat, but not mouse, tumors.

The apparent success for examination of mammary tissue from animals under explant conditions has prompted several investigators to study human breast tissues under similar conditions. Among the first studies was that of Barker et al.,[56] in which it was found that addition of insulin to the medium resulted in marked morphological changes of ductal epithelium including proliferation, hypertrophy, and foci resembling squamous metaplasia. Although microscopically normal, these tissues came from a variety of patients — of different ages with different breast diseases — and the effects of insulin on ductal cells were quite consistent. Ceriani et al.[57] obtained explants of normal breast tissue from women who had mammary fibroadenomas and examined the effects of a variety of hormones on growth and differentiation in vitro. Full maintenance of the cells, with epithelial proliferation in some of the stimulated ducts, was observed when insulin was the only hormone present in the chemically defined medium. Interestingly, partial maintenance was obtained in the absence of any added hormones, a situation unlike that seen in mice and other mammals.[58] Wellings and Jentoft[59] examined a number of human breast biopsy specimens, including fibroadenoma, mammary dysplasia, scirrous carcinoma, and colloid carcinoma, and failed to note any effect of insulin on survival or cell proliferation in vitro. However, Elias and Armstrong[60] found that insulin, at 10μg/mℓ or higher, caused hyperplastic and squamous metaplastic changes in the epithelium in biopsies of fibroadenomas and dysplasias. The apparent differences in the results of these latter two groups may be due to the level of insulin used; in the former report,[59] 5 μg/mℓ insulin was the highest level studied, whereas in the latter report,[60] more consistent effects of insulin were seen at 10 μg/mℓ or higher. Recently, Welsch and colleagues[55,61] examined the effects of insulin on DNA synthesis in benign and malignant human breast tumors. Although there was considerable variation in the thymidine incorporation per unit of DNA among the samples studied, insulin caused an average increase of 176% for carcinomas and about 200% for samples of fibroadenoma and fibrocystic disease. In the case of benign lesions, insulin was found to consistently increase the mean number of thymidine-labeled epithelial cells as well as the mean number of epithelial cells demonstrating mitotic figures. Thus, from the foregoing studies of human breast tissues in vitro, it would seem that insulin has the capacity to stimulate proliferation of the epithelial cells in normal and in benign or malignant specimens. It is also apparent that insulin plays a facilitative role in relation to other hormones, and these relationships will require further elucidation.

Another approach for the study of hormone action employs established cell lines that can be shown to possess characteristic markers of the tissue of origin. Recently, one breast cancer cell line, MCF-7, which was developed from a pleural effusion of a postmenopausal breast cancer patient, has been extensively examined as a potential model for elucidation of hormone action in vitro. This cell line, originally described by Soule et al.,[62] has been characterized for the presence of hormone receptors and mammary gland protein constituents as well as its morphological features; these parameters have been investigated to ascertain if any changes occurred during continuous culture.[63] For the purpose of this review, only those studies related to insulin will be noted.

Studies to determine the effects of insulin in vitro were conducted by measurement of labeled precursor incorporation into macromolecules in MCF-7. In cells that had been incubated for 24 hr in serum-free medium prior to addition of insulin, Osborne et al.[64] reported that thymidine and uridine incorporation were stimulated by $10^{-11}M$ insulin with a maximal stimulation seen at $10^{-8}M$ insulin. The reported lag periods, i.e., time between addition of insulin and significant stimulation of incorporation, after addition of $10^{-8}M$ insulin to the cells were 3 hr for uridine and 10 hr for thymidine incorporated into total trichloroacetic acid-precipitable macromolecules. Leucine incorporation into macromolecules was observed to be stimulated by as little as $5 \times 10^{-11}M$ insulin, was maximal at $10^{-9}M$ insulin, and maximal stimulation was seen at 3 hr after addition of $10^{-8}M$ insulin. An increase in the number of cells per dish was found at 3 days after the addition of either 10^{-10} or $10^{-8}M$ insulin (about 500%), although it should be noted that the cell number increased by 200% in control dishes, which contained cells cultured in serum-free medium. This latter finding indicates that MCF-7 cells are not insulin dependent, but rather are insulin responsive. The ability of insulin to stimulate growth of MCF-7 cells was also observed by Shafie and Brooks[65] who also reported that insulin was able to overcome the lethal effects of estradiol in vitro. Other than the preservation of viability brought about by the combined effect of insulin and estrogen, a most striking effect of these two hormones was the restoration of the epithelioid morphological characteristics of the cells and the generation of domes. The formation of domes in these monolayer cultures strongly suggests a conservation of certain differentiated characteristics of mammary epithelial cells.[62] MCF-7 cells were unable to form domes after confluence if grown in serum- or hormone-free (chemically defined medium) or in chemically defined medium supplemented with various concentrations of estradiol-17β. With the addition of insulin alone to chemically defined medium, these cells formed only a few domes. However, in the presence of $10^{-8}M$ estradiol-17β, cells grown in chemically defined medium supplemented with 10 µg/ml insulin were capable of forming domes at a comparable frequency to that of control cells grown in medium supplemented with serum. These findings lend support for a proposed role of insulin in the differentiation of this cell culture line, a role which might act via estrogen receptor regulation. This postulated relationship between insulin and estrogen through mechanisms of hormone receptors arose from several observations. In MCF-7 cells, Shafie and Brooks[66] reported that estrogen receptor levels declined when the cells were kept in chemically defined medium for 18 days, but supplementation with insulin restored the estrogen receptor level. Similar results demonstrating a decline in estrogen receptor levels in experimental mammary tumors after induction of diabetes were reported by Gibson and Hilf,[47] Shafie et al.,[42] and Shafie and Hilf.[43]

Other human cell lines have been recently investigated by Lippman and colleagues, and some of their results have been summarized.[67] Osborne et al.[68] have examined insulin binding and response in these cell lines, all of which were originally obtained from pleural effusions of breast cancer patients with metastatic disease. It was observed that two of these cell lines, EVSA-T and MDA-231, showed little or no response to insulin (maximum concentration used was $10^{-8}M$ insulin), with respect to incorporation of leucine into proteins, thymidine into DNA or acetate into fatty acids. In contrast, MCF-7 and ZR-75-1 responded in somewhat varying degrees to the addition of insulin in vitro (10^{-11} to $10^{-8}M$ insulin) in the above-mentioned three end points measured. Curiously, when examining insulin binding to these cell lines, they observed no correlation between the amount of insulin bound and the cells' ability to respond to insulin. In fact, MCF-7, which showed the most responsiveness in terms of labeled precursor incorporation, had the lowest specific insulin binding and the greatest ability to degrade insulin. As is often the case with hormone-ligand interactions, caution is required when attempting to interpret the significance of the initial interaction in relation to a meaningful event for the cell.

Finally, specific insulin binding to human breast carcinomas and nonmalignant breast tissues has recently been demonstrated.[69] In this series, 43/48 malignant specimens showed specific binding for insulin (difference between total and suppressible binding was at least 1000 cpm or 1% of the labeled ligand added); the binding demonstrated an average K_a of $\sim 2 \times 10^9$ ℓ/mol. Specificity of binding, as judged by competition with various analogs of insulin, was as expected on the basis of biological activity. Autoradiographic studies indicated that insulin was bound to tumor cells rather than to fat or fibrous tissue. Thus, there now appears to be confirmation of the existence of insulin receptors in human breast tumors, a finding that lends further credence to the results obtained from studies with rodent mammary tumors.[28]

V. EPIDEMIOLOGICAL STUDIES

Numerous epidemiological studies have examined the empirically observed relationship between diabetes and various forms of cancer. These studies have attempted to define this relationship by determining the incidence of various forms of cancer in patients previously diagnosed to be diabetic. Alternatively, the incidence of diabetes in patients diagnosed to have cancer has also been examined. The main objective of this review is to examine the relationship of insulin (or the lack of insulin) specifically to breast cancer. For the broader discussion of diabetes and cancer in general, we refer the reader to the reviews by Kessler.[70,71]

Pertinent to the discussion of a possible relationship between insulin and breast cancer is the clinical evidence which demonstrates a positive association between cancer and abnormal glucose metabolism. Several theories have been proposed to explain how a neoplasm could produce a hypoglycemic state.[72-74] These include: (1) ectopic secretion of an insulin-like substance leading to an imbalance in the insulin-glucose relationship; (2) increased utilization of glucose by the tumor, resulting in glucose deprivation of other tissues; (3) decreased degradation of insulin caused by tumor secretion of an "insulinase" inhibitor; and (4) metastatic invasion of the liver, adrenal glands, or other organs of the endocrine system. The assumption made by these theories is that the cancer causes the glucose intolerance and not the reverse.

Epidemiologists who have specifically examined the proportion of breast cancer patients with diabetes have observed similar trends. In England, Harnett[75] found that 1.1% of primary breast cancer patients were diabetic. In a 10-year study of breast cancer patients in Grand Rapids, Michigan, Repert[76] reported that 4.9% of the patients were also diabetic and compared this percentage to the incidence of diabetes in the general population, which was 0.67%. Abnormal thyroid function was observed to be ten times more prevalent in the breast cancer patients than in the general population.

Glicksman and co-workers[77,78] compared the incidence of diabetes in breast cancer patients to all other cancer patients and found a lower incidence in breast cancer patients. Recently, Muck et al.[79] utilized 510 women with benign breast afflictions and 327 women with breast cancer in a prospective study. Matched-pairs analysis was conducted to correct for diabetogenic factors such as age and body weight. They concluded that manifest diabetes mellitus was twice (21% vs. 10%) as frequent in breast cancer patients as in patients with benign histological findings. It is interesting to note that only 34% of the carcinoma patients were aware of the diabetes prior to the study, while 75% of the women with benign afflictions were aware of the disorder. In a second study, Muck et al.[80] evaluated 792 women with breast disease, again corrected for age and body weight. They found the frequency of diabetes in breast cancer patients to be 22%; in patient groups with fibroadenoma, fibrocystic disease, and lipoma to be 1 to 3%; in patients with proliferative processes, including carcinoma *in situ*, to be 7%; and in patients with papilloma to be 14%. However, they noted that women with papilloma tended to be of a higher age and were more frequently obese than the other patients in the study. Thus, it appears that women with breast cancer have a higher incidence of diabetes than either the general population or women with benign breast disease, but they apparently have a lower incidence of diabetes when compared to patients with other forms of cancers.

Another method of investigating the relationship between cancer and diabetes has been to examine the cancer risk among diabetics. In a study of 182 autopsied cases of diabetes at the Mayo Clinic from 1925 to 1936, Dry and Tessmer[81] reported 38 cases had cancer. The most frequent sites for cancer in this small study were large intestine, pancreas, stomach, and breast. Lancaster[82] and Lancaster and Maddox[83] also reported on the cancer risk to diabetic patients admitted to the diabetic clinic of the Royal Prince Alfred Hospital, Sydney, Australia, from 1932 to 1947. They compared the number of cancer deaths in the diabetic group vs. the general population and concluded that there was an increased risk of cancer in the diabetic population. They computed observed/expected ratios for the more frequently occurring cancers. They found the largest ratios for pancreatic cancer in both male and female diabetics. Also, in female patients a large ratio was obtained for uterine cancer (including cervical cancer) and breast cancer. Unfortunately, both of these studies suffer from a limited number of patients. In studies conducted on patients from the Joslin Clinic,[84] no increased risk of breast cancer was observed in diabetic patients.

Upon evaluation of the results of studies examining the cancer risks in a diabetic population, one realizes that the conclusions of a particular study may be predetermined by the source of the data and the methods used for computation. In general, clinical studies seem to suggest a positive association between cancer and diabetes while the reverse is suggested in most autopsy-based investigations. The design of an epidemiological investigation must include an evaluation of the results according to the known variables of the diseases. Thus, age, race (or national origin), and weight are three obvious variables which must be corrected for in an analysis of risk factors involved in breast cancer or diabetes. It has been observed that two age groups have the highest frequency of breast cancer, women from 45 to 55 years of age and women from 65 to 70 years of age; the incidence of diabetes increases monotonically after age 40. Race or national origin has also been related to the risk of either breast cancer or diabetes. Women of North America and western Europe have an extremely high risk of breast cancer relative to women from Asia. Certain groups of people are more susceptible to diabetes. For example, caucasian populations in the U.S. or in western Europe show an incidence of diabetes of 5% in people over 65, while diabetes is very rare in Athabascans and Eskimos of Alaska. In the Pima Indians of Arizona, diabetes occurs in 60% of the people over 65. Increased weight, a third factor related to these diseases, has been clearly shown to increase the incidence of both diabetes and breast cancer. Hence, it becomes necessary to use matched-pair analysis (which corrects for age, weight, and demographic variables) to verify if a relationship exists between these diseases.

Many of the studies have failed to include the criteria used to diagnose diabetes or the type of diabetes which the patients in the study were prone to have. The majority of diabetics have either juvenile or mature onset diabetes. These vary in the age of onset of the diabetes and the treatment required to maintain glucohomeostasis. Juvenile diabetes usually is diagnosed in patients below 20 years of age, has a very rapid onset, and requires insulin administration. Mature onset diabetes occurs in patients of 40 years or older and can generally be controlled with diet and/or oral pancreatic stimulating compounds. Both of these forms of diabetes can be diagnosed by a glucose tolerance test and can be controlled by insulin therapy, either directly or indirectly, as insulin secretion is diminished or is absent. However, there are other forms of diabetes which are not exemplified by diminished insulin levels but rather elevated insulin levels. These diseases are referred to as insulin resistant. Therefore, relationships between diabetes and cancer can be made only when it has been determined if the observer was comparing patients with altered insulin or glucose levels. Additionally, when utilizing the results of glucose tolerance tests, one must verify that the cause of the alteration from normal has not been caused by another disease such as liver disfunction, malnutrition, infection, or thyroid diseases.

There are a number of other criteria that must be taken into consideration when designing an epidemiological study to ascertain if a relationship exists between diabetes and breast cancer. These include the time of onset of diabetes vs. the diagnosis of cancer, the genetic susceptibility to either disease, the size of the tumor, the method of maintaining glucohomeostasis, the life expectancy of a diabetic which has been corrected for death by other causes, the number of cases in the study, and the methods of selecting patients for participation in the study.

Because none of the studies presented above meet all the criteria necessary, a definitive statement cannot be made concerning the relationship between diabetes and breast cancer.

VI. CLINICAL STUDIES

Since the isolation of insulin in 1921, there have been several clinical evaluations of insulin therapy for cancer patients. In 1926, Silberstein et al.[85] treated 21 advanced cancer patients with insulin. Using insulin concentrations bordering on the limits of tolerance, they observed that further tumor growth was minimized and, in a few cases, primary and secondary tumor regression was observed. They suggested that insulin therapy may be a useful adjunct with surgery to prevent recurrence of the disease and to improve the condition of the patient. Neufeld,[86] working under the hypothesis that cancer patients suffer from dietary insufficiencies caused by the tumor, administered maximally tolerated doses of insulin to seven patients with advanced carcinoma. Treatment was continued for up to 48 days. Clinical improvement was reported in all cases, although the period of observation and the effect of the treatment on the tumors was not indicated. Koroljow[87] proposed that insulin administration could be utilized to produce hyperoxygenation, which might be detrimental to malignant cells. He treated two patients with metastatic cancer (cervix and melanoma) with a sufficient amount of insulin to induce hypoglycemic shock. Both patients showed complete remission of the disease with no recurrences observed nearly 2 years later. Thus, it appears that, by whatever mechanism, high levels have been shown to induce tumor regression in some cases.

There have also been several clinical evaluations of carbohydrate disturbances in breast cancer patients. In 1972 and 1973, Rhomberg[88] treated 130 women (30 of whom had clinical or subclinical diabetes mellitus) for progressive, metastasizing breast carcinoma with hormones and cytostatic drugs. He reported that the cancer in patients with diabetes took a protracted course. He suggested that diabetic women with breast cancer may be more responsive to hormonal therapy (estrogen, androgen, or ovariectomy) than the nondiabetic patients, since 18 of 24 diabetic patients went into objective remission whereas only one third of the remaining patients went into remission after hormonal therapy. Pearson and co-workers[89] measured the insulin levels in 23 patients with metastatic mammary carcinoma. Of the 23 patients, 12 were found to have diabetic-type glucose tolerance curves. During glucose loading, a delayed rise in serum insulin levels was observed in those subjects with diabetic-type glucose curves. Additionally, the levels of insulin reached in these patients after glucose ingestion were much lower than those in the noncancer patients. The authors suggest that there may be a decreased pancreatic insulin reserve in cancer patients. Carter and co-workers[90] examined glucose tolerance, hormone secretion, and metabolic response to growth hormone in breast cancer patients and normal women. They observed glucose intolerance, delayed and prolonged insulin secretion (but not decreased levels as Pearson has reported), increased basal growth hormone levels, and insensitivity of adipose tissue to growth hormone in the breast cancer patients. These differences could not be accounted for by differences in age, weight, stress, or nutritional status. They propose that these metabolic abnormalities may characterize host susceptibility to breast cancer or may be indicative of host response to the cancer. Hence, there is clinical evidence to suggest that breast cancer patients do have altered carbohydrate metabolism. From the work of Muck et al.,[80] it appears that this abnormality in metabolism is associated with breast cancer rather than other breast dysplasia. The suggestion by Rhomberg[88] that this metabolic imbalance may alter the course of the disease as well as the patient's response to hormonal therapy is very intriguing and surely requires further investigation.

VII. CONCLUSIONS

There is a growing interest in the role of insulin in breast cancer, and there are now several reports that have been directed towards elucidation of the effects of insulin on the growth and metabolism of experimental rodent mammary tumors. If these experimental tumors are models for some portion of the clinical disease, then it appears that insulin has to be considered as another hormonal factor in breast cancer, a factor that could result in enhancement of tumor growth or inhibition of tumor growth. In this sense, insulin would resemble other hormones, such as estrogen or perhaps prolactin, in presenting a biphasic response that may depend on dose or target cell population. The mechanisms by which such effects are noted need to be identified, and a logical initial approach is to examine those responses known to occur in normal tissues. Thus, investigation of the effects of insulin on substrate transport and subsequent effects on metabolism, protein, and DNA synthesis should shed light on how insulin may alter the growth of these tumors.

A new aspect of studies with hormones deals with hormone receptors and their regulation. Certainly, the absence of a receptor would impair the response of that cell to the hormone and this has now been demonstrated for estrogen receptors in breast cancers. For insulin, whose receptor is located in the cell membrane, either its absence or an alteration in structure could account for a lack of response. However, data obtained so far indicate that insulin receptors are present in mammary cancers, implying that the initial event of hormone-receptor interaction can occur. It would appear that if there is a defect in response, it is probably distal to the initial event. Also to be considered is the regulation of receptors either by autoregulation of the receptor or regulation by other hormones. In a multihormonal system, such as the mammary gland, regulation of one hormone receptor by a different hormone has been proposed and this may also apply for insulin. Recent studies in our laboratory suggest an insulin-estrogen relationship for regulation of receptors.

Finally, there is a suggestion from the clinical literature that abnormalities in carbohydrate metabolism are seen in women with breast cancer, who demonstrate a diabetic-type response to a glucose load. The frequency of diabetes may be higher in women with breast cancer compared to age-matched women with benign breast diseases, but the question of cause or effect remains to be answered. The difficulties with interpretation of the older epidemiological studies lie in the criteria used for classifying a patient as diabetic and there is a need to distinguish the incidence of cancer in the juvenile-onset diabetic vs. the mature-onset diabetic and the role of therapy in these situations. The employment of insulin as a therapeutic agent in conjunction with other hormonal agents might be considered should additional data become available that insulin acts to enhance response to other forms of therapy.

ACKNOWLEDGMENTS

Studies cited from the authors' laboratory were supported by USPHS Grants CA16660, CA12836, and CA11198 from the National Cancer Institute, National Institutes of Health.

REFERENCES

1. Beatson, G. T., On the treatment of inoperable cases of carcinomas of the mamma. Suggestion for a new method of treatment with illustrative cases, *Lancet,* 2, 104, 1896.
2. Lyons, W. R., Li, C. H., and Johnson, R. E., The hormonal control of mammary growth and lactation, *Recent Prog. Horm. Res.,* 14, 219, 1958.
3. Kumareson, P. and Turner, C. W., Effect of graded levels of insulin on lactation in the rat, *Proc. Soc. Exp. Biol. Med.,* 119, 415, 1965.
4. Martin, R. J. and Baldwin, R. L., Effects of alloxan diabetes on lactational performance and mammary tissue metabolism in the rat, *Endocrinology,* 88, 863, 1971.
5. Ahren, K. and Jacobson, D., Mammary gland growth in hypophysectomized rats injected with ovarian hormones and insulin, *Acta Physiol. Scand.,* 37, 190, 1956.
6. Ahren, K. and Etienne, M., Stimulation of mammary glands in hypophysectomized male rats treated with ovarian hormones and insulin, *Acta Endocrinol.,* 28, 89, 1958.
7. Ahren, K., The effect of various doses of oestrone and progesterone on the mammary glands of castrated hypophysectomized rats injected with insulin, *Acta Endocrinol.,* 30, 435, 1959.
8. Topper, Y. J. and Oka, T., Some aspects of mammary gland development in the mature mouse, in *Lactation. A Comprehensive Treatise,* Vol. 1, Larson, B. L. and Smith, V. R., Eds., Academic Press, New York, 1974, 327.
9. von Bruchhausen, F., Action of insulin on some organs and on differentiation, *Handb. Exp. Pharmakol.,* 32 (part 2), 1975.
10. Goranson, E. S. and Tilser, G. J., Studies on the relationship of alloxan-diabetes and tumor growth, *Cancer Res.,* 15, 626, 1955.
11. Salter, J. M., Meyer, R., and Best, C. H., Effect of insulin and glucagon on tumour growth, *Br. Med. J.,* 2, 5, 1958.
12. Heuson, J. C., Coune, A., and Heimann, R., Cell proliferation induced by insulin in organ culture of rat mammary carcinoma, *Exp. Cell Res.,* 45, 351, 1967.
13. Huggins, C., Grand, L. C., and Brillantes, F. P., Mammary cancer induction by a single feeding of polynuclear hydrocarbons and its suppression, *Nature* (London), 189, 204, 1961.

14. **Heuson, J. C. and Legros, N.**, Study of the growth-promoting effect of insulin in relation to carbohydrate metabolism in organ culture of rat mammary carcinoma, *Eur. J. Cancer*, 4, 1, 1968.

15. **Heuson, J. C. and Legros, N.**, Effect of insulin and of alloxan diabetes on growth of the rat mammary carcinoma *in vivo*, *Eur. J. Cancer*, 6, 349, 1970.

16. **Heuson, J. C. and Legros, N.**, Influence of insulin deprivation on growth of the 7,12-dimethylbenz(a)anthracene-induced mammary carcinoma in rats subjected to alloxan diabetes and food restriction, *Cancer Res.*, 32, 226, 1972.

17. **Heuson, J. C., Legros, N., and Heimann, R.**, Influence of insulin administration on growth of the 7,12-dimethylbenz(a)anthracene-induced mammary carcinoma in intact oophorectomized and hypophysectomized rats, *Cancer Res.*, 32, 233, 1972.

18. **Cohen, N. D. and Hilf, R.**, Influence of insulin on growth and metabolism of 7,12-dimethylbenz(a)anthracene-induced mammary tumors, *Cancer Res.*, 34, 3245, 1974.

19. **Harmon, J. T. and Hilf, R.**, Insulin binding and glucose transport in the R3230AC mammary adenocarcinoma, *J. Supramol. Struct.*, 4, 233, 1976.

20. **Cohen, N. D. and Hilf, R.**, Effect of estrogen treatment on DMBA-induced mammary tumor growth and biochemistry in intact and diabetic rats, *Proc. Soc. Exp. Biol. Med.*, 148, 339, 1975.

21. **Elbrink, J. and Bihler, J.**, Membrane transport: its relation to cellular metabolic rates, *Science*, 188, 1177, 1975.

22. **Harmon, J. T. and Hilf, R.**, Effect of insulin on glucose transport in DMBA-induced mammary tumors, *Eur. J. Cancer*, 12, 933, 1976.

23. **Cohen, N. D. and Hilf, R.**, Influence of insulin on estrogen-induced responses in the R3230AC mammary carcinoma, *Cancer Res.*, 35, 560, 1975.

24. **Cuatrecasas, P.**, Membrane receptors, *Annu. Rev. Biochem.*, 43, 169, 1974.

25. **Cuatrecasas, P., Hollenberg, M. D., Chang, K. J., and Bennett, V.**, Hormone receptor complexes and their modulation of membrane function, *Recent Prog. Horm. Res.*, 31, 37, 1975.

26. **Roth, J., Kahn, C. R., Lesniak, M. A., Gordon, P., De Meyts, P., Megyesi, K., Neville, D. M., Jr., Gavin, J. R., Soll, A. H., Freychet, P., Goldfine, I. D., Bar, R. S., and Archer, J. A.**, Receptors for insulin, NSILA-s and growth hormone: applications to disease state in man, *Recent Prog. Horm. Res.*, 31, 95, 1975.

27. **Kahn, C. R.**, Membrane receptors for hormone and neurotransmitters, *J. Cell Biol.*, 70, 261, 1976.

28. **Harmon, J. T. and Hilf, R.**, Identification and characterization of the insulin receptors in the R3230AC mammary adenocarcinoma of the rat, *Cancer Res.*, 36, 3993, 1976.

29. **Gavin, J. R., Roth, J., Neville, D. M., Jr., DeMeyts, P., and Buell, D. N.**, Insulin-dependent regulation of insulin receptor concentrations: a direct demonstration in cell culture, *Proc. Natl. Acad. Sci. U.S.A.*, 71, 84, 1974.

30. **DeMeyts, P., Roth, J., Neville, D. M., Jr., Gavin, J. R., and Lesniak, M. A.**, Insulin interactions with its receptors: experimental evidence for negative cooperativity, *Biochem. Biophys. Res. Commun.*, 43, 400, 1973.

31. **Boeymaems, J. M. and Dumont, J. E.**, The two-step model of ligand-receptor interaction, *Mol. Cell. Endocrinol.*, 7, 33, 1977.

32. **Jacobs, S. and Cuatrecasas, P.**, The mobile receptor-hypothesis and ''cooperativity'' of hormone binding, application to insulin, *Biochim. Biophys. Acta*, 433, 482, 1976.

33. **Narakara, H. J. and Ozard, P.**, Studies on tissue permeability. IX. The effect of insulin on the penetration of 3-O-methylglucose-³H in frog muscle, *J. Biol. Chem.*, 238, 40, 1963.

34. **Czech, M. P., Lawrence, J. C., and Lynn, W. S.**, Hexose transport in isolated human fat cells. A model system for investigating insulin action on membrane transport, *J. Biol. Chem.*, 249, 5421, 1974.

35. **Harmon, J. T. and Hilf, R.**, Effect of insulin to decrease glucose transport in dissociated cells from the R3230AC mammary adenocarcinoma of diabetic rats, *Biochim. Biophys. Acta*, 443, 114, 1976.

36. **Hissin, P. J. and Hilf, R.**, Characteristics of proline transport into R3230AC mammary tumor cells, *Biochem. Biophys. Acta*, 508, 401, 1978.

36a. **Hissin, P. J. and Hilf, R.**, α-Aminoisobutyrate transport into cells from R3230AC mammary adenocarcinoma. Evidence for sodium ion-dependent and -independent carrier mediated entry and effects of diabetes, *Biochem. J.*, 176, 205, 1978.

37. **Finerman, G. A. M. and Rosenberg, L. E. E.**, Amino acid transport in bone. Evidence for separate transport systems for neutral amino acids, *J. Biol. Chem.*, 241, 1487, 1966.

38. **Gazzola, G. S., Franchi, R., Saibene, V., Ronchi, P., and Guiddotti, G. G.**, Regulation of amino acid transport in chick embryo heart cells. I. Adaptive system of mediation for neutral amino acids, *Biochim. Biophys. Acta*, 266, 407, 1972.

38a. **Hissin, P. J. and Hilf, R.**, Effects of insulin *in vivo* and *in vitro* on amino acid transport into cells from the R3230AC mammary adenocarcinoma and their relationship to tumor growth, *Cancer Res.*, 38, 3646, 1978.

38b. Hilf, R., Hissin, P. J., and Shafie, S. M., Regulatory interrelationships for insulin and estrogen action in mammary tumors, *Cancer Res.*, 38, 4076, 1978.

39. Lesniak, M. A. and Roth, J., Regulation of receptor concentration by homologous hormone. Effect of human growth hormone on its receptor in IM-9 lymphocytes, *J. Biol. Chem*, 251, 3720, 1975.

40. Harrison, L. C., Martin, F. I. R., and Melick, R. A., Correlation between insulin receptor binding in isolated fat cells and insulin sensitivity in obese human subjects, *J. Clin. Invest.*, 58, 1435, 1976.

41. Lockwood, D. H., Livingston, J. N., and Amatruda, J. J., Relation of insulin receptors to insulin resistance, *Fed. Proc. Fed. Am. Soc. Exp. Biol.*, 34, 1564, 1975.

42. Shafie, S. M., Gibson, S. L., and Hilf, R., Effect of insulin and estrogen on hormone binding in the R3230AC mammary adenocarcinoma, *Cancer Res.*, 37, 4641, 1977.

43. Shafie, S. M. and Hilf, R., Relationship between insulin and estrogen binding to growth response in 7,12-dimethylbenz(a)anthracene-induced rat mammary tumors, *Cancer Res.*, 38, 759, 1978.

44. Mukherjee, A. S., Washburn, L. L., and Banerjee, M. R., Role of insulin as a permissive hormone in mammary gland development, *Nature* (London), 246, 159, 1973.

45. Smith, R. D., Hilf, R., and Senior, A. E., Prolactin binding to R3230AC Mammary carcinoma and liver in hormone-treated and diabetic rats, *Cancer Res.*, 37, 595, 1977.

46. Smith, R. D., Hilf, R., and Senior, A. E., Prolactin binding to 7,12-dimethylbenz(a)anthracene-induced mammary tumors and livers in diabetic rats, *Cancer Res.*, 37, 4070, 1977.

47. Gibson, S. L. and Hilf, R., Influence of hormonal alteration of host on estrogen binding capacity in 7,12-dimethylbenz(a)anthracene-induced mammary tumors, *Cancer Res.*, 36, 3736, 1976.

48. Elias, J. J., Effect of insulin and cortisol on organ cultures of adult mouse mammary gland, *Proc. Soc. Exp. Biol. Med.*, 101, 500, 1959.

49. Topper, Y. J., Multiple hormone interactions in the development of mammary epithelial cells, *Recent Prog. Horm. Res.*, 26, 287, 1970.

50. Rivera, E. M. and Bern, H. A., Influence of insulin on maintenance and secretory stimulation of mouse mammary tissues by hormones in organ-culture, *Endocrinology*, 69, 340, 1961.

51. Stockdale, F. E., Juergens, W. G., and Topper, Y. J., A histological and biochemical study of hormone dependent differentiation of mammary gland tissue *in vitro*, *Dev. Biol.*, 13, 266, 1966.

52. Elias, J. J. and Rivera, E. M., Comparisons of the responses of normal precancerous and neoplastic mouse mammary tissues to hormones *in vitro*, *Cancer Res.*, 19, 505, 1959.

53. Turkington, R. W. and Hilf, R., Hormonal dependence of DNA synthesis in mammary carcinoma cells *in vitro*, *Science*, 160, 1457, 1968.

54. Pasteels, J. L., Heuson, J. C., Heuson-Stiennon, J., and Legros, N., Effects of insulin, prolactin, progesterone and estradiol on DNA synthesis in organ culture of 7,12-dimethylbenz(a)anthracene-induced at mammary tumors, *Cancer Res.*, 36, 2162, 1976.

55. Welsch, C. W., de Iturri, G. C., and Brennan, M. J., DNA synthesis of human, mouse and rat mammary carcinomas *in vitro*, *Cancer*, 38, 1272, 1976.

56. Barker, B. E., Fanger, H., and Faires, P., Human mammary slices in organ culture. I. Method of culture and preliminary observations on the effect of insulin, *Exp. Cell Res.*, 35, 437, 1964.

57. Ceriani, R. L., Contesso, G. P., and Nataf, B. M., Hormone requirement for growth and differentiation of the human mammary gland in organ culture, *Cancer Res.*, 32, 2190, 1972.

58. Forsyth, I. A., Organ culture techniques and the study of hormone effects on the mammary gland, *J. Dairy Res.*, 3, 419, 1971.

59. Wellings, S. R. and Jentoft, V. L., Organ cultures of normal, dysplastic, hyperplastic and neoplastic human mammary tissues, *J. Natl. Cancer Inst.*, 49, 329, 1972.

60. Elias, J. J. and Armstrong, R. C., Hyperplastic and metaplastic responses of human mammary fibroadenoma and dysplasias in organ culture, *J. Natl. Cancer Inst.*, 51, 1341, 1973.

61. Welsch, C. W. and McManus, M. J., Stimulation of DNA synthesis by human placental lactogen or insulin in organ cultures of benign human breast tumors, *Cancer Res.*, 37, 2257, 1977.

62. Soule, H. D., Vasquez, L., Long, A., Albert, S., and Brennan, M., A human cell line from a pleural effusion derived from a breast carcinoma, *J. Natl. Cancer Inst.*, 51, 1409, 1973.

63. Lippman, M., Hormone-responsive human breast cancer in continuous culture, in *Breast Cancer: Trends in Research and Treatment*, Heuson, J. C., Mattheiem, W. H., and Rozencweig, M., Eds., Raven Press, New York, 1976, 111.

64. Osborne, C. K., Bolan, G., Monaco, M. E., and Lippman, M., Hormone responsive human breast cancer in long-term tissue culture: effect of insulin, *Proc. Natl. Acad. Sci. U.S.A.*, 73, 4536, 1976.

65. Shafie, S. M. and Brooks, S. C., The relationship of insulin to the regulation of breast cancer cells by 17β-estradiol, *Cancer Res.*, submitted for publication.

66. Shafie, S. M. and Brooks, S. C., The relationship of insulin to the regulation of breast tumor cells by 17β-estradiol, *Fed. Proc. Fed. Am. Soc. Biol.*, 35, 1628, 1976.

67. Lippman, M. E., Osborne, C. K., Knazek, R., and Young, N., In vitro model systems for the study of hormone-dependent human breast cancer, *N. Engl. J. Med.*, 296, 154, 1977.

68. Osborne, C. K., Monaco, M. E., Lippman, M. E., and Kahn, C. R., Correlation among insulin binding, degradation, and biological activity in human breast cancer cells in long-term tissue culture, *Cancer Res.,* 38, 94, 1978.
69. Holdaway, I. M. and Friesen, H. G., Hormone binding of human mammary carcinoma, *Cancer Res.,* 37, 1946, 1977.
70. Kessler, I. I., Cancer mortality among diabetics, *J. Natl. Cancer Inst.,* 44, 673, 1970.
71. Kessler, I. I., Cancer and diabetes mellitus. A review of the literature, *J. Chronic Dis.,* 23, 579, 1971.
72. Lowbeer, L., Hypoglycemia-producing extra pancreatic neoplasma, *Am. J. Clin. Pathol.,* 35, 233, 1961.
73. Sachs, B. A., Endocrine disorders produced by nonendocrine malignant tumors, *Bull. N. Y. Acad. Med.,* 41, 1069, 1965.
74. Unger, R. H., The riddle of tumor hypoglycemia, *Am. J. Med.,* 40, 325, 1966.
75. Harnett, W. L., A Survey of Cancer in London, Report of the Clinical Cancer Research Committee, British Empire Cancer Campaign, London, 1952.
76. Repert, R. W., Breast carcinoma study: relation to thyroid disease and diabetes, *J. Mich. State Med. Soc.,* 51, 1315, 1952.
77. Glicksman, A. S., Myers, W. P. L., and Rawson, R. W., Diabetes mellitus and carbohydrate metabolism in patients with cancer, *Med. Clin. North Am.,* 40, 887, 1956.
78. Glicksman, A. S. and Rawson, R. W., Diabetes and altered carbohydrate metabolism in patients with cancer, *Cancer (Philadelphia),* 9, 1127, 1956.
79. Muck, B. R., Trotnow, S., and Hommel, G., Cancer of the breast, diabetes and pathological glucose tolerance, *Arch. Gynaekol.,* 220, 73, 1975.
80. Muck, B. R., Trotnow, S., Egger, H., and Hommel, G., Altered carbohydrate metabolism in breast cancer and benign breast affections, *Arch. Gynaekol.,* 221, 83, 1976.
81. Dry, T. J. and Tessmer, C. F., Postmortem findings in cases of diabetes, *Minn. Med.,* 24, 96, 1941.
82. Lancaster, H. O., The mortality in Australia from cancer of the pancreas, *Med. J. Aust.,* 1, 596, 1954.
83. Lancaster, H. O. and Maddox, J. K., Diabetic mortality in Australia, *Australas. Ann. Med.,* 7, 145, 1958.
84. Joslin, E. P., Lombard, H. L., and Burrows, R. E., Diabetes and cancer, *N. Engl. J. Med.,* 260, 486, 1959.
85. Silberstein, F., Freud, J., and Revesz, T., Versuche, inoperable Carcinome mit Insulin zu behandeln, *Z. Gesamte Exp. Med.,* 55, 78, 1927.
86. Neufeld, O., Insulin therapy in terminal cancer: a preliminary report, J. Am. Geriatr. Soc., 10, 274, 1962.
87. Koroljow, S., Two cases of malignant tumors with metastases apparently treated successfully with hypoglycemic coma, *Psychiatr. Q.,* 36, 262, 1962.
88. Rhomberg, W., Metastasierendes Mammakarzinom and Diabetes mellituseine prognostisch günstige Krankheitskombination, *Dtsch. Med. Wochenschr.,* 100, 2422, 1975.
89. Pearson, O. H., Llerena, O., Samaan, N., and Gonzalez, D., Serum growth hormone and insulin levels in patients with breast cancer, in *Prognostic Factors in Breast Cancer,* Forrest, A. P. M. and Kunkler, P. B., Eds., Williams & Wilkins, Baltimore, 1968, 421.
90. Carter, A. C., Lefkon, B. W., Farlin, M., and Feldman, E. B., Metabolic parameters in women with metastatic breast cancer, *J. Clin. Endocrinol. Metab.,* 40, 260, 1975.

Chapter 6

THYROID HORMONES AND TUMOR DEVELOPMENT

B. A. Eskin

TABLE OF CONTENTS

I. INTRODUCTION

Historically, publications relating thyroid hormones with cancer development appeared in the last century. Because of clinical correlations that thyroid secretions or lack of them might be involved in the etiology of cancer, a voluminous literature exists; however, it has only been within the last decade that research on thyroid hormone and/or iodine action has effectually shown intracellular changes to occur.

Most of the older data depended on chance or retrospective observations of clinical case histories and employed thyroid function tests which were difficult to interpret. While the newer radioimmune assays and competitive protein binding procedures are more precise, they are predicated on measuring serum and thyroid levels of free and bound thyronines, not end-organ responses. Experimental animal data provide evidence of tumorigenesis in many tissues when altered thyroid or iodine conditions are employed as primary or secondary carcinogens. Once again, the data seem inconclusive.

An analysis of the effects of thyroid hormones on tumor development requires consideration of both the epidemiologic clinical data and the available biochemical impact of these hormones on the affected end organs. Tumorigenesis resulting from thyroid hormone alterations has been suspected in various tissues and organs. Within tissue cells many changes have been described as directly influenced by the thyroid hormones, triiodothyronine and thyroxine. However, in addition to these known active effluents, the thyroid gland has major control over the total metabolism of body iodine and, in so doing, regulates quantitatively and qualitatively the iodine and iodine salts available in the serum and distributed to other tissues. The thyroid gland is an endocrine gland which is centrally regulated and which responds to many physiological barometers.

The physiologic effects of thyroid hormones have been described in many tissues in animals and humans.[1] Specific intracellular responses have been experimentally studied in several tissues, particularly bone and brain.[2,3] However, in reviewing the existing literature, few tumors have been described in tissues where iodine is not demonstrated by radioactive iodine uptakes. Areas where moderate quantities of iodine have been measured in humans and experimental animals by such studies are the salivary glands, liver, skin, ovary and other female reproductive organs, testes, gastric mucosa, and the mammary glands.[4-6] Descriptive data have been published on all of these tissues, but much of the recent work, both basic and clinical, has been related to the mammary glands.

Thus, tumor development associated with thyroid hormones may result from (1) abnormal thyroid hormone action directly on cell biochemistry, (2) disturbances in iodine metabolism, or (3) variations in pituitary or hypothalamic secretions as a response to thyroid or iodine alterations.

In this chapter, the clinical and basic research studies that seem pertinent will be cited. There are several reviews of the early data and the reader who wishes extensive bibliography is referred to them.[7,8,11,12] There have been many conflicting theories involving thyroid and iodine metabolism in the etiology of tumors. This chapter will attempt to review the existing data available and present a plausible theory of how thyroid may cause tissue neoplasia.

II. THYROID ENDOCRINOLOGY

A. The Thyroid Gland

The sequence of biochemical steps in the thyroid gland is complex, but it results in the secretion of two primary hormones: tetraiodothyronine (thyroxine, T_4) and triiodothyronine (T_3). Calcitonin, which retards bone absorption, is secreted as well; however, the action of this hormone does not seem pertinent to tumorigenesis. The thyronines are notably implicated and the endocrinology of these thyroid hormones will be described in this section. Further details may be obtained from several texts on the subject since only information pertinent to tumorigenesis is included.[9-11]

The thyroid gland consists of two butterfly-shaped lobes joined by an isthmus, weighs 20 to 25 g in the human adult, and is attached to the anterior aspect of the trachea. The thyroid gland stores its hormonal products as thyroglobulin in colloid-containing, epithelial-lined vesicles. Thyroglobulin contains two groups of iodinated compounds: (1) iodotyrosines: monoiodotyrosine (MIT) and diiodotyrosine (DIT), and (2) iodothyronines: T_3 and T_4 (Figure 1). Follicular colloid contains the amino acid thyroxine in the form of thyroglobulin molecules with up to 115 tyrosyl residues.

Thyrogenesis first occurs about the 16th to 18th day after fertilization providing only exocrine functions. The early development of the thyroid gland is presumably independent of pituitary influence, but as the gland begins to form colloid (14th week) further thyroid development and regulation require pituitary control since a direct correlation exists between thyroid follicular cell height and levels of thyroid stimulating hormone (TSH). Maternal chorionic TSH from the placenta has been measured, but its effect is not known.

B. Iodine Metabolism

Nutritional iodine is reduced to iodide and absorbed by the gastrointestinal glands, particularly the upper tract, where it is made available to the blood stream. Carried by the blood vessels, it appears to be taken up by several organs such as the salivary glands, stomach mucosa, ovaries, testes, and mammary tissues, but the iodide-trapping mechanism in the thyroid is many times more efficient. Of the total body iodine, 90% is concentrated in the thyroid pool. This is in the form of organic iodide in the thyroglobulin and has a turnover rate of 1% daily.

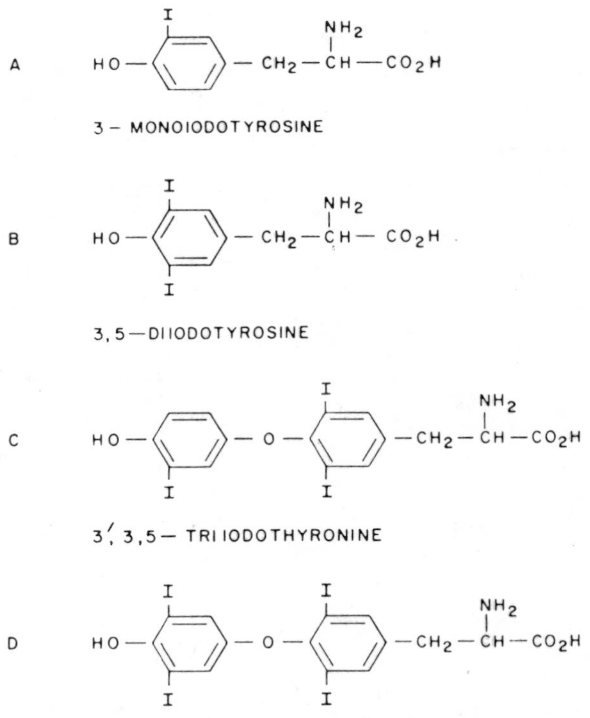

FIGURE 1. The iodotyrosines (A and B) and iodothyronines — thyroid hormones (C and D).

The organs that show evidence of iodine transport appear to also mimic the intracellular biology seen in the thyroid gland. It is in these tissues that tumor development has been described in the literature as allegedly due to changes in thyroid hormones.

The processes involved in hormone synthesis in the thyroid gland are primarily that of iodine transport, organification, and release. The progression has been subdivided by most thyroidologists[10] into several steps: (1) iodide transport, (2) iodine oxidation, (3) iodination, (4) colloid resorption, (5) thyroglobulin proteolysis, (6) deiodination of iodotyrosines, and (7) hormone secretion and blood distribution (Figure 2). In some of the extrathyroidal tissues, which show the presence of iodine by biochemical analyses or radioactive uptakes, evidence of transport, oxidation, and iodination have been described.[5,6,12-14] These events have been shown to occur also in tissues where there is tumor development. A short description of these biochemical sequences leading to thyroid hormone formation follows.

1. Iodide Transport and Organification

Iodide transport is the biochemical process of rapid iodide intake through the cell membranes of the thyroid gland from the extracellular fluid. This unique mechanism involves iodide movement against an electrolyte concentration gradient with subsequent rapid diffusion into the follicular lumens. The activity of this "trapping mechanism" is easily assessed by the use of agents such as perchlorates, thiocyanates, nitrites, dinitrophenols, and cardiac glycosides which inhibit iodide. The diffusion reaction requires an energy source, intact cell membranes and organelles, and the ability to transport sodium (Na^+) and potassium (K^+) through an adenosine triphosphatase system. TSH secretion and iodide ingestion cause increased iodide concentration.

Iodide is converted to iodine in the thyroid by an oxidizing system, considered to be a peroxidase. Iodide thus metabolized is removed from the iodine pool and can no

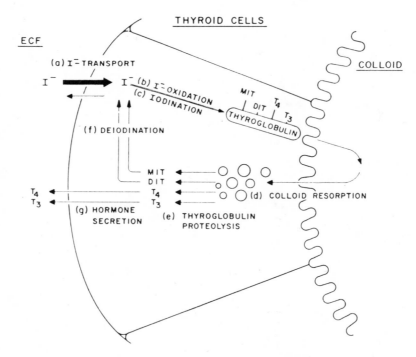

FIGURE 2.   The pathways of iodine metabolism in the thyroid. (From Werner, S. C. and Ingbar, S. H., *The Thyroid,* Harper & Row, New York, 1971. With permission.)

longer be discharged by thiocyanate, perchlorate, or other inhibitors of iodide transport. The reaction catalyzed by peroxidase in vitro has many properties of the iodination reaction in vivo, including inhibition by antithyroid agents (propylthiouracil) and by high concentrations of iodide (Wolff-Chaikoff effect).

Tyrosyls are iodinated when exposed to iodine in the cell strata. By means of an iodinase enzyme, iodination of certain tyrosyl moieties within the thyroglobulin takes place. In an euthyroid individual, equal amounts of MIT and DIT are formed. In iodine deficiency, a decrease in the elaboration of DIT leads to a preferential synthesis of T_3, the biologically more effective hormone. Hence, clinical euthyroidism is maintained in the face of iodine deficiency.

2. Thyroxine and Triiodotyrosine Formation

MIT and DIT molecules proximated within the thyroglobulin enzymatically couple into T_3 and T_4 at the cell colloid interface. When small amounts of antithyroid are given, inhibition of coupling occurs with increased MIT and DIT remaining. T_3 and T_4 are released by pinocytosis from the thyroglobulin colloid and enter the epithelial follicular cells. TSH activates membrane adenyl cyclase with the release of the second messenger, cAMP. By these processes the biologically active compounds T_4 and T_3 are released into the parafollicular capillaries along with small amounts of thyroglobulin and minute amounts of MIT and DIT. TSH also stimulates glucose metabolism and oxygen consumption from which presumably energy and cofactors are derived which are essential for thyroid hormonigenesis. There is presently good evidence that surface phospholipids may be iodinated and organified.

In the follicle cell, deiodinase enzymes remove iodine from the iodotyrosines but not from iodothyronines. The iodine released in this step is quantitatively important in synthetic processes and constitutes over one half of the iodine used for the iodination of thyroglobulin-tyrosyl molecules.

C. Thyroid Hormones and Distribution

Extrathyroidal tissues appear to be responsible for the peripheral conversion of T_4 to T_3. Both thyroid hormones T_4 and T_3 are carried by the blood serum reversibly but firmly bound to serum proteins. The major carrier is thyroid binding globulin (TBG), a glycoprotein, while thyroid binding prealbumin (TBPA) and albumin (TBA) bind to a lesser extent. TBG and TBPA binding sites are saturable, whereas those of albumin are not. Structural relationships determine the binding affinities of T_4 and T_3 to the binding proteins, and T_3 is not appreciably bound to TBPA. The affinity of T_3 for TBG is weaker than that of T_4 and is, therefore, readily displaced by the latter.

Biological activities as well as degradation of the thyroid hormones are influenced by the binding affinities to carriers. Of circulating T_4, 0.4% exists in the free form and 99.6% is distributed as follows: 60% bound to TBG, 30% to TBPA, and the remainder to albumin. The proportion of free T_3 is ten times greater than T_4 (i.e., 4.0% is free and 96.0% is protein bound). The rapid onset of action of T_3 is due to its looser affinity for protein binding. The intrinsically greater biologic activity of T_3, compared with T_4, cannot be ascribable to differences in binding affinity.

D. Extrathyroidal Regulation

There are two major regulatory mechanisms for thyroid activity: hypothalamic-pituitary control and intrathyroidal autoregulation. TSH influences thyroid gland structure, hormonigenesis, and quantity of stored colloid. TSH stimulates intrathyroidal metabolic processes which include glucose oxidation, phospholipid synthesis, and RNA synthesis.

The release of TSH from the pituitary depends on the serum levels of free T_4 and T_3 (Figure 3). The pituitary influence seems more effective in the pituitary-thyroid axis than in the other target organs regulated by trophic hormones. TSH secretion is inversely proportional to the metabolic effects of T_4 and T_3 in the pituitary.

The hypothalamus exerts a modulating influence on pituitary TSH secretion through the thyrotropin releasing hormone (TRH), but TRH does not appear to be the final regulator of this feedback control for the pituitary-thyroid axis. TRH, however, has been found to have a peripheral effect on the pituitary by increasing the secretion of prolactin.[15] Thus, many believe that TRH may be the prolactin releasing hormone (PRH).

Recent studies have shown that intrathyroidal mechanisms exist which buffer the level of hormones stored within the thyroid independent of TSH secretion. Large pulses of iodide depress the organic binding and coupling reactions within the gland and thereby prevent acute massive increases in hormone synthesis (Wolff-Chaikoff). Acute iodine deficiency causes extracellular depletion of iodide but induces an increase in iodide clearance and uptake by the thyroid. However, under chronic conditions the thyroid content of organic iodine is inversely related to the ability of the iodide transport system. Decreased levels of thyroid hormone stores initiate changes in glandular function and in the responses to TSH. The iodide transport mechanism of the thyroid is more responsive to TSH in a gland depleted of iodide than in a gland rich in iodide.[16] These changes increase thyroid hormone synthesis. On the other hand, when there are increased hormone stores, TSH released by the pituitary is inhibited, and the biosynthetic steps are suppressed.

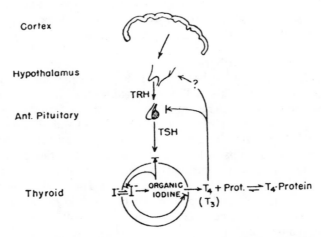

FIGURE 3.   Diagram of the factors that regulate thyroid function. Thyroid hormones (T_4 and T_3) in the pituitary, as reflected by their unbound concentrations in blood, inhibit secretion of thyroid stimulating hormone (TSH). The TSH releasing hormone (TRH) sets the threshold in the pituitary at which this negative feedback occurs. Factors regulating the secretion of TRH are uncertain, but may include influences from higher centers and a stimulatory effect of the thyroid hormones. Autoregulatory control of thyroid function is also shown. High concentrations of intrathyroid iodide decrease the rate of release of thyroid iodine. In addition, the magnitude of the organic iodine pool inversely influences the iodide transport mechanism and the response to TSH. (From Williams, R. H., *Textbook of Endocrinology*, 5th ed., W. B. Saunders, Philadelphia, 1974, chap. 4. With permission.)

III. INTRACELLULAR METABOLISM

The effect of thyronines on the peripheral cell has been a concern of many workers, and several acceptable theories have evolved. Even so, no single regulatory reaction explains the multiple end-organ effects of thyroid hormones.

As recently described, the actions of all hormones fall into two general classes: they either influence cytoplasmic and nuclear processes through secondary messengers, notably of the adenyl cyclase system, as a consequence of their primary interactions with highly specific receptors on plasma membranes (protein hormones and biogenic amines) or they enter the cell, engage with cytoplasmic receptors, and thereafter enter the nucleus where they directly influence gene expression.[17]

As yet, reproducible evidence that T_4 acts according to a combination of these mechanisms has not been developed. The alanyl side chains present in the T_4 and T_3 molecules confer remarkable biologic activity to the molecule. If the iodine is replaced by another halogen, a decrease in the level of intracellular activity occurs, since the iodines provide stability by preventing free rotation about the ether oxygen.[10] The necessary configuration for attachment to target receptors may require these spatial positions.

One theory that has evolved considers T_4 and its analogs as essential amino acids, which respond accordingly at the cell membrane. According to the amino acid hypothesis, thyronines would be expected to act along one or another of the anticipated hormonal paths as are other individual amino acids and their derivatives in the course of expressing control functions in metabolism. However, the encompassing role of T_4 itself is explained, at least at the first level, by its identification with the general biologic role of amino acids and amino acid analogs.[17,18]

In tumor formation there would be concern over the mechanism of receptor responses and potential abnormalities in RNA replication that would result. These changes can occur by an error in thyroid hormone synthesis. If, on the other hand, the cause of tumor growth and development in the tissue involved is an abnormality in the intrinsic cell processes that cause a defect in transport or organification of iodide or iodine, the condition seems more approachable.

Evidence has been presented for the metabolic mechanisms within the cells of bone, brain, and fetal nervous systems as a response to protein action by the thyronines;[19] as yet, these tissues have not been implicated as tumorigenic under conditions of altered thyroid hormone synthesis. In the breast and stomach glands, abnormal iodine metabolism has shown dysplastic and neoplastic effects.[20-22] In these examples the iodine and not the tyrosyl protein material appears to be responsible for the tissue changes that occur. Thus, it is difficult to assign definitive biochemical end-organ responses for all the actions of thyroid hormones. *There may be more than one intracellular sequence available, and the choice is dependent on the metabolic function to be served.*

Using these basic data, a discussion of the effect of thyroid hormones on tumor development will be presented.

IV. MAMMARY GLAND

A. Introduction

During the last several decades a large number of publications have alluded to abnormal thyroid function as a causative factor of mammary tumor growth and development in animals and humans. The early findings, in general, were inconsistent and seemed to represent the sum of multiple factors rather than simple responses to altered thyroid hormones. More recent studies employ fewer variables and gain consistency by measuring the iodine and thyroid hormone available, in both the clinical and experimental programs. The results have stimulated biochemical intracellular research as well as implicating sex hormone interaction in the growth of dysplasias and neoplasias.

B. Clinical Studies

Many articles have shown that altered clinical conditions of the thyroid place the patient at risk for breast cancer. Conversely, breast cancer statistics are employed to show a remarkable incidence of thyroid disease among these patients. While thyroid hormone-mammary gland interaction was implied before the turn of the century,[23] most of the publications utilizing adequate populations for statistical evaluation have appeared only since 1950.[7] In the following sections many of these clinical studies are described. Although not exhaustive, they are representative of the huge literature that has accumulated suggesting a possible clinical interrelationship between these two disease states.

1. Epidemiologic Studies

A correlation between thyroid and breast cancer has been considered and presumably investigated since 1890,[23] but no formal clinical or animal experiments about a relationship between thyroid and mammary gland response was published until the early 1940s.[24] Available statistics indicate high rates of breast cancer in regions of known endemic goiter and lower rates where goiter was not endemic. The incidence of breast cancer is high in Mexico and Thailand, both of which are regions of endemic goiter, while the incidence of breast carcinoma is low in Japan and Iceland where goiter is not endemic.[8,25-27] Higher incidence rates of breast cancer have been published concerning specific regions of endemic goiter in Poland, Switzerland, Australia, and the Soviet Union.[28,29] In the U.S. an amazingly close correspondence exists between regions of high breast cancer mortality and areas of endemic goiter as described by literature from the World Health Organization.[30] Some observations suggest that the factor or factors responsible for parallel differences in the rates of breast cancer in different regions of the world are environmental rather than genetic.

Workers have argued that the death rate in breast cancer remains unaltered although a remarkable decline in the incidence of goiter in the U.S. has occurred.[31] However, iodine deficiency is not always reflected by a goiter. It has been shown that iodine deficiency is not always reflected by a goiter. It has been shown that iodine deficiency, particularly when inadequately treated with iodine replacement, may metabolically remain in the presence of a normal-sized gland.[32]

2. Breast Cancer in Thyroid Disease

Repert[33] and Loesser[34] showed that patients with thyroid dysfunction had breast cancer ten times more commonly than expected in a similarly controlled population. Hypothyroid patients particularly had a higher incidence of breast cancer than normal women. Thyroid extract was responsible for a reduction in the incidence of breast cancer recurrence following radical mastectomy in one series.[34] Ellerker[35] reported a higher incidence (6%) of breast cancer in thyroidectomized women as compared with the general population (2%) and conversely a higher incidence of goiter (7%) in a large population with breast cancer.

Sommers[36] noted that only 14% of the breast cancer patients had normal thyroid glands; 65% of his controls showed a histologically normal thyroid. In a negative study, Wynder et al.[37] used a controlled population of women and concluded that hyperthyroidism was less likely to be found in breast cancer patients than in the normal group of women. Bogardus and Finley[25,27] showed that over half of the patients in their series with breast cancer had goitrous thyroid glands but none were hyperthyroid. In 18.5% of breast cancer patients in a series described by Backwinkel and Jackson,[31] hypothyroidism was present. The population employed was not paired for age or geographical location.

Patients who have had thyroidectomy for hyperthyroidism or nontoxic goiter did not develop breast carcinoma after a control period of 5 years.[38] Benign cystic disease of the breast was found to be greatly increased in patients with thyroid disease. The presence of breast changes occurred more often in hypothyroid than hyperthyroid women.[39]

Chalstrey and Benjamin[40] investigated the incidence of breast cancer in female patients treated for thyroid cancer during a 20-year period. The report gives evidence of an association between thyroid disease and breast cancer. Liechty et al.[41] studied 3290 patients who were thyrotoxic, euthyroid, or myxedematous and found a decrease in incidence of cancer in the thyrotoxic group as compared with those who were euthyroid or myxedematous. The development and growth of malignant disease appeared more common in hypothyroidism, although thyrotoxic women with carcinoma of the breast survived longer than myxedematous patients.

Itoh and Maruchi[42] studied 1810 women over age 30 in a large thyroid clinic who had Hashimoto's thyroiditis. These patients were matched by age, sex, marital status, and residency with women who had myxedema, benign nodular goiter, or hyperthyroidism. The incidence of breast cancer for the thyroiditis group was significantly higher (three to ten times) than expected which suggests that patients with Hashimoto's thyroiditis are at high risk for breast cancer.

A publication that has provoked much recent controversy concerned the safety of thyroid medication for women.[43] Conclusions reached were that (1) thyroid supplementation increases the incidence of breast cancer; (2) the longer the treatment is maintained, the greater the incidence of breast cancer; and (3) the cancer rate found in nulliparous women who have been on thyroid medication for more than 15 years is three times greater than the control population. The authors state that the increased incidence of breast cancer in their patients is either a function of hypothyroidism itself or of the thyroid supplements used for therapy. A selected bibliography presented by the Education Committee of the American Thyroid Association in answer to this article described briefly the state of knowledge in this area.[44] It concluded that hypothyroid patients, properly diagnosed, should continue to receive indicated medication and that more support for related research is required.

3. Thyroid Disease in Breast Cancer

In patients with breast cancer, studies have been done to determine whether thyroid disease exists. The results have been somewhat inconclusive mainly because it is difficult to objectively recognize the manifestations of the endocrinopathies by the past or present laboratory studies. Measurement of serum levels of the thyronines does not necessarily reflect the end-organ response or deficiencies. As previously stated by Hayward,[7] these many reports seem to contribute little to our understanding of the problem.

Patients with localized breast cancer were found to be clinically euthyroid while patients with metastatic disease had diminished thyroid activity.[45] When serum protein-bound iodine (PBI) levels were used, postmenopausal normal women and patients who had been successfully treated for early breast cancer also appeared to show no difference, although patients with disseminated disease had higher PBI levels than the earlier localized group.[46] Using ^{131}I uptakes, no difference was seen between women with active and those with no breast cancer, although an extremely low ^{131}I uptake was seen[47] in a small group of patients with large necrotic tumors. No abnormality in thyroid function was seen in patients with breast cancer.[48,49] Operable breast cancer patients were observed to have higher ^{131}I uptakes than controls at both 3 and 24 hr after ^{131}I administration.[50]

A lower incidence of local recurrence in women with thyroid history (6.8%) than in the controls (13.8%) was recorded,[38] while a longer survival time in patients dying from breast cancer who were hypothyroid than those who were euthyroid was also observed.[31] In order to assess this difficult area of prognosis by determination of thyroid status, breast cancer patients were followed for 5 years with ^{131}I uptake determinations and plasma PBI, but no correlation was seen.[51] The authors attributed the negative results to the use of inappropriate methods for measuring thyroid activity. A retrospective study of thyroid disease and breast cancer showed no evidence that a relationship existed between these parameters using the then available serum studies for thyroid function: PBI, butanol-extractable iodine (BEI), uptakes, and serum T_4 by column.[52] If a relationship existed, it was felt it must involve peripheral mechanisms or some cellular manifestation which was overlooked.

C. Basic Research — Thyroid and Breast Tumor Development

Histologic evidence that breast changes occurred in laboratory rodents and domestic animals when thyroid secretions were altered was described in 1941.[24] Because variables such as species, age, and hormone levels differed between investigators, the results appeared inconclusive. Most of the earlier basic studies concern the histologic changes in breast tissues caused by a lack of available thyroid hormone produced by antithyroid drugs.[24,53] Iodine deficiency likewise has been shown to result in dysplastic changes which were assigned initially to the hypothyroid state often produced by chronic iodine deprivation.[20] Hypothyroidism and iodine deficiency appear, however, to be separate states in which levels of each may exist with the other depending on the ability of the biomechanisms to adjust.

The responses occurring at the cellular level in the breast tissues under the conditions produced are significantly unknown. Tumor development by the thyroid hormones on the breast may be basically divided into direct carcinogenic action and secondary enhancement of a carcinogen.

1. Thyroid Hormones as Carcinogens

When antithyroid substances, such as thiourea, are given to mice, remarkable tissue changes occur in the breast.[53, 54] A conclusion drawn was that a special local systemic "milk factor" was responsible for mammary cancer and alveolar hyperplasia development. Low estrogen found with hypothyroidism appeared to be involved as well, and this "milk factor" was influenced by "inherited hormonal influences."[54] Using ovariectomized rats it was soon shown that thyroid hormone was a limiting factor in mammary gland growth even when estrogen and progesterone secretions were adequate. When T_4 secretion rate (TSR) is optimal, then estrogen and progesterone availability may limit growth.[55]

In mild hyperthyroidism, by exogenous T_4 given to normal pregnant rats, limited attainment of maximal mammary gland proliferation occurs. It was shown that DNA decreased in the fat-free breast tissues when T_4 was given.[56] Graded doses of T_4 on mammary growth in hypothyroid, ovariectomized rats treated with estrogen and progesterone were determined by DNA content. Cell proliferation apparently increased as a dose response to a maximum level under thyroxine stimulation. The possibility of a lactogen response was presented.[57] Normally aging rats have abrupt increases in the rate of development of mammary tumors at the 500th and 600th day of life.[58] Both total mammary tumor incidence and rate were the same for parous rats as for virgin controls. Thyroidectomy did not reduce the life span incidence of mammary tumors but did postpone slightly those mammary tumors arising late in life.

In experimental Sprague-Dawley rats both hypothyroidism (propylthiouracil-induced) and dietary iodine deficiency cause atypia in the female breasts.[20] While each therapy produced what appeared to be different changes in the histopathology of the breast, the combination caused remarkably enhanced changes that broadened the dysplasia seen in clinical sections. There was an enhancement of the atypia when estrogen or testosterone was given concurrently.

The anatomic alterations of the breast in rats receiving propylthiouracil (PTU), iodine-deficient diets, and estrogen, singly or in combination, were studied. A strong resemblance was noted between the experimental lesions that occurred and those of naturally occurring fibrocystic disease of the breast of women. The most severe pathologic changes were seen when the three agents acted concomitantly.[59]

When perchlorate is used as an iodine-blocking agent in Sprague-Dawley rats, breast atypia results. Perchlorate treatment is supplemented by T_4 therapy in order to maintain an euthyroxinemic state, thereby, presumably, limiting the blockade to the iodine transporting tissues such as the breast.[60] Tissues considered to transport iodine, such as salivary glands, gastric mucosa, and ovaries, respond specifically to perchlorate ions by preventing iodine from entering the cells, which is the basis for its use in these experiments.[61,62] Estrogen affected the atypia in increasing the cellular hyperplasia and increasing the number of foci of abnormal cells. Thus, altering the thyroid hormone or iodine levels in experimental mice or rats seems to cause tissue modifications resembling breast tumorigenesis.

2. Thyroid Hormones as Cocarcinogens

Several carcinogens have been studied which induce breast carcinoma in rodents. The most commonly employed are 3-methylcholanthrene (MCA), 2-acetylaminofluorene (AAF), and 7,12-dimethylbenz(a)anthracene (DMBA). Breast carcinoma incidence with these chemicals is described variously from 40% in AAF to 100% in DMBA. Studying the onset, number, size, and growth of tumors has provided information on the cocarcinogenicity of many substances including thyroid hormones.

When MCA was given to thyroidectomized rats, a decrease in the incidence of breast cancer was found when compared with control animals. This result was attributed to consequent smaller caloric intake since nutrition has been shown to have marked effects on the genesis of spontaneous and induced tumors.[63] The dietary factor was studied in rats using MCA, where both hypothyroidism (PTU-induced) and T_4 therapy were employed. Under the circumstances regardless of the dietary intake, hypothyroidism appeared to inhibit carcinogenesis. When T_4 was given to reverse the thyroidal status, the incidence and latency of appearance of mammary cancer were not different from control rats treated with MCA only. These data suggest that the effects of MCA administration on thyroid function may be partially but not entirely due to decreased food intake by the treated animals.[64]

Another study showed that in rats concomitantly made hypothyroid (PTU-induced) at the onset of DMBA therapy singly or on a weekly basis, fewer mammary tumors developed.[65] The incidence of DMBA-induced breast cancer was shown to increase significantly in rats made hypothyroid by ^{131}I thyroid ablation. The mechanism considered was a summation effect on the release of trophic hormones in the anterior pituitary dependent upon the presence of ovarian hormones.[66] When a subsequent study was done it also showed that restoration of an euthyroid state was not followed by tumor regression and that the effect of ^{131}I is primarily that of producing hypothyroidism.[66]

The effects of surgical thyroidectomy and of exogenous T_4 on the induction of mammary cancer with repeated doses of MCA in Wistar female rats and with single doses of DMBA in Sprague-Dawley female rats were described as minimal. These few effects were most evident in the MCA induction system when T_4 inhibited tumor appearance slightly, and the inhibitory effect of thyroidectomy was attributable once again to reduced food intake. The DMBA-induced system was not affected by these procedures.[67]

These findings would appear to be explained when it was shown that the responses of both altered thyroid states and iodine deficiency depended on when the carcinogen was given. [8,68] In these experiments, dietary intake was carefully evaluated by pairing the rats. If the condition existed prior to the carcinogenic insult the effect was significant, while if given simultaneously with therapy the results were minimal. Hypothyroidism and iodine deficiency led to earlier onset of tumors and increased numbers while hyperthyroidism did not change the induction characteristics in dietary pairing. Concomitant iodine replacement with dietary iodine deficiency is effective in neutralizing this change; however, tumors in rats already iodine deficient only decrease slightly. When thyroid (T_4) medication is given to chronically iodine-deficient animals, the histologic findings become more atypical. [66,69] Using PTU-induced hypothyroidism did not appear to interfere with the initiation phase of DMBA carcinogenesis in rats but seemed to inhibit the growth of adenocarcinomas due to MCA subsequent to their initiation. [70]

Greater incidences of gross tumors were seen in rats treated with ^{131}I ablation as compared with those made iodine deficient by Remington diet. The conclusion was that the increased incidence of DMBA-induced breast cancers, in rats over controls treated with ^{131}I (90.4%), as compared with Remington diet (64.4%), was the consequence of radiation injury to breast tissue rather than the associated hypothyroidism. It is of note that the iodine-deficient rats had hyperplastic thyroid glands with little or no colloid; the thyroid glands of the ^{131}I-treated rats were essentially destroyed. [71] In a review, data involving thyroid/iodine alterations were correlated with dysplasia, atypia, and cancer production from rat and human breast studies. Iodine metabolism appeared responsible for the breast changes seen and, while thyroid alterations also caused tissue abnormalities, the responses were specific. A consideration of intracellular action and biochemical interaction was introduced. Human changes were recognized by prospective studies. [8] When methiazone was used to induce hypothyroidism in rats and a concomitant pulse dose of DMBA was given, breast cancer induction was suppressed during an observation period which would be sufficient for a 100% tumor incidence if the carcinogen were used alone. An excellent review of the multiplicity of results obtained by many authors using MCA and DMBA is included in this article. [72]

Jabara and Maritz [73] stated that hypothyroidism, alone or combined with progesterone, significantly decreased DMBA mammary tumorigenesis relative to controls. However, the decrease was less in the progesterone-treated group, and statistical analysis showed that progesterone enhanced tumorigenesis to the same extent in hypothyroid animals as in the controls. Most tumors in hypothyroid progesterone-treated rats were adenocarcinomata; in the absence of the steroid, most tumors were benign. However, the difference between the tumor types in the two treatments was not statistically significant. The higher tumor yield in the hypothyroid progesterone-treated rats may have been due to higher circulating levels of prolactin in this group compared with those in the hypothyroid group which received no hormone. The effect of decreased food intake could not be excluded completely. [73]

Some laboratory studies have been done in mice using transplantable tumors and determining the response of altered thyroid/iodine states on these tumors. Using various doses of thyroid and thyroid hormone analogs on C3H/HeN mice given a single transplant injection, no response was obtained. [74] Evidence of mammary tumor growth in mice was seen when either PTU was given or ^{131}I ablation was effected. [75] A recent paper used transplanted estrogen-responsive and independent tumors in GR mice. The uptake of ^{125}I was remarkably greater in the hormone-responsive (HR) tumors than in the hormone-independent (HI) transplants. This shows evidence of an independent iodine effect. [76]

3. Iodine and Breast Tumors

The thyroid gland and mammary glands may be associated because of the common link of iodine metabolism. Both organs have iodine reservoirs and under certain physiologic conditions both have the capability of organifying this element.[13,14] Additionally, laboratory and clinical studies show that a relationship may exist between iodine metabolism and breast and thyroid tumors.[8,27,42]

Basic research evidence has been presented showing that iodine deficiency, either from dietary restriction or blockade of iodine by perchlorate, produces histologic changes in rat breasts.[20,60] These findings have usually consisted of dysplastic changes either atrophic or hyperplastic and often atypical. In the presence of estrogen treatment the responding microanatomy approaches that of a neoplastic state.[77] Concomitantly with this work, the possibility that these dysplastic changes were secondary to hypothyroidism caused by iodine deprivation was tested by inducing hypothyroidism in the presence of adequate iodine. The histologic changes seen in the breast of the hypothyroid rat appear to have distinct differences from those seen in the breast of the iodine-deficient animal which was euthyroid as indicated by serum thyroid function studies.[20,59] From these results it appears likely that iodine may be responsible for an end-organ effect.

With increasing age of the rats, the breasts of iodine-deficient animals show even more evidence of atypical changes in the epithelium than in young rats.[22] This is seen in many foci in the older age groups. With the chronicity of iodine deprivation by perchlorate blockade we have seen statistically significant increases in periductal fibrous overgrowth in trapping adjacent lobules with aberrant ductular proliferation, sclerosing adenosis, and microcyst formation. All are strongly reminiscent of the analagous fibrocystic disease in the human female.[59,78] Additionally, there are areas of atypical lobules showing hyperchromatism, enlargement of nuclei, altered nuclear-cytoplasmic ratios, increased mitosis, and loss of polarity of the epithelium. Some of the lobules exhibit papillomatosis with poorly polarized epithelium and foci of neoplastic epithelium.[22] These appear to be transformations of the lobules to histologically malignant patterns completely apart from the adenosis.

Iodine deficiency, as described previously, has been shown to produce an earlier onset of DMBA-induced breast cancer in rats with an increase in size and number of lesions. This requires that the deficiency state be present prior to the pulse dose of the carcinogen. Perchlorate blockade of the breast appears to have the same effect as the various dietary regimens in this experiment.[8,68] Further study of these changes by Kellen[72] showed acceleration of mammary tumorigenesis in DMBA-treated rats under these specific conditions.

Using GR mice transplanted with HR or HI mammary tumors, Thorpe[76] found that the uptake of ^{125}I by HR mammary tumors was greater than HI mammary tumors. In the presence of progesterone and estrogen the difference was 20 times greater between HR and HI tumors. The ^{125}I uptake by HR tumors was greatly reduced by simultaneous injection of either perchlorate or an excess of nonradioactive iodide.

4. Intracellular Metabolism of Iodine

The presence of intracellular breast iodine in rats was confirmed by the utilization of autoradiography employing radioactive ^{125}I.[79] The distribution of radioactive iodine in the cells appeared random and in multiple foci. It appears that iodine tissue saturation in the breast is not complete in the length of time employed before the rats were sacrificed or that reception of iodine by the cells occurs in a casual manner.

Relative iodine content in the soluble cytosol of breast tissue of rats under various iodine or thyroid hormone treatments was determined. The ^{125}I uptakes appeared to be more affected by reduced available serum iodide than by hyper- or hypothyroidism. In iodine deficiency, where there was a decreased cytosol uptake in the breast tissues, dysplasia characteristically resulted. Perchlorate treatment showed a similar response, apparently due to its chemical action of restricting iodide movement into the breast cells similar to its action in the thyroid.[60,62]

Early studies have indicated that normal and lactating mammary glands, as well as salivary, gastric, and thyroid glands, are able to concentrate iodine.[8] Thus, the effect of iodine and thyroid hormones in breast tumor development may depend on intracellular breast iodine metabolism. Basic to this hypothesis of intracellular action is the question of whether extravascular organification of iodine occurs in the breast.

Studies have implied that mammary gland tissues concentrate iodine and that organification of iodine takes place within breast tissues under certain physiologic conditions (Figure 4). Mammary gland tissue slice studies in rats[14] using trichloracetic acid (TCA) techniques showed that both nonlactating and lactating rat breasts organify iodine and that MIT, DIT, and other thyronines can be identified by chromatographic separation. The work of Brown-Grant[13,80] showed that iodination of breast tissues seems to occur perhaps in a manner similar to the responses described in salivary glands, stomach secreting cells, and certain specific tumors. The ability of the lactating breast to concentrate and secrete iodide in vivo has been reported in rats by several authors[81-83] and in mice by Thorpe.[76] Recent work from our laboratory[12] uses tissue solubilization techniques, subsequent electrophoresis with amylamite gels, and chromatography by molecular exclusion columns. This method has confirmed a marked presence of such activity in lactating breasts and shows a lesser response in the normal breast.

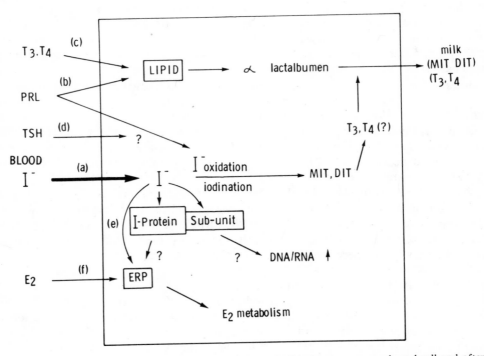

FIGURE 4.   Intracellular metabolism of iodine. Blood iodide (a) enters parenchymal cell and after oxidation and iodination results in MIT, DIT (T_3,T_4?) secretion with milk. T_3,T_4 entering breast (c) reacts with PRL and lipid to form a lactalbumin for secretion as milk. Additionally iodide iodinates small protein (20,000 daltons) which may act on DNA/RNA increases or changes in estrogen receptor protein effect with estrogen (f).

Additionally, a small protein (20,000 daltons) was found which appears to be directly involved in this iodination process. Further research is being done to isolate this protein and determine its involvement in this pathway.

Radioactive iodine uptakes by the breast tissues indicate the amount of iodine transported into the breast parenchyma. However, total breast ^{125}I uptakes in the rat represent both vascular and cellular iodine fractions. The specific uptake in the breast parenchyma can be calculated by subtracting the ^{125}I activity in the serum as estimated by ^{51}Cr serum dilution studies from the total breast count.[84] The calculated vascularity of the rat breast appears to be 0.015 ml/g of tissue. Radioactive iodine uptakes increase in the breast tissue of iodine-deficient rats. Other iodine uptakes were determined in rats under modified iodine and thyroid conditions and varied with the available iodine. In rat breast tissues showing foci of dysplastic changes, uptake was increased, a fact utilized for clinical diagnostic research.[4]

Using radioactive T_4-^{125}I comparison of control and perchlorate-blocked rats showed no differences in ^{125}I counts per milligram in the parenchyma and cytosol of the breasts. After interpolation of the data by the ^{51}Cr technique to account for serum iodine, no significant difference was seen.[85] By this study thyroxine does not appear to change the intracellular iodine characteristics in the rat breast. Addition of T_4 or T_3 to cultures of mammary gland explants in specific media results in a selective enhancement of the activity of the milk protein, alpha-lactalbumin.[86] Added to the media were insulin, hydrocortisone, and prolactin. This end-organ response by thyroid hormones on the synthesis and secretion of milk for lactation implicates a direct effect. It also may suggest that thyroid hormones react with prolactin since the secretion of milk is an accepted result of prolactin stimulation.

The DNA content in breast tissues treated with graded T_4 doses was studied in hypothyroid, ovariectomized rats.[57] DNA content did not differ between breasts of rats receiving estradiol and progesterone and those to which thyroid hormone was also added. One interesting finding was that pituitary lactogen concentration was 28 to 143% greater in rats receiving additional T_4. Thus, T_4 appeared to influence production and secretion of lactogenic hormone (PRL) and enhancement of mammary growth, which was postulated to be due, in part, to an increased secretion of the lactogen. The DNA/RNA ratio measured as micrograms per milligram of dehydrated fat-free tissue (DFFT) has been studied in breasts of iodine-deficient and hypothyroid rats.[8,87] Iodine deficiency shows elevated RNA and DNA while hypothyroidism data indicate a remarkable increase in DNA but not RNA.

Preliminary laboratory data show that estrogen receptors as measured by sucrose gradients are changed qualitatively in the cytosol of breasts of iodine-deficient rats when compared with normal.[87] This work shows that receptor protein size may be affected in a manner similar to the changes seen in experimental neoplastic mammary tissue exposed to high plasma estrogen.[88] This finding, in light of the estrogen effects described later, permits speculation on the possibility that iodine may be involved in the breast cells in the estrogen metabolic pathway. Estrogen appears to increase the secretion of prolactin from the pituitary as well as its own action on breast tissue and in gonadotropin rebound effects on the pituitary.[89] Its interaction in tumor regression seems profound in secondary sexual tissues of the female, clinically and experimentally.

5. Hypothalamic-Pituitary Stimulation

There has been a good deal of recent interest in the hypothalamic-pituitary-thyroid axis as it relates to breast cancer (Figure 5). However, it has been shown that breast cancer patients as a group have a level of thyroid function which is lower than that found in women in hospitals with conditions unrelated to the breast and that this lowered function is of primary thyroid and not of pituitary or hypothalamic origin as

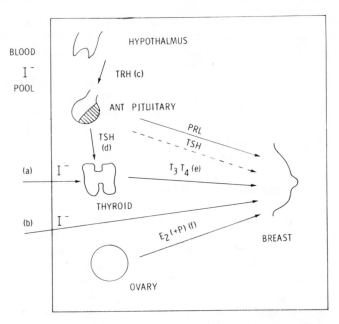

FIGURE 5.   Endocrine influences on the breast. (a) Iodide enters
the thyroid for metabolic actions leading to final secretion (e) of T_3, T_4
hormones. This is mediated by TRH (c) and TSH (d). In the breast
iodide (b) enters from the blood. TRH (c) releases both PRL and TSH
to the breast for secretory activity. Ovarian secretion of both estrogen
and progesterone (f) stimulates breast tissue.

shown by TSH values.[90] On the other hand, women with breast cancer may exhibit
higher resting levels of TSH and a greater TSH response to TRH than women admitted
with disorders unrelated to the breast.[91]

Breasts of hypophysectomized rats show no breast tissue changes in hypothyroidism
or iodine deficiency from controls.[8] However, giving TSH to these rats resulted in the
altered breast pathology already described in intact animals. Thus, a pituitary factor
is required for these thyroid/iodine responses to occur and it appears to be TSH.[8] The
response of TSH in breast tissues would be likely to be effective if the intracellular
responses in the breast showed the organification and coupling seen in the thyroid
gland. Trophic hormone responses on tissues other than the target endocrine glands
have been seen with several hormones including gonadotropins and growth hormone.
However, at this time the intracellular metabolism still requires further clarification.

PRL has been described as a mammotrope responsible for breast tissue responses
in both normal and abnormal lactation. The availability of accurate serum determinations of PRL has renewed research interest in this hormone as a potential breast carcinogen[89] although, as yet, no direct evidence has been found. Particularly lacking is
how it responds within the breast cell cytosol although tissue culture studies have been
done in mice. It has been shown that alpha-lactalbumin is secreted when PRL is present, enhanced by T_3 and T_4 in the presence of cortisone and insulin.[86] The beneficial
effect of thyroid hormone and thyroid active substances upon lactation has been
known for many years.[55]

An important connection here is the research that has shown that TRH acts in rats
and humans as a prolactin activator on the pituitary cells.[15] TRH may then be the
intermediate secretion for thyroid interaction on the breast. Hypothyroid patients and
rodents have an elevated serum prolactin due to the rebound elevation of TRH. In our
study, PRL and TSH were given to hypothyroid and iodine-deficient rats. Histological

differences in the breast tissues examined were recognizable between the groups.[92,93] The variability appeared to be qualitative and not quantitative although further evaluation of the intracellular changes is warranted. The difficulty encountered was the dose response of PRL under the conditions that were used. It is necessary that the levels be maintained for a period of time that permits breast tissue changes to occur.[93]

6. Estrogen Effects

There is ample evidence that ovarian hormones, particularly estrogens, play a key role in determining breast cancer risk. Age at menarche and at natural menopause are related to risk, as is surgical menopause at an early age. Further, it has been known for a long time that nulliparous women are at high risk of breast cancer; conversely, grand multiparous women have a low rate of disease.[94]

How estrogen and thyroid hormones might interact on breast tissues has been difficult to determine. It has been shown that estrogen secretion from the ovary is disturbed in hypothyroidism. Conversely, elevated serum estrogen values lend to increased thyroid hormone binding, requiring an increase in thyroid gland secretions. The latter effect often leads to hypothyroidism, if the gland is incapable of producing the additional hormones, as in thyroiditis. It has been noted that breast cancer patients were more likely to have hyperplastic changes in ovaries, endometrium, uninvolved breast, pituitary, and adrenal cortex than controls at postmortem examination.[36] Possibly all of these changes may be mediated by estrogen secretion.

An hypothesis for dietary iodine and risk of breast cancer has been presented in which it is suggested that relatively low dietary iodine intake might produce an evanescent, intermittent primary hypothyroidism which would lead to changes in the hypothalamic-pituitary pool. This thesis assumes that abnormal estrogen secretion would result and, hence, be the etiology for breast and endometrial carcinoma. It was concluded that women in areas of the world where iodine intake is relatively low should be encouraged to increase their iodine intake.[95,96] While a steady state of estrogen secretion has been shown to be a possible cause of endometrial carcinoma, no conclusive data are available proving that breast cancer is so affected.[97]

Early research showed that breast dysplasia in rat breasts that resulted from hypothyroidism or dietary iodine deficiency was worsened by estrogen.[20] Progesterone per se was not effective in these rat models. When perchlorate blockade of the breast is employed in rats the added estrogenic effect was less.[77]

Qualitative changes in estrogen receptor were found in iodine-deficient rat breasts as compared with the normal euthyroid animal.[87] These recent findings may imply potential action for iodine in the synthesis of the estrogen receptor proteins.

Thus, in chemically blocked, iodine-deficient breast tissue the estrogen receptors may be inhibited in its action, reducing the estrogen effect on the breast. It is important to note that with perchlorate therapy T_4 replacement was given to the rats to provide euthyroxinemia. Particularly evident is the finding that in DMBA rats, which have estrogen-independent tumors, estrogen does not inhibit growth in iodine-deficient rats.[8] Perhaps the receptor changes are significant in causing this observation.

Significantly, when estrogen-responsive and independent tumors were transplanted to mice, radioactive uptake studies showed that estrogen-responsive tumors had higher iodine uptakes than estrogen-independent transplants.[76] Additionally, nonradioactive iodine or perchlorate greatly reduced the uptake in HR tumors. Considering the use of measuring estrogen receptors to determine estrogen-dependent cancer in metastatic lesions of women,[89] this response by the tumors would agree with the previously stated theory that an interaction between iodine metabolism and estrogen may exist within the cells.

In ovariectomized rats the perchlorate influence on the breast tissues is reduced. There appears to be a need for intrinsic estrogen to obtain these abnormalities.[60] These results would cause further speculation on the interaction with prolactin response which is increased in the presence of estrogen.

D. Diagnostic Findings

Several studies have shown that mammary gland tissues concentrate iodine and that organification of iodine takes place within breast tissue.[13,14] The presence of breast iodine was confirmed by the utilization of autoradiography employing radioactive [125]I. Findings indicated that in iodine deficiency there was, in fact, a decrease in the iodine in the breast tissues, and iodine diminished further in the chronic deficiency state leading to dysplastic changes. The same response occurred in perchlorate blockade of tissues, and iodine again did not enter the breast tissue itself.[79]

Thus, it was considered that radioactive iodine uptake by the breast tissue could be confirmatory in indicating the amount of iodine present within the limits of the breast tissues. The iodine uptake in breasts were determined in rats under varying physiological and pharmacologic conditions of iodine availability.[77,99] Using radioactive uptake studies, it was apparent that the uptake of iodine in breast tissues varied with the overall status of iodine in the rat, and it became apparent that in rat breast tissues with dysplasia the uptake was increased.[59] This utilizes the fact that when radioactive iodine is given, uptake is greatest in deficient areas.

Counts obtained in measuring radioactive iodine in the breast include serum (vascular) iodine as well as cellular iodine counts. To obtain relative and absolute values for breast parenchyma, ^{125}I rat uptakes were done on both breast tissues and blood serum. Radioactive ^{51}Cr was given and counted in a similar manner.[89] The preliminary studies show a residual value in the breast which is measurable.

A number of experiments have utilized radioactive nuclides in the diagnosis and management of breast carcinoma. Until recently the use of these procedures was restricted to diagnosis of distant metastases at an advanced state of the disease.[100,101] Visualization of a breast neoplasm with ^{99m}Tc has been reported. Images of the breast have been noted in six patients, and localization of the radionuclide in breast masses correlated with clinical examination, mammography, and pathological diagnosis using [99m]Tc.[103] Carrier-free gallium[67] citrate given intravenously localized in a variety of neoplasms and was detectable in scans.

Concentration of gallium[67] in breast carcinoma has been erratic and not sufficiently dependable to make gallium[67] scanning useful in the diagnosis of breast neoplasia. Utilization of iodine as a therapeutic agent in breast disease has long been described. Most recently, several works have utilized Lugol's solution procedure for detection of breast neoplasms and other basic iodine preparations in breast diseases with impressive success.[104]

From data collated, it was possible to determine the breast uptake of an administered tracer dose of radioactive iodine (^{123}I). After experimenting with several techniques, reproducible results were obtained. Radioactive iodine uptakes were greater in malignant or atypical breasts than in normal breasts.[4] Statistical analysis shows that (1) thyroid uptakes and breast uptakes appear to be dependent and to vary directly with one another, (2) iodine and estrogen appear to interact by the fact that radioactive iodine uptake is higher in postmenopausal breasts than it is in premenopausal breasts, and (3) gestational status and breast feeding do not seem to change the uptake of the breasts.

Computerized tomography breast scanners (CT/M) are being employed in the diagnosis of not only breast cancer but possible precancerous lesions in the breast.[105] By using contrast medium enhancement techniques not only morphological changes but also quantitative measurement of iodine concentration have been described in breast tissues. Breast cancer and severe ductal epithelial hyperplasia show significant contrast medium enhancement.

E. Thyroid Hormones as Treatment for Breast Cancer

Thyroid hormones were suggested as therapy initially in 1892 when thyroid extract was given for metastatic disease with apparent remission.[23] More recently it was proposed as a prophylactic measure after mastectomy.[34] Desiccated thyroid with or without prednisone was employed. It was difficult to distinguish between the remissions due to thyroid and those due to prednisone. When clinical hypothyroidism was controlled by T_3 in randomly selected patients with advanced breast cancer, the compound appeared to have no therapeutic effect.[106]

Recent literature presents data to show that thyroid medication may be involved in the etiology of breast carcinoma.[43] At present, neither thyroid nor iodine therapy appears to be clinically applicable.

F. Summary

Major efforts have been made on research concerning the effects of thyroid hormone and iodine on mammary glands in both humans and experimental animals. The most promising results have been seen in the intracellular and peripheral endocrine studies. How these function to permit a cohesive theory of end-organ action will be described in the chapter summary.

V. FEMALE REPRODUCTIVE TUMORS

Thyroid hormone secretion affects the serum levels of ovarian and testicular steroids, and conversely thyroid hormone production responds to sex steroid variations. As stated, both T_3 and T_4 signal the hypothalamic-pituitary axis to provide feedback thyrotropic secretion. There is evidence that, additionally, both serum estrogen and prolactin are elevated when thyroid conditions result in inadequate T_4 or T_3, producing increased TRH and TSH secretions. How this series of events affects the breast tissues has been discussed; however, the effect of these changes on the endometrium and ovaries also seems to be measurable.

A relatively high prevalence of goiter/hypothyroidism among women with endometrial cancer (10%) has been reported.[107] The incidence rates for breast and endometrial cancer parallel each other in geographic areas associated with high prevalences of goiter.[108] Implications that there are parallel prevalences of ovarian and endometrial carcinoma permit speculation that goiter is more common in the geographic distribution of ovarian cancer as well. These epidemiologic data would thus imply a higher risk of both endometrial and ovarian cancer in hypothyroidism or endemic goiter.[95]

Another thyroid hormone effect on ovarian activity has been seen in menstrual disorders. Thyroid alterations promote dysfunctional changes of both ovary and endometrium which is considered as a premalignant effect by some in perimenopausal and menopausal women.[107] While this hypothesis has been presented, no direct basic or clinical prospective studies have resulted.

It appears that endometrial cancer is markedly affected by estrogen levels; however, how this response occurs is speculative. Some studies have been made to clinically define a higher risk characteristic by the estrone/estradiol ratios,[109] with less estradiol being secreted in the cancer patients. Recent data concerning women given estrogen for menopausal symptoms or for birth control showed a significant increase in endometrial carcinoma.[97] Prolactin and estrogen titers are elevated in breast and endometrial cancer in humans and rodents.[110]

T_4 and T_3 metabolism are affected by the increases in thyroid binding proteins which occur when serum estradiol is raised. Increased binding causes a total serum thyroid hormone to elevate. In normal physiologic conditions (i.e., menstrual cycle, pregnancy) the feedback mechanisms are activated, and the hypothalamic-pituitary-thyroid axis is maintained, releasing a normal level of "free" iodothyronines from the thyroid gland. How the extrathyroidal synthesis of T_4 to T_3 acts under these conditions is still not certain.

Since the availability of estrogen receptor determinations, measurement of the effect of estrogen in responsive tissues has been possible.[98] A linkage between this intracellular characteristic with thyroid/iodine alterations has only been seen in rodents. Estrogen receptor proteins appear to have a qualitative shift in iodine-deficient rat breasts.[87] The characteristics seen are suggestive of receptors seen in atypical rat endometrium[88] and in rabbits where remarkable differential characteristics in estrogen receptors occur depending on available sex steroids.

Statistically, multiple foci of cancer in the breast, endometrium, and ovary occur in women more often than anticipated, which led to a consideration of common etiology.[26] The mortality rate of endometrial-ovarian cancer in Japanese-American women is higher than for Japanese women living in Japan.[111] Thus, these observations may be evidence of an environmental, endocrine, or metabolic factor. The factors that have been considered deal with the availability of iodine. Dietary changes occur in the transitions seen in the Japanese population among which are the ingestion of seafood and iodine-rich seaweed. Since increased endometrial and ovarian cancer have been seen in other countries where there is endemic goiter, this epidemiologic factor must be considered.

The effect of the administration of l-thyroxine and methylthiouracil alone, together, and in combination with stilbestrol (DES) on the induction of cervicovaginal tumors using local DMBA was investigated in intact and castrate rats. The rate of sarcomatosis and epithelial neoplasm induction was accelerated by methylthiouracil and reduced by l-thyroxine. The influence of the thyroactive compounds on the induction of tumors is not correlated with their effect on body weight or on growth of the stroma.[112]

There is no consistent published factor concerning the effect of thyroid hormones on the male reproductive system, although changes in the male breast (hyperthyroidism), testes (hypothyroidism), and seminal vesicles (reduced T_3) have been referenced. A minimal literature is available concerning abnormalities of thyroid secretions as they relate to tumor formation in the reproductive tract of females.

In summary, thyroid hormones quantitatively affect estrogen and prolactin secretion. The changes on the ovary, endometrium, and breast cause irregularities histologically and intracellularly which appear to be precancerous. Epidemiologic data are presented which show evidence that these may result in increased neoplasia.

VI. INTEGUMENTARY TUMORS

The influence of thyroid hormones on the development of integumentary tumors has been described in several research articles. Kreyberg[113] observed that thyroid administration accelerated skin tumor formation in mice, while Silverstone and Tannenbaum[114] found that thyroid extracts had little or no effect on benzpyrene-induced skin tumors in mice. Epitheliomatous proliferation in a rabbit's ear due to tarring was reported to be inhibited by thyroidectomy.[115] The carcinogenic effect of dibenzanthracene was diminished by coadministration of T_4 and augmented by thiouracil,[116] but methylcholanthrene-induced sarcomas in rats were not influenced by thyroid extracts or thyroidectomy.[117]

As noted by Meites,[118] development and growth of other skin tumors have been reported to be enhanced, diminished, or not affected by administration of thyroid substances. In his experimental studies with DMBA, T_4 or thiouracil was given to mice. Little or no growth of individual tumors resulted in the T_4-fed mice whereas most of the tumors in the controls, and particularly in thiouracil-fed mice, grew in size during the period of treatment. Most of the tumors appeared to be papillomas as determined by gross and histological examination.

Experimental evidence has shown that thyroid hormone can alter the hair cycle in a direction opposite to the effect of cortisone; whereas cortisone was shown to cause inhibition of hair growth, thyroid was shown to cause stimulations.[119] In a summary article, liothyronine administration has been shown to affect the hair cycle and chemically induced epidermal carcinogenesis in mice.[120] Experiments were designed in a manner to permit the study of the action of this preparation on hair changes and to study the relationship, if any, between the effect of the preparation on hair growth and its effect on tumor development. The phases of the hair cycle were ascertained by means of dyeing the fur according to previous techniques. Definite stimulation of hair growth was observed in all groups of animals which had received liothyronine. No decrease in tumor incidence, however, was obtained under the influence of liothyronine administration. Indeed, under certain experimental conditions an unexpected increase occurred after the administration.

In summary, experimental studies to date have shown that responses by skin to various carcinogens are modified by the presence of thyroid hormones. None of the reported studies suggested a mechanism of action for the changes seen. In some, evidences of vitamin A interference were considered, but the question seems unresolved.

VII. LIVER

The induction of liver tumors in rats fed 2-acetylaminofluorene (AAF) is partially inhibited by concurrent treatment with thiouracil.[121] The result was later confirmed; however, the theory that reduced food intake in the goitrogen-treated animals accounted for the strikingly lower tumor incidence was excluded by pair feeding.[119] Paschkis et al.[122] presented evidence that the anticarcinogenic effect might be attributable to disordered uracil metabolism.

Bielschowsky and Hall[120] showed that these changes were due to chronic hypothyroidism by using surgically thyroidectomized rats. The inhibition of liver carcinogenesis by thyroidectomy in their experiments was absolute; neither AAF nor 2-aminofluorene (AF) treatments resulted in a single liver tumor in the completely thyroidectomized animal. However, virtually all of their intact controls, which received the same total dose of carcinogen, developed malignant hepatomas. The treatment produced extrahepatic tumors (of secretory glands, breast, lung, and other tissues) with approximately the same frequency in both the thyroidectomized and intact animals. With respect to the liver, the degree of thyroid deficiency was bound to be crucial, since even a very small thyroid remnant permitted the development of a small but significant number of tumors.[124] These results have been confirmed. An equally powerful and specific inhibition of carcinogenesis by azo dyes as well as by AF and AAF has been demonstrated in completely hypophysectomized rats and adrenalectomized rats.[125]

These experiments raised several important problems which are still unresolved, such as the identity of the hormones involved as permissive agents in liver carcinogenesis. Additionally the questions of why the anticarcinogenic protective effect of the endocrine ablation is effective only in the liver and also at what stage of carcinogenic process the inhibitory effect of the endocrine deficiencies are exerted remain unanswered. Goodall[126] confirmed that the protective effect of thyroidectomy against the induction of liver tumors by AAF in rats is confirmed. Evidence was presented which indicated that the effect of thyroidectomy may be attributable to blockade of liver carcinogenesis at or before the stage of initiation rather than to retardation of tumor progression in such animals.

On the other hand, several workers have been concerned with whether hyperthyroidism alters the effectiveness of carcinogenic agents. Conflicting effects are reported by authors using rodents exposed to tar,[127] 3,4-benpyrene,[128] or AAF.[121] Since the hyperthyroid state might be expected to alter either the metabolism of the carcinogen or the reactions leading to the development or suppression of tumors, the net response would be a variant depending on dose, caloric intake, and time of exposure.

Using an azo dye, *p*-dimethylamino azo benzene (DAB), the basal metabolic rates of rats were studied as well as the incidences of rat liver carcinoma.[129] Hyperthyroid animals receiving DAB had a low survival rate with a high incidence of tumors. Additionally, work by Leathem and Oddis[130] showed that liver tumor incidence, weight, and total protein were significantly greater following the combination of AAF and thyroid than with either drug alone.

Notable research has been done in the action of thyroid compounds with carcinogens on liver tissues; however, presently no acceptable thesis has been able to withstand the pressure of time.

Stroev and Nikulin[131] found in experiments with a transplanted strain of alveolar-mucus cancer of the liver that thyroid hormones regulated the activity and content of the lactate and malate dehydrogenase isocompounds. There was a similarity in the thyroid hormone regulation of dehydrogenase activity in normal and tumor cells, a less labile transformation in metabolism of the latter occurring after alterations of the serum hormone level. T_4 induced a synthesis of lactic dehydrogenase H (LDH) subunits. With regard to this fact, it was suggested that uniform changes in the LDH spectrum in different tumors are caused by suppression of a corresponding locus. Specific hormone regulation of genetic processes in the transformed cells is maintained when there is unchanged activity of chromatin regulatory elements.

In summary, liver metabolic responses by thyroid hormones are usually considered as resulting from changes in decreased oxygen consumption, decreased cholesterol in the biliary tract, and decrease of glycogenesis. If thyroid secretion is altered, tissue changes reflecting these physiologic responses could provide intracellular biochemical errors. The results of studies described show changes within these parameters, although how the hormone reacts at the liver cell remains clouded.

VIII. GASTRIC AND SALIVARY GLANDS

The tissues that have not been described as yet which have an "iodine transport" mechanism are the gastric mucosal glands and salivary glands.[72] Several references have been made to tissue changes within these areas when treated with perchlorate[53] or in iodine deficiency,[5,6] but no evidence of a response towards tumor development was found in a literature search.

Japanese statistics show remarkably high stomach cancer morbidity and mortality.[41] Elevated iodine uptakes have been seen in the gastric mucosal tissues of biopsied specimens. This may reflect a Wolff-Chaikoff effect with a reversed iodine response causing an overreaction in these cells. In rats, while it has been seen that perchlorate blockades the uptake of ^{131}I in the gastric and salivary glands,[54] no studies on the induction of tumors in these organs have been made. The absorption of iodine by these glands appears to be variable, making an interpretation of the present data difficult.

In patients with stomach cancer there appears to be a statistically increased incidence of low-serum thyroid hormone. Studies of ^{131}I uptake and clinical evaluation show evidence of reduced thyroid activity.[21]

In summary, more information is needed concerning the potential action of both thyroid hormones and iodine metabolism on the salivary and gastric mucosal glands. Both have remarkable quantities of iodine and are affected quantitatively by iodine deprivation and perchlorate blockade.

IX. SUMMARY

An association between thyroid hormones and tumorigenesis has been considered for over 75 years. In that time, a large and diversified research literature has accumulated which has shown conflicting results. Initial studies were primarily clinical and epidemiologic observations. The difficulty has been the omnipresence of thyroid hormone activity in all cells and tissues. Thyroid hormones have metabolic intracellular responses, such as oxygen consumption and calorogenesis, mitochondrial activation, amino acid incorporation in ribosomes, and several enzymatic conversions. Under these circumstances the intracellular changes caused by the hormones could be initially indistinguishable from the milieu seen in neoplastic changes.

Similarly, if an alteration of thyroid hormone activity on an end organ were to occur, abnormal changes in the tissues involved could result in tumorigenesis. Some biochemical studies already described have shown that these events can occur. In addition, centrally mediated abnormalities of thyroid function appear to cause end-organ restrictions in the normal activities of the circulating thyroid hormone.

When studying thyroid hormone activity, the influences of iodine metabolism are apparent since the thyroid gland transports over 90% of all iodine found in the body and is the regulatory center for iodine in the body. Any abnormalities of iodine intake or utilization would be reflected by the thyroid gland and eventually in the secretion of thyroid hormones. Consideration of the end-organ responses of iodine is essential.

The effect of thyroid hormones on tumorigenesis has been researched in the breast more than any other tissue. The breast is a complicated secretory gland responding cyclically to the sex steroids, estrogen and progesterone. Under the endocrine conditions relevant to the postpartum period, all the intracellular activities respond to prepare and secrete milk. The milk contains large amounts of iodides, iodinated tyrosyls, and iodothyronines derived from the mother's blood content of these substances. In a similar way, there are other organs where thyroid hormone accepts a role in secretion or growth and development. Organs such as gastric glands, salivary glands, and liver receive iodides and appear to actively utilize this element within the cell.

In the breast, it is most apparent that thyroid hormones are utilized in the preparation of milk for secretion and, perhaps through amino acid synthesis, assist in growth and development. Iodine is required for breast tissue normality and acts through iodination, oxidation, and organification and, by an interaction with receptor systems, with the cellular activities of estrogen. Iodine is not provided by deiodination of T_4 as seen when ^{125}I-T_4 is used in breast ^{125}I uptake studies.

Thus, in the breast at least two distinct intracellular systems are involved (Figure 5) which are supported by central endocrine secretions (Figure 4). The first intracellular pathway involves thyroid hormone combined with prolactin (and other hormones: insulin, cortisone) to provide lactalbumin secretion in the estrogen-progesterone-prepared lactating mammary gland cell. Secondly, iodine reacts within the cell to oxidize and iodinate a protein measuring 10,000 to 20,000 daltons in the cytosol. This iodinated protein may be involved in the qualitative changes in estrogen receptor and increased intracellular DNA and RNA seen in iodine-deficient states.

This thesis would provide sufficient basis for the conflicting results seen in many research programs. In order to maintain normal breast tissues, both adequate thyroid hormone and iodine must be present in the blood. In some preliminary studies, the response from alterations of each system has been separated by histologic techniques.

In rodents, focal hyperplasia and atypia occur in the glandular structures of the breast in hypothyroidism or iodine deficiency. These changes qualitatively and quantitatively differ according to the type and chronicity of the altered condition. Other variables include age of animal, steroid treatment (especially estrogen), and diet. Altered thyroid and iodine status change the onset, size, duration, and histology of chemically induced carcinogenesis.

The breast in lactating shows iodide transport, oxidation, organification, and even secretion in milk which contains both T_4 and its precursors. The amount of organification in nonlactating breasts appears modest as compared with lactating breasts (Figure 5). Prolactin has been shown to be the hormone responsible for formation of the milk in the secretory cells of the breast. Other hormones responsible are insulin, cortisone, T_3, and T_4. In addition, prolactin has been considered as an activator of both benign and malignant breast tumors.

Endocrine research has shown that elevated TRH results in increased serum PRL as well as TSH secretion from the pituitary (Figure 4). Both TRH and TSH are increased in hypothyroidism. An additional fact, which seems to fit into this scheme, is that TSH must be present for the atypical breast changes to occur in hypothyroid or iodine-deficient rats. Thus, TRH may control both the secretion of PRL and TSH, which appear to share in normal and abnormal breast physiology. This link may be a pathway for some precancerous and cancerous lesions.

When considering the thyroid hormone effects on tumorigenesis, other systems which seem closely linked to the breast changes are endometrial and ovarian tissues. The findings, both clinical and experimental, have been associated with breast malignancy. Intracellular studies of the endometrium have shown that estrogen receptor (ERP) systems are remarkably influenced by tumorigenesis, which should perhaps be correlated with the ERP changes seen in the iodine-deficient breast of rats. The interaction of clinical hypothyroidism due to iodine deficiency or thyroid pathology (thyroiditis) with estrogen as a cause of breast malignancy has been described.

The gastric and salivary glands may respond similarly to the breast and, thus, provide further evidence to support this thesis. These glands have been shown to be involved with iodine metabolism and seem to show evidence of neoplasia under certain altered thyroid states.

While implications that thyroid hormones may affect integumentary tumors have been described, critical research in these tissues has been limited. In the liver, however, considerable research has been published and early cocarcinogenesis experimentation showed specific changes in liver cancer when thyroid hormone alterations occurred. The complexities of hepatic tumors make much of the data difficult to interpret at this time.

Continuation of research on the effect of thyroid hormones on tumorigenesis, particularly in the mammary glands, would be rewarding. This experimentation could yield information useful in diagnosis, therapy, and prevention of neoplasia since thyroid and iodine alterations can generally be corrected. The close analogy of the results from animal models with clinical data makes this research medically significant.

REFERENCES

1. Nicoloff, J. T., Low, J. C., Dussault, J. H., and Fisher, D. A., Simultaneous measurement of thyroxine and triiodothyronine peripheral turnover kinetics in man, *J. Clin. Invest.*, 51, 473, 1972.
2. Oppenheimer, J. H., Surks, M. I., and Schwartz, H. L., The metabolic significance of exchangeable cellular thyroxine, *Recent Prog. Horm. Res.*, 25, 381, 1969.
3. Dratman, M. B., Crutchfield, F. L., Axelrod, J., Colburn, R. W., and Thoa, N., Localization of triiodothyronine in nerve ending fractions of rat brain, *Proc. Natl. Acad. Sci. U.S.A.*, 73, 941, 1976.
4. Eskin, B. A., Parker, J., Bassett, J. G., and George, D., Human breast uptake of radioactive iodine, *Obstet. Gynecol.*, 44, 398, 1974.
5. Honour, A. S., Myant, M. B., and Rowlands, E. N., Secretion of radioiodine in digestive juices and milk in man, *Clin. Sci.*, 11, 447, 1952.

6. Schiff, L., Stevens, C. D., Molle, W. R., Steinberg, H., Kumpe, C. W., and Stewart, P., Gastric and salivary gland excretion of radioiodine in man, *J. Natl. Cancer Inst.*, 7, 349, 1947.
7. Hayward, J., *Hormones and Human Breast Cancer*, Springer-Verlag, New York, 1970, 139.
8. Eskin, B. A., Iodine metabolism and breast cancer, *Trans. N.Y. Acad. Sci.*, 32, 911, 1970.
9. Williams, R. H., *Textbook of Endocrinology*, 5th ed., W. B. Saunders, Philadelphia, 1974, 95.
10. Werner, S. C. and Ingbar, S. H., *The Thyroid*, Harper & Row, New York, 1971, 26.
11. Bacchus, H., *Essentials of Gynecologic and Obstetric Endocrinology*, University Park Press, Baltimore, 1975, 145.
12. Sparks, C., Eskin, B. A., LaMont, B., and Kolansky, D., Organification of iodine by rat breast tissues, *Proc. Endoc. Soc.*, 160, A394, 1978.
13. Brown-Grant, K., The iodide concentrating mechanism of the mammary gland, *J. Physiol. (London)*, 135, 644, 1957.
14. Freinkel, N. and Ingbar, S. H., The metabolism of ^{131}I by surviving slices of mammary tissue, *Endocrinology*, 58, 51, 1956.
15. Hill-Samli, M. and MacLeod, R. M., Interaction of thyrotropin-releasing hormone and dopamine on the release of prolactin from the rat anterior pituitary *in vitro*, *Endocrinology*, 95, 1189, 1974.
16. Ingbar, S. H., Autoregulation of the thyroid. Response to iodide excess and depletion, *Mayo Clin. Proc.*, 47, 814, 1972.
17. Dratman, M. B., On the mechanism of action of thyroxin, an amino acid analog of tyrosine, *J. Theor. Biol.*, 46, 255, 1974.
18. Carter, W. J. and Faas, F. H., Thyroxine stimulation of protein synthesis *in vitro* in the absence of mitochondria, *J. Biol. Chem.*, 246, 4973, 1971.
19. Larsen, P. R., Direct immunoassay of triiodothyronine in human serum, *J. Clin. Invest.*, 51, 1939, 1972.
20. Eskin, B. A., Bartuska, D. G., Dunn, M. R., Jacob, G., and Dratman, M. B., Mammary gland dysplasia in iodine deficiency, *JAMA*, 200, 691, 1967.
21. Pankov, A. K., Hormonal activity of the thyroid gland in patients with stomach cancer, *Vopr. Onkol.*, 20, 93, 1974.
22. Krouse, T. B. and Eskin, B. A., Age-related changes in iodine-blocked rat breasts, *Proc. Am. Assoc. Cancer Res.*, 18 (Abstr. 314), 79, 1977.
23. Beatson, G. T., Adjuvant use of thyroid extract in breast cancer therapy, *Lancet*, 2, 162, 1896.
24. Leonard, S. L. and Reece, R. P., The relationship of the thyroid to mammary gland growth in the rat, *Endocrinology*, 28, 65, 1941.
25. Finley, J. W. and Bogardus, G. W., Breast cancer and thyroid disease, *Rev. Surg. Obstet. Gynecol.*, 17, 139, 1960.
26. Buell, P., Epidemiological study of breast cancer statistics in Japanese women, *J. Natl. Cancer Inst.*, 51, 1479, 1973.
27. Bogardus, G. W. and Finley, J. W., Breast cancer and thyroid disease, *Surgery*, 49, 461, 1961.
28. Koszarowski, T., Gadomska, H., Warda, B., and Drozdzweska, Z., Prevalence of malignant neoplasms of the breast in Poland in selected areas (1962—1965), *Pol. Tyg. Lek.*, 23, 933, 1968.
29. Zhivetskii, A. V., Distribution of breast cancer in a goiter district of Northern Bukovina, *Vrach. Delo*, 7, 37, 1968.
30. Kelly, F. C. and Snedden, W. W., Prevalence and geographical distribution of endemic goiter, *WHO Monogr. Ser.*, 44, 27, 1960.
31. Backwinkel, K. and Jackson, A. S., Some features of breast cancer and thyroid deficiency. Report of 280 cases, *Cancer* (Brussels), 17, 1174, 1964.
32. Delange, F., Thilly, C., and Ermans, A. M., Iodine deficiency; a permissive condition in the development of endemic goiter, *J. Clin. Endocrinol. Metab.*, 28, 114, 1968.
33. Repert, R. W., Breast carcinoma study; relation to thyroid disease and diabetes, *J. Mich. State Med. Soc.*, 51, 1315, 1952.
34. Loeser, A. A., A new therapy for prevention of post-operative recurrence in genital and breast cancer: six-year study of prophylactic thyroid treatment, *Br. Med. J.*, 2, 1380, 1954.
35. Ellerker, A. G., Thyroid disorders in breast cancer, a causal connection?, *Med. Press*, 235, 280, 1956.
36. Sommers, S. C., Endocrine abnormalities in women with breast cancer, *Lab. Invest.*, 4, 160, 1955.
37. Wynder, E. L., Bross, I. J., and Hirayama, T., The study of the epidemiology of cancer of the breast, *Cancer (Brussels)*, 13, 559, 1960.
38. Humphrey, L. J. and Swerdlow, M., The relationship of breast disease to thyroid disease, *Cancer (Brussels)*, 17, 1170, 1964.
39. Daro, A. F., Gollin, H. A., and Samos, F. H., The effect of thyroid on cystic mastitis, *J. Int. Coll. Surg.*, 41, 58, 1964.
40. Chalstrey, L. J. and Benjamin, B., High incidence of breast cancer in thyroid cancer patients, *Br. J. Cancer*, 20, 670, 1966.

41. Liechty, R. D., Hodges, R. E., and Burket, J., Cancer and thyroid function, *JAMA*, 183, 116, 1963.
42. Itoh, K. and Maruchi, N., Breast cancer in patients with Hashimoto's thyroiditis, *Lancet*, 2, 1119, 1975.
43. Kapdi, C. C. and Wolfe, J. N., Breast cancer: relationship to thyroid supplements for hypothyroidism, *JAMA*, 236, 1124, 1976.
44. Gorman, C. A., Becker, D. B., Greenspan, F. S., Levy, R. P., Oppenheimer, J. H., Rivlin, R. S., Robbins, J., and VanderLaan, W. P., Breast cancer and thyroid therapy, *JAMA*, 237, 1459, 1977.
45. Edelstyn, G. A., Lyons, A. R., and Welbourn, R. B., Thyroid function in patients with mammary cancer, *Lancet*, 1, 670, 1958.
46. Carter, A. C., Feldman, E. B., and Schwartz, H. L., Levels of serum PBI in patients with metastatic carcinoma of the breast, *J. Clin. Endocrinol.*, 20, 477, 1960.
47. Stoll, B. A., Breast cancer and hypothyroidism, *Cancer (Brussels)*, 18, 1431, 1965.
48. Reeve, T. S., Rundle, F. F., Hayles, I. B., Myhill, J., and Croydon, M., Thyroid function in the presence of breast cancer, *Lancet*, 1, 632, 1961.
49. Capelli, L. and Margottini, M., Thyroid function in cancer patients, *Acta Unio Int. Contra Cancrum*, 20, 1493, 1964.
50. Bignazzi, D. B. and Veronesi, U., Thyroid function in patients with cancer of the breast, *Surg. Gynecol. Obstet.*, 20, 1132, 1965.
51. Sicher, K. and Waterhouse, J. A. H., Thyroid function in relation to prognosis in mammary cancer, *Br. J. Cancer*, 21, 512, 1967.
52. Schottenfeld, D., The relationship of breast cancer to thyroid disease, *J. Chronic Dis.*, 21, 303, 1968.
53. Morris, H. P., Dubnik, C. S., and Salton, A. J., Effect of prolonged ingestion of thiourea on mammary glands and the appearance of mammary tumors in adult C3H mice, *J. Natl. Cancer Inst.*, 7, 159, 1946.
54. Vazquez-Lopez, E., The effects of thiourea on the development of spontaneous tumors on mice, *J. Endocrinol.*, 12, 401, 1949.
55. Moon, R. C. and Turner, C. W., Thyroid hormone and mammary gland growth in the rat, *Proc. Soc. Exp. Biol. Med.*, 103, 149, 1960.
56. Griffith, D. R. and Turner, C. W., Thyroxine and mammary gland growth in rat, *Proc. Soc. Exp. Biol. Med.*, 106, 873, 1961.
57. Moon, R. C., Influence of graded thyroxin levels on mammary gland growth, *Am. J. Physiol.*, 203, 942, 1962.
58. Durbin, P. W., Williams, M. H., Jenug, N., and Arnold, J. S., Development of spontaneous mammary tumors in Sprague-Dawley rat: influence of ovariectomy, thyroidectomy, and adrenalectomy-ovariectomy, *Cancer Res.*, 26, 400, 1966.
59. Aquino, T. I. and Eskin, B. A., Rat breast structure in altered iodine metabolism, *Arch. Pathol.*, 94, 280, 1972.
60. Eskin, B. A., Shuman, R., Krouse, T., and Merion, J., Rat mammary gland atypia produced by iodine blockade with perchlorate, *Cancer Res.*, 35, 2332, 1975.
61. Schonbaum, E., Sellers, E. A., and Gill, M. J., Some effects of perchlorate on the distribution of ^{131}I, *Acta Endocrinol. (Copenhagen)*, 50, 195, 1965.
62. Yamada, T., Effects of perchlorate and other anions on thyroxine metabolism in the rat, *Endocrinology*, 81, 1285, 1967.
63. Jull, J. W. and Huggins, C., Influence of hyperthyroidism and of thyroidectomy on induced mammary cancer, *Nature (London)*, 188, 73, 1960.
64. Newman, W. C. and Moon, R. C., Chemically induced mammary cancer in rats with altered thyroid function, *Cancer Res.*, 28, 864, 1968.
65. Helfenstein, J. E., Young, S., and Currie, A. R., Effect of thiouracil on the development of mammary tumors in rats induced with DMBA, *Nature (London)*, 191, 1108, 1962.
66. Grice, O. D., Fairchild, S., and Thomas, C. G., The effect of hypothyroidism on induced cancer of the breast, *Cancer Res.*, 7 (Abstr.), 26, 1966; 8 (Abstr.), 23, 1967.
67. Gruenstein, M., Meranze, D. R., Acuff, M., and Shimkin, M. B., The role of the thyroid in hydrocarbon-induced mammary carcinogenesis in rats, *Cancer Res.*, 28, 471, 1968.
68. Eskin, B. A., Murphey, S. A., and Dunn, M. R., Induction of breast cancer in altered thyroid states, *Nature (London)*, 218, 1162, 1968.
69. Eskin, B. A., Aquino, T., and Dunn, M. R., Replacement therapy with iodine and thyroxine in breast neoplasias, *Int. J. Gynaecol. Obstet.*, 8, 232, 1970.
70. Shellabarger, C. J., Hypothyroidism and DMBA rat mammary carcinogenesis, *Proc. Am. Assoc. Cancer Res.*, 10, 79, 1969.
71. Davidson, A., Owen, J., and Thomas, C. G., Further studies on the role of altered thyroid functions on experimentally induced breast cancer, *Proc. Am. Assoc. Cancer Res.*, 10, 17, 1969.
72. Kellen, J. A., Effect of hypothyroidism on induction of mammary tumors in rats by DMBA, *J. Natl. Cancer Inst.*, 48, 1901, 1972.

73. Jabara, A. G. and Maritz, J. S. Effects of hypothyroidism and progesterone on mammary tumors induced by DMBA, *Br. J. Cancer*, 28, 161, 1973.

74. Wilkins, R. H. and Morton, D. L., The influence of thyroid hormone analogues on an isotransplanted spontaneous mammary adenocarcinoma in mice, *Cancer (Brussels)*, 16, 558, 1963.

75. Shoemaker, J. P., Bradley, R. L., and Hoffman, R. V., Increased survival and inhibition of mammary tumors in hypothyroid mice, *J. Surg. Res.*, 21, 151, 1976.

76. Thorpe, S. M., Increased uptake of iodide by hormone-responsive compared to hormone-independent mammary tumors in GR mice, *Int. J. Cancer*, 18, 345, 1976.

77. Eskin, B. A., Merion, J. A., Krouse, T. B., and Shuman, R., Blockade of breast iodine by perchlorate in estrogen deficiency, in *Thyroid Research*, Robbins, J. and Braverman, L., Eds., Excerpta Medica, Amsterdam, 1976.

78. Marcuse, P. M., Fibrocystic disease of the breast, correlation of morphologic features with the clinical course, *Am. J. Surg.*, 103, 428, 1962.

79. Eskin, B. A., Merion, J. A., and Stamieszkin, I., Estrogen-iodine interaction in breast dysplasia, *Proc. Am. Assoc. Cancer Res.*, 17 (Abstr. 675), 169, 1976.

80. Brown-Grant, K., Extrathyroidal iodide concentrating mechanisms, *Physiol. Rev.*, 41, 189, 1961.

81. Honour, A. J., Myant, M. B., and Rowlands, E. N., Secretion of radioiodine in digestive juices and milk in man, *Clin. Sci.*, 11, 447, 1952.

82. Van Middlesworth, L., Tuttle, A. H., and Haney, D. F., Iodination of milk proteins by iodide, *Fed. Proc. Fed. Am. Soc. Exp. Biol.*, 13, 157, 1954.

83. Grosvenor, C. F., Secretion of ^{131}I into milk by lactating rat mammary glands, *Am. J. Physiol.*, 199, 419, 1960.

84. Eskin, B. A. and LaMont, B., Measurement of rat breast vascularity by ^{51}Cr uptakes, in manuscript.

85. Merion, J. A. and Eskin, B. A., unpublished data, 1973.

86. Vonderhaar, B. K., A role of thyroid hormones in differentiation of mouse mammary gland *in vitro*, *Biochem. Biophys. Res. Commun.*, 67, 1219, 1975.

87. Eskin, B. A., Jacobson, H. I., Bolmarich, V., and Murray, J. A., Breast atypia in altered thyroid states: intracellular changes, *Senologia*, 4, 114, 1977.

88. Lee, C. and Jacobson, H. I., Uterine estrogen receptor in rats during pubescence and estrus cycle, *Endocrinology*, 88, 596, 1971.

89. Furth, J., *Prolactin and Carcinogenesis*, Boynes, A. R. and Griffith, K., Eds., Alpha Omega Alpha Publishing, Cardiff, 1972.

90. Mittra, I. and Hayward, J. L., Hypothalamic-pituitary-thyroid axis in breast cancer, *Lancet*, 2, 885, 1974.

91. Mittra, I. and Hayward, J. L., Hypothalamic-pituitary-prolactin axis in breast cancer, *Lancet*, 2, 889, 1974.

92. Eskin, B. A., Shuman, R., and Wiley, S., The effects of prolactin on iodine-blocked rat breasts — morphology, *Endocrinology*, 56 (Abstr. 357), A234, 1974.

93. Eskin, B. A., Merion, J., Shuman, R., and Krouse, T., The influence of prolactin, thyrotropin, and TRH on perchlorate-blocked breast tissues, *Endocrinology*, 57, A350, 1975.

94. MacMahon, B., Cole, P., and Brown, R., Etiology of human breast cancer. A review, *J. Natl. Cancer Inst.*, 50, 21, 1973.

95. Stadel, B. V., Dietary iodine and cancer risk — an hypothesis, *Lancet*, 1, 89, 1976.

96. Eskin, B. A., Dietary iodine and cancer risk, *Lancet*, 2, 807, 1976.

97. Lipsett, M. B., Estrogen use and cancer risk, *JAMA*, 237, 1112, 1977.

98. McGuire, W. L., Carbone, P. P., and Vollmer, E. P., *Estrogen Receptors in Human Breast Cancer*, Raven Press, New York, 1975, 17.

99. Eskin, B. A., The influence of estrogen and testosterone on radioactive iodine uptakes in the rat breast, *Endocrinology*, 53, A192, 1971.

100. Quinn, J. L., III, Use of diagnostic nuclear medicine procedures in breast cancer, *Cancer (Brussels)*, 28, 1659, 1971.

101. Whitley, J. E., Witcofski, R. L., Bolliger, T. T., and Maynard, C. D., Tc^{99m} in the visualization of neoplasms outside the brain, *Am. J. Roentgenol.*, 96, 706, 1966.

102. Cancroft, E. T. and Goldsmith, S. J., ^{99m}Tc-pertechnetate scintigraphy as an aid in the diagnosis of breast masses, *Radiology*, 106, 441, 1973.

103. Edwards, C. L. and Hayes, R. L., Scanning malignant neoplasms with gallium,[67] *JAMA*, 212, 1182, 1970.

104. Silverberg, E. and Holleb, A., *Cancer Statistics 1971*, American Cancer Society, New York, 1971.

105. Chang, C. H. J., Sibala, J. L., Lin, F., Jewell, W. R., and Templeton, A. W., Pre-operative diagnosis of potentially precancerous breast lesions by computed tomography breast scanner, *Radiology*, 131, 459, 1978.

106. Emery, E. W. and Trotter, W. R., Triiodothyronine in advanced breast cancer, *Lancet*, 1, 358, 1963.

107. Wynder, E. L., Escher, G. C., and Mantel, N., An epidemiological investigation of cancer of the endometrium, *Cancer (Brussels)*, 19, 489, 1966.
108. MacMahon, B., Risk factors for endometrial cancer, *Gynecol. Oncol.*, 2, 122, 1974.
109. Hansknecht, R. V. and Gusberg, S. B., Estrogen metabolism in patients at high risk for endometrial carcinoma, *Am. J. Obstet. Gynecol.*, 116, 981, 1973.
110. Dickinson, L. E., MacMahon, B., Cole, P., and Brown, J. E., Estrogen profiles of Oriental and Caucasion women of Hawaii, *N. Engl. J. Med.*, 291, 1211, 1974.
111. Haenszel, W. and Kurihara, M., Studies of Japanese migrants. I. Mortality from cancer and other diseases among Japanese in the United States, *J. Natl. Cancer Inst.*, 40, 43, 1968.
112. Cherry, C. P. and Glucksmann, A., The influence of thyroactive substances on the induction of cervico-vaginal tumors in intact and castrate rats, *Br. J. Cancer*, 24, 510, 1970.
113. Kreyberg, L., The influence of intrinsic factors on the development of induced tumors in animals, *Acta Pathol. Microbiol. Scand. Suppl.*, 37, 317, 1938.
114. Silverstone, H. and Tannenbaum, A., Influence of thyroid hormone on the formation of induced skin tumors in mice, *Cancer Res.*, 9, 684, 1949.
115. Shibata, S., Influence of thyroidectomy on the production of epitheliomatous proliferation in the rabbit's ear due to tarring, *Acta Dermatol. Kyoto, Engl. Ed.*, 14, 129, 1929.
116. Bather, R. and Frankcs, W. R., Further studies on the role of thyroxine in chemical carcinogenesis, *Cancer Res.*, 12, 247, 1952.
117. Smith, D. L., Wells, J. A., and D'Amour, F. E., The relationship of the endocrine system to carcinogenesis, *Cancer Res.*, 2, 40, 1942.
118. Meites, J., Effects of thyroxine and thiouracil on induction of skin tumors in mice by 9,10-dimethyl-1,2,benzanthracene and croton oil, *Cancer Res.*, 18, 176, 1958.
119. Morrell, S. D. and Hermann, F., Influence of systemically administered cortisone on hair growth in mice, *J. Invest. Dermatol.*, 37, 243, 1961.
120. Sherwin-Weidenreich, R. and Herrmann, F., Hair cycle and chemically induced epidermal carcinogenesis in mice receiving tri-iodothyronine, *J. Invest. Dermatol.*, 40, 225, 1963.
121. Paschkis, K. E., Cantarow, A., and Stasney, J., Influence of thiouracil on carcinoma induced by 2 AAF, *Cancer Res.*, 8, 257, 1948.
122. Paschkis, K. E., Cantarow, A., and Stasney, J., Competitive action of 2-thiouracil and uracil in AAF-induced cancer of the liver, *Science*, 114, 264, 1951.
123. Bielschowsky, F. and Hall, W. H., Carcinogenesis in the thyroidectomized rat, *Br. J. Cancer*, 7, 358, 1953.
124. Leathem, J. H. and Barken, H. B., Relationship between thyroid activity and liver tumor induction with 2AAF, *Cancer Res.*, 10, 231, 1950.
125. Perry, D. J., Effect of adrenalectomy on the development of tumors induced by 2 AAF, *Br. J. Cancer*, 15, 284, 1961.
126. Goodall, C. M., Hepatic carcinogenesis in thyroidectomized rats: apparent blockade at the stage of initiation, *Cancer Res.*, 26, 1880, 1966.
127. Kreyberg, L., Influence of dinitrolerisol on the development of tar tumors in mice, *Am. J. Cancer*, 36, 51, 1939.
128. Tannenbaum, A. and Silverstone, H., Effect of low environmental temperature, dinitropherol, or sodium fluoride on the formation of tumors in mice, *Cancer Res.*, 9, 403, 1949.
129. Miller, W. L. and Baumann, C. A., Basal metabolic rate and liver tumors due to azo dyes, *Cancer Res.*, 11, 634, 1951.
130. Leathem, J. H. and Oddis, L., Hyperthyroidism and hepatic tumor induction, *Proc. Am. Assoc. Cancer Res.*, 3, 243, 1961.
131. Stroev, E. A. and Nikulin, A. A., Hormone regulation of the enzyme content of cells of transplantable liver cancer in rat, *Vopr. Onkol.*, 20, 56, 1974.

Chapter 7

THE ROLE OF PROLACTIN IN TUMOR DEVELOPMENT

P. A. Kelly, F. Labrie, and J. Asselin

TABLE OF CONTENTS

I. INTRODUCTION

Prolactin, the "mammotropic hormone," was first isolated from sheep pituitary glands in the 1930s.[1,2] Although prolactin was identified and purified in a number of other species in the subsequent years, there was a serious question regarding the existence of a separate human prolactin molecule since human growth hormone was shown to possess, in addition to its growth-promoting activity, substantial bioassayable "prolactin activity."[3] In fact, a 1970 publication by Bewley and Li,[4] stated that the "hormonal control of lactation and growth in the human is effected through a single pituitary hormone, namely hGH."

There was, however, mounting evidence supporting the existence of a separate prolactin in the primate. Frantz and Kleinberg[5] used an in vitro bioassay to measure elevated lactogenic activity in serum of patients with abnormal lactation, while in the same samples, growth hormone levels were normal. Friesen's group then made the important observations that pregnant monkey pituitaries produce a protein immunologically different from human growth hormone, but which cross-reacts with an antiserum to ovine prolactin,[6] and that incubations of human pituitaries actively synthesize and secrete prolactin.[7]

Independently, human prolactin was isolated and purified in the laboratories of Lewis[8] and Friesen.[9] A specific radioimmunoassay was developed by Friesen's group[10] and subsequently a number of other laboratories developed homologous and heterologous radioimmunoassays to measure circulating prolactin. With interest rekindled by the identification of human prolactin, there has been, in the succeeding years, a plethora of data appearing on the secretion, control, and mechanism of action of prolactin.

In this chapter, we will review some of the data on the physiological control of prolactin secretion as well as describe some of the numerous functions ascribed to prolactin and placental lactogens. One of the most recent aspects has been the identification of specific receptors for prolactin in various target tissues. These receptors will be discussed as a means of modulating hormone action. Finally, the role of prolactin as a promoter of tumor development will be described with special emphasis on mammary carcinoma.

II. MEASUREMENT OF PROLACTIN

The ability of an extract of pituitary glands to stimulate the crop sacs of hypophysectomized doves was the initial assay method utilized to measure prolactin (PRL) activity.[1,2] Using this pigeon-crop sac assay system, Riddle et al.[2] successfully isolated, purified, and named prolactin. Probably the most widely known action of prolactin in mammals is its effect on the mammary gland. In addition, prolactin is luteotropic in rodents, thus being a primary hormone involved in the maintenance of the corpus luteum.[11] Although these and other bioassay techniques have been successfully applied to the measurement of prolactin in pituitary extracts, none of the assays was suitable to measure normal circulating levels of prolactin, since the assay sensitivity was between 200 and 10,000 ng of prolactin. As was mentioned in Section I, the identification of human prolactin was not made until 1971. This delay was due in part to the inherent lactogenic activity of the growth hormone molecule. Another assay technique, namely, in vitro bioassays using mammary tissue explants from mice or rabbits, was important in the identification of human prolactin as a separate molecule.[5] These assays, which measure activity between 2 to 100 ng/mℓ plasma, are much more sensitive than those previously utilized. However, a major drawback is the amount of work and time required to assay only a few samples.[12]

Yalow and Berson[13] revolutionized endocrinology in 1959 with the development of a radioimmunoassay to measure plasma insulin. In the years that followed, specific radioimmunoassays for numerous protein as well as nonprotein hormones were developed, including radioimmunoassays for prolactins of cow, sheep, goat, pig, mouse, rat, and dog.

The initial radioimmunoassays for human prolactin were heterologous and used the cross-reaction of prolactin from one species with an antiserum of another. The first such assay utilized the cross-reaction of primate prolactins with antiserum to ovine prolactin.[6] With the subsequent isolation and purification of human prolactin, specific homologous radioimmunoassays were developed.[10,14] This development of a simple and reliable means of measuring human prolactin enabled a great expansion of knowledge of both the physiological and pathological control of prolactin secretion.

A recent advance in methodology is the development of a radioreceptor assay (RRA) to measure prolactin and lactogenic hormones.[15,16] This assay utilizes specific, high-affinity receptors for prolactin in rabbit mammary glands (see Section VI). A major advantage of the prolactin RRA is that it is not species specific as are most radioimmunoassays, since presumably the biologically active part of the molecule binds to the receptor. This assay can and has been used to screen active fragments of the prolactin molecule in the search for smaller active peptides. The other advantages of the RRA are that it is simple and quick (samples can be assayed in 6 hr) and the reaction is highly specific to hormones with lactogenic activity. This includes prolactin, primate growth hormones, and placental lactogens (PL). The RRA has in fact been successfully applied to identify and quantitate PL in species which before had not been recognized as possessing PL activity.[17] Data on PL activity in a number of species have recently been reviewed.[18] It should be mentioned that the ability of the receptor to recognize all three types of lactogenic hormones necessitates, when the levels are sufficiently high to interfere, measuring the level of the other two hormones by RIA. This is not a problem when measuring human placental lactogen, however, since hPL levels often exceed 2000 to 3000 ng/mℓ, whereas hGH levels are usually below 5 ng/mℓ and PRL levels below 30 ng/mℓ, and not higher than 200 ng/mℓ at term.

III. CIRCULATING FORMS OF PROLACTIN

For many years, hormones circulating in the blood were thought to exist with a single molecular size, that is, with the molecular weight of the purified hormone. A number of polypeptide hormones have been reported to be heterogeneous, that is, they appear in the circulation in more than one form, including insulin,[19] parathyroid hormone,[20] gastrin,[21] adrenocorticotropic hormone,[22] and growth hormone.[23]

Native human prolactin has a molecular weight of approximately 21,000 daltons.[8,9] In normal subjects, two forms of human prolactin were first separated by gel filtration using a column of the molecular sieve Sephadex® G-100. The first two forms identified were "little" human PRL, which accounted for 80 to 90% of the total activity and the "big" form which was less than 20%.[24] Aubert et al.[25] reported a third form, "big-big" prolactin, which constituted between 0.8 to 7.9% of the total prolactin activity.

The molecular form of prolactin varies under different physiological conditions and following various stimuli. The greatest amounts of "big" prolactin (up to 31%) are found during pregnancy.[24] In a study reported by Kataoka et al.,[26] the major circulating form of human prolactin was "big", and following stimulation with thyrotropin releasing hormone (TRH), the predominant form was "little". Suh and Frantz,[24] however, failed to observe any change in the distribution of human prolactin following TRH injection nor with breast stimulation or L-dopa inhibition.

The distribution pattern in serum of patients with pituitary-secreting tumors is altered compared to that of normal patients, in that there is a shift to the larger molecular weight forms "big" and "big-big".[24,25] Freezing and thawing, urea or mercaptoethanol treatments have been reported to convert some of the "big" prolactin to the "little" form.

Aubert et al.[25] compared the forms of human PRL by radioimmunoassay and radioreceptor assay and reported that "big" prolactin had 25% less activity in the RRA than when measured by radioimmunoassay (RIA). Guyda[27] failed to confirm this, reporting comparable immunologic and receptor activity for all forms of human prolactin.

These data indicate that prolactin is found in the circulation in several forms, albeit the major form is "little" prolactin. During periods of increased secretion, such as during pregnancy or in patients with tumors, a larger proportion of the bigger forms is found. These larger forms may be storage or precursor forms of production, suggesting the possibility that prolactin is secreted as a prohormone.

IV. REGULATION OF PROLACTIN SECRETION

A number of excellent reviews on the control of prolactin secretion in animals[28-30] and humans[31,32] have been published in the last several years. It is not within the scope of this chapter to present a complete review on the control of prolactin secretion. However, it is important to understand the complexity of the physiology of prolactin secretion in viewing its overall involvement in tumor development.

In a number of species, plasma prolactin levels fluctuate during the reproductive cycle. In the rat, for example, a tremendous surge in plasma prolactin occurs in the late afternoon of proestrus, coincident with the preovulatory surge in luteinizing hormone (LH) and follicle-stimulating hormone (FSH) that occurs at this time.[33] In humans, on the other hand, there is still some question as to the existence of a midcycle peak, but if one occurs at all, it is of a very small magnitude.[32] Normal plasma levels are less than 30 ng/ml.[10]

The proestrous peak of prolactin in rats is mediated by estrogens, as ovariectomy abolishes the peak, and estrogen administration to rats ovariectomized in proestrus causes a rise in prolactin the next day.[34] The administration of estrogen to either male or female rats, in fact, increases basal plasma prolactin levels[35] and estradiol administration to ovariectomized rats induces spontaneous diurnal prolactin peaks.[36,37]

Prolactin levels are low during pregnancy, increasing just before term in a number of species.[29] Several species also possess a placental lactogen which is present in much higher concentrations than the prolactin of pituitary origin.[17] In humans, plasma PRL levels begin to rise at approximately 8 weeks of gestation with a continual increase until term, attaining levels of 200 ng/ml.[10] In amniotic fluid, the concentration of human prolactin increases to exceedingly high levels (1 to 15 μg/ml) compared to either maternal or fetal levels.[38]

Overall, prolactin levels are lower in male rats than in females and the pronounced cyclic fluctuations seen in females is not present in males.[39] Prolactin secretion in humans is episodic, that is, it shows bursts of variable height and duration[40] and these irregular bursts have been reported to be higher in women than in men.[32]

In addition to the peak of prolactin which occurs on proestrus, Koch et al.[41] observed a diurnal rhythm or prolactin secretion in both male and female rats, with values approximately twice as high in the late afternoon as in the morning. More recently, an early morning (4 a.m.) peak or nyctohemeral rhythm has also been observed in rats.[42] In humans, this nyctohemeral rhythm is absent, but sleep, whether it occurs in day time or night time, is associated with significant elevations of human prolactin concentrations.[40,43]

Stress has been reported to be a potent stimulator of prolactin secretion in rats.[34] In humans, psychic and physical stress result in marked elevations in prolactin secretion.[44] Therefore, the method of sampling used for either animals or humans is an important consideration, so that artificially elevated levels are not obtained.

A resume of the proposed factors controlling the secretion of prolactin from the anterior pituitary is shown in Figure 1. In 1954, Everett[45] established that the hypothalamus exhibits an overall inhibitory effect on prolactin secretion. This was shown by removal of the pituitary from the sella turcica and transplantation beneath the kidney capsule which resulted in a continuous secretion of prolactin, indicated by a maintenance of luteal function, whereas secretion of the other anterior pituitary hormones was diminished as was evidenced by an atrophy of the target organs and a decreased rate of body growth. Later, Chen et al.[46] measured plasma prolactin levels in rats receiving one to four transplanted pituitaries and showed a progressive increase in

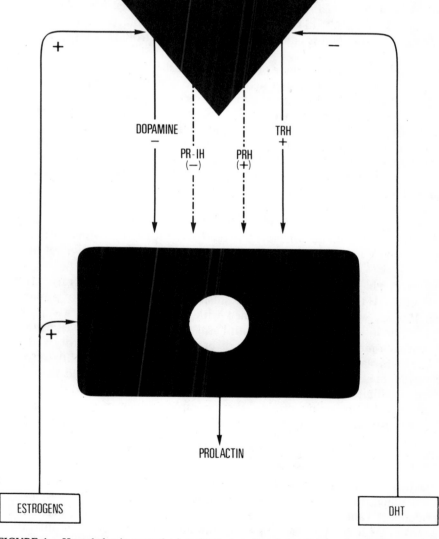

FIGURE 1. Hypothalamic control of prolactin secretion from the anterior pituitary and the influence of peripheral steroid hormones.

prolactin secretion, the more pituitaries that were present. As a result of reports such as this, a negative control or "prolactin inhibiting factor" (PIF) was proposed. This is indicated by the broken line PR-IH or prolactin-release-inhibiting hormone in Figure 1. The existence of a separate PR-IH is clouded by the potent inhibitory effect of dopamine on prolactin secretion.[30]

The site of the dopamine inhibition on prolactin secretion has been studied. L-Dopa, a dopamine precursor, has been shown to inhibit prolactin secretion in man via a proposed dopamine stimulation of PIF activity. The existence of dopamine receptors in the hypothalamus is in question,[48,49] but recently dopamine receptors have been identified and characterized in the anterior pituitary gland,[50] which raises the possibility that dopamine is the PR-IH since it can act directly at the pituitary level. Using an in vitro model system of anterior pituitary glands in primary culture, Caron et al.[50] have also shown the ability of dopamine and its agonists to markedly inhibit prolactin secretion and, interestingly, the ability of the catecholamines studied to inhibit prolactin secretion was strongly correlated with its affinity for the dopamine receptor.

One of the important dopamine agonists, due to its reduced toxicity in humans, which has been developed is an alkaloid of the naturally occurring ergots, 2-bromoergocryptine (CB-154). CB-154 is a potent inhibitor of prolactin secretion in both animals[51] and humans[52] and is clinically important in controlling cases of hyperprolactinemia.

Thyrotropin-releasing hormone (TRH) was first shown in vitro to increase prolactin release,[53] and was later demonstrated in vivo in a number of species,[54-56] including man,[57] to be a potent stimulator of prolactin secretion. TRH receptors have, in fact, been identified in the plasma membrane of pituitary cells,[58] and TRH receptors in rat pituitaries are increased by estrogen administration[59] and fluctuate with the estrous cycle.[60] Estrogens (Figure 1) are a potent stimulator of prolactin secretion in rats[61] and man.[62] The fact that TRH receptors are elevated during periods of increased prolactin secretion[59,60] indicates that TRH may have an important role in the physiological control of prolactin secretion.

The existence of a separate prolactin releasing hormone (PRH) is at present uncertain (Figure 1). The most direct evidence for such a factor is that elevations of prolactin secretion can occur with no coincident increase in thyroid stimulating hormone (TSH). However, such a factor, which acts only to release prolactin, has not yet been identified.

Testosterone has been reported to stimulate prolactin secretions in rats.[29] If dihydrotestosterone (DHT) is used rather than testosterone, no stimulation of prolactin is observed. Rather, when DHT is combined with estrogen treatment, a suppression of plasma prolactin levels is observed, both basal morning levels[63] as well as the spontaneous estrogen-induced afternoon peak of prolactin.[64] The stimulatory action of testosterone on prolactin secretion is, therefore, probably due to its ability to form estrogenic metabolites. Such conversion does not occur with DHT, and the only effect observed is inhibitory (Figure 1). A number of catecholamines and drugs have been reported to affect prolactin secretion. For a complete review of the effect of catecholamines on prolactin secretion, see Chapter 6 by Cave and MacLeod.

V. FUNCTIONS OF PROLACTIN

Prolactin has more reported actions than any other hormone. In fact, at least 85 proposed functions have been ascribed to prolactin when the entire Vertebrate Class is considered.[65] Table 1 outlines some of the reported actions that prolactin may have in mammals. Of course, prolactin is most commonly known for its stimulatory action on the mammary gland, including mammogenesis, lactogenesis, and galactoporesis. It

TABLE 1

Some Reported Actions of Prolactin in Mammals

Action	Target organ
Mammary development	Mammary gland
Mammogenesis	
Lactogenesis	
Galactopoiesis	
Maintenance of luteal function	Corpus luteum
Luteolysis	Corpus luteum
Stimulation of secondary sex glands	Prostate, seminal vesicles
Glycogenolysis	Liver
Increased free fatty acids	Mammary gland, liver
Stimulation of somatomedin production	Liver
Reduction of blood glucose	Blood
Increased fluid ion transport	Intestine
Osmoregulation	Kidney
Elevation of cardiac output	Heart
Reduction of blood volume	Circulatory system
Stimulation of estrogen receptors	Mammary gland, liver
Stimulation of prolactin receptors	Liver, mammary gland, mammary tumor, prostate
Stimulation of LH receptors	Ovary, testis

is important, however, to remember that prolactin produces its effects on the mammary gland by a synergism with estrogen, progesterone, corticosteroids, insulin, and growth hormone.[66]

In addition to the well-known effects at the level of the mammary gland, prolactin has also been characterized as a luteotropic hormone involved in the maintenance of the corpus luteum.

Examination of the various actions of prolactin as well as the target organs involved is important, for any tissue which is prolactin responsive could also develop a prolactin-responsive tumor. The biochemical identification of such prolactin-responsive tissues is described in the next section.

VI. PROLACTIN RECEPTORS

A. Assay of Prolactin Receptors

For the quantification of receptor levels in a tissue, crude plasma membrane fractions are prepared by differential centrifugation, and ovine prolactin is iodinated to a low specific activity (20 to 60 μCi/μg). Prolactin binding is assayed using a fixed quantity of membrane preparation (200 μg) with a fixed quantity of [^{125}I] ovine prolactin (approximately 100,000 counts/min.). The difference in the counts per minute of tubes incubated in the absence (total binding) or presence (nonspecific binding) of excess unlabeled prolactin yields the prolactin specifically bound to the binding sites. Dividing the specific binding by the number of counts per minute added to the incubation results in the "percent specific binding". In addition to these "single-point assays", saturation curves or displacement curves can be carried out on representative membrane preparations and the data transformed into Scatchard plots[67] yielding affinity constants and binding capacities of the membranes.

B. Tissue Distribution

Binding of polypeptide hormones to specific receptors located in the plasma membrane of the cell is the first event in the action of these hormones in their target tissues. Specific receptors for a large number of polypeptide hormones have already been identified.[68]

Specific prolactin binding has been identified in plasma membrane fractions of these tissues as follows:[69-72]

- Liver
- Kidney
- Mammary gland
- Mammary tumor
- Adrenal
- Ovary
- Testis
- Prostate
- Seminal vesicle
- Uterus

Surprisingly, one of the tissues which bound the greatest quantity of prolactin was the liver. The presence of prolactin binding sites in the liver is not restricted just to one or two species, as is illustrated in Figure 2. Prolactin binding was observed in pigeons as well as a number of mammals.[73] Undoubtedly, the list will grow as other species are investigated.

SPECIES DISTRIBUTION OF LIVER PROLACTIN OR GROWTH HORMONE BINDING SITES

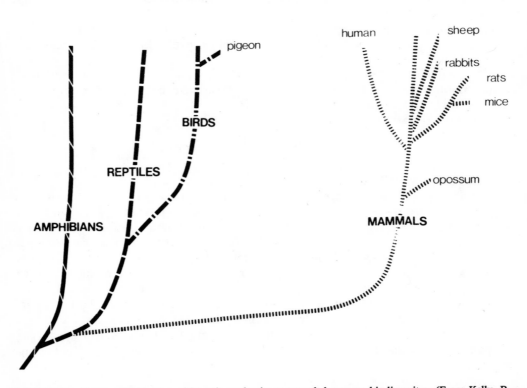

FIGURE 2. Species distribution of hepatic prolactin or growth hormone binding sites. (From Kelly, P. A., Ferland, L., Labrie, F., and DeLean, A., in *Hypothalamus and Endocrine Functions*, Labrie, F., Meites, J., and Pelletier, G., Eds., Plenum Press, New York, 1976, 321. With permission.)

C. Regulation of Prolactin Receptors

The concept that hormone receptors are not static systems, but rather change according to the physiological state of the animal, has many interesting implications in terms of control of cellular activity. We initially chose as a model system for our study the prolactin receptor in rat liver. These binding sites have been shown to be specific for lactogenic hormones, i.e., prolactin, primate growth hormones, or placental lactogens.[69] The first interesting observation was that the level of these binding sites is very low in male rats and quite high in female animals. Furthermore, when these binding sites were studied as a function of the developmental state of the rat, we observed a marked increase of receptor levels following puberty and during pregnancy.[74] In addition, we demonstrated a fluctuation in the concentration of these binding sites during the estrous cycle as well as a reduction after ovariectomy and a rapid decline following hypophysectomy.[75]

In rats, prolactin has specifically been reported to affect hepatic free fatty acid synthesis[76] and RNA synthesis[77] and stimulate somatomedin production[78] as well as estrogen receptor levels[79] in the liver. Although a coupling of prolactin binding to one of these events has not yet been established, prolactin binding sites in rat liver do conform to the other requirements which define a hormone receptor, namely, they are specific for only prolactin or prolactin-related hormones and they have an affinity constant of a magnitude sufficient to bind circulating of levels of hormones (Ka $\sim$ 1.5 nM^{-1}). We have conclusively shown, however, that these sites are not sites associated with the degradation of the prolactin molecule.[69,74]

1. Stimulatory Effect of Estrogens

A schematic representation of the hormonal control of the prolactin binding site in rat liver is shown in Figure 3. Since binding sites were higher in females than males and increased following puberty and during pregnancy,[69,74] and these periods are normally associated with increased production of ovarian steroids, the effects of estrogen and progesterone on prolactin binding were examined. Estradiol (50 μg) injected daily for 8 days to male rats increased liver prolactin binding to levels observed in females, whereas progesterone was without effect.[80] The fact that prolactin binding can be stimulated by estrogens, fluctuates with the estrous cycle, and is reduced by ovariectomy implies a direct physiological involvement of estradiol. A confirmation of this involvement was obtained using the antiestrogenic compounds tamoxifene or nafoxidine, which were capable of reducing estrogen-stimulated prolactin binding in male rats.[75] In females, we have recently found that a highly potent antiestrogen, RU16117 (11α-methoxyethinyl estradiol), a product of Roussel-UCLAF, Paris, is capable of reducing estrogen-stimulated prolactin binding by 30 to 70% with doses 1000 times less than those required for the other antiestrogens.[73]

2. Stimulatory Effect of Prolactin

The loss of prolactin binding in rat liver following hypophysectomy implied the importance of a pituitary factor in the maintenance of these binding sites.[75,80] A direct effect of prolactin on its own receptor was first implied when we demonstrated that prolactin binding to rat liver in hypophysectomized rats, given a pituitary implant under the kidney capsule, began to increase approximately 3 days following the increase in serum prolactin levels.[81] Costlow et al.[82] have also shown that direct administration of 2 mg prolactin to hypophysectomized female rats increased prolactin binding in rat liver.

Another method of demonstrating a direct effect of prolactin on its own receptor is to study prolactin receptor levels in animals bearing prolactin-secreting tumors. The tumor chosen in this case was MtT/F4, which secretes prolactin, growth hormone, and ACTH. Six weeks after transplantation, at a time when tumors were well developed,

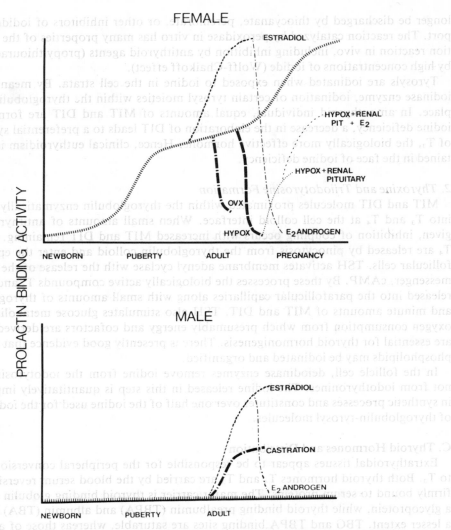

FIGURE 3.   Endocrine control of liver prolactin binding sites in male and female rats.

the animals were sacrificed and livers removed. For both intact and adrenalectomized rats, presence of the prolactin-secreting tumor was associated with significant stimulation of prolactin binding.[73] These results are similar to those reported by Posner[83] for MtT/F4, MtT/F45, and MtT/W5 tumors.

Although prolactin is capable of increasing prolactin binding in hypophysectomized animals, it is not able to increase binding to levels found in intact female animals. Costlow et al.[82] found that even with replacement of a number of other anterior pituitary hormones, binding was never greater than 30% of intact levels. This positive effect of prolactin on the maintenance of its own receptor levels is contrary to what is observed for a number of other hormones, such as GH, insulin, and LH, for which increased plasma hormone levels result in a down regulation of the receptor. We have, in fact, recently shown a desensitization of testicular LH receptors with exogenously administered human chorionic gonadotropin or by increasing the endogenous level of LH by injection of a potent luteinizing hormone-releasing hormone agonist.[84]

3. Inhibitory Effect of Androgens

The effect of androgen administration to both males and females results in a reduction of prolactin binding to rat liver.[64,73] Testosterone and DHT reduced basal- as well as estrogen-stimulated prolactin binding without affecting plasma prolactin levels. Recently, we have found that the afternoon peak of prolactin induced in ovariectomized rats by estrogen administration[36,37] is inhibited when estrogen treatment is combined with DHT injections.[64] However, the fact that DHT reduces prolactin binding in males without affecting plasma prolactin levels indicates that this androgen may have a direct effect on prolactin receptors.

4. Mechanism of the Stimulatory Effect of Estradiol

Since estrogen administration increases plasma prolactin levels,[29] it is also important to examine the mechanism by which estrogens increase prolactin receptor levels in rat liver. At the outset of this discussion, it should be mentioned that estrogen administration to hypophysectomized rats has no effect on the level of hepatic prolactin receptors.[80] In an attempt to examine the stimulatory effect of estradiol, a dose response was carried out for both prolactin binding as well as the level of plasma prolactin in ovariectomized rats. As little as 0.05 μg estradiol injected twice a day for 7 days significantly increased prolactin binding, while plasma prolactin increased significantly in rats receiving the dose of 3.2 μg. Although these animals were sacrificed in the morning prior to the afternoon peak, it is still unlikely that with the 60-fold difference between the dose-response curve for prolactin binding and plasma prolactin level that the increase in prolactin binding following estradiol treatment is only mediated by an increase in circulating prolactin levels.[73]

The concept that estrogen stimulates the prolactin receptor directly is strengthened by a study which showed that the prolactin-lowering drug CB-154 injected together with estradiol was capable of reducing the plasma prolactin levels, but had no inhibitory effect on the level of prolactin binding. This is true for animals sacrificed both in the morning and at the time of the afternoon peak.[37,73]

A consideration of the various factors modulating the level of prolactin receptor in the female rat is illustrated in Figure 4. It is unquestionable that the presence of the pituitary is necessary for maintenance of prolactin receptor levels. This positive effect of prolactin is probably exerted by a direct interaction with the receptor. Also, the anterior pituitary exerts a positive influence on the ovary, which in turn (along with the adrenal) secretes estrogens, which via an interaction with a cytoplasmic receptor also have a positive effect in the maintenance of prolactin receptors.

D. Dissociation of Endogenously Bound Prolactin

As a result of elevated plasma levels of prolactin or other lactogenic hormones, often exceeding 1000 ng/mℓ, occurring, for example, during pregnancy[17] or during a spontaneous afternoon surge,[36,37] a certain fraction of the prolactin receptors in a target cell might be occupied with endogenous prolactin. This situation is illustrated in Figure 5. Although the procedure of homogenization and plasma membrane fractionation offers the opportunity for prolactin to dissociate from its binding sites, a large portion of the prolactin still remains bound to the receptors at the end of the preparation. It thus became of interest to develop a technique to remove this endogenously bound prolactin.

Two possible approaches have evolved. The first involved an in vivo desaturation of the prolactin receptor by lowering the circulating level of plasma prolactin for a short period prior to removal of the tissue. We have successfully applied this approach to the quantitation of prolactin receptors in the mammary gland of the rabbit during pregnancy.[85] It was effective because the rabbit does not produce a placental lactogen.[17,18] A quantitation of prolactin receptor levels in rat mammary glands revealed a

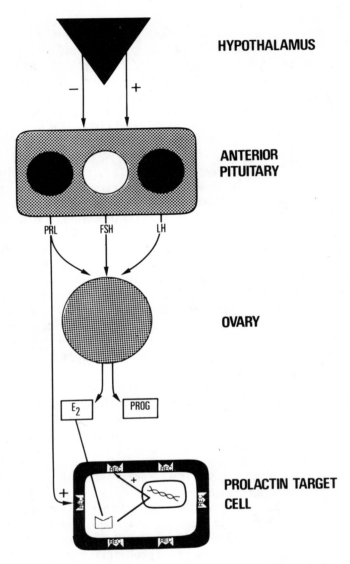

FIGURE 4.   Interaction of prolactin and estradiol in the regulation
of prolactin receptors.

low level of receptors during pregnancy with a marked increase during lactation. If,
however, the source of placental lactogen was removed by surgical removal of the
placenta, the level of prolactin binding approached that observed during lactation.[86]

The level of placental lactogen in the rat during the second half of pregnancy is
approximately 800 ng/mℓ.[15,87] Holdaway et al.,[88] using rats infused with ovine prolactin, demonstrated that when levels exceeded 300 ng/mℓ, receptor concentrations in
both mammary tumor and liver began to decline. Therefore, the hypothesis that placental lactogen was occupying a majority of the prolactin receptor sites and lowering
available receptor levels is reasonable.

The second technique involves an in vitro desaturation of the hormone from the
receptor. Several chiotropic agents were examined including high molar concentrations
of magnesium chloride, ammonium thiocyanate, and sodium trifluoroacetate as well
as urea or acidic or basic pH. Most of these agents were capable, with more or less

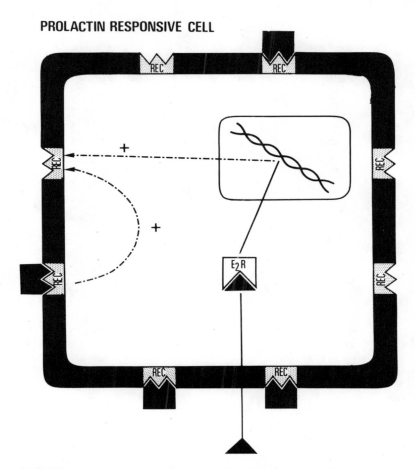

FIGURE 5. A prolactin-responsive cell with 50% occupancy of receptors by endogenous prolactin.

effectiveness, of removing [^{125}I]-labeled prolactin from the receptors. Few, however, maintained the integrity of the receptor. Figure 6 shows that 4 to 5 M magnesium chloride is capable of removing 90 to 95% of the labeled hormone from rabbit mammary gland prolactin receptors. When the receptors are reexposed to fresh labeled prolactin, they retain their ability to specifically bind the prolactin. Ammonium thiocyanate was less effective both in dissociating and rebinding.

Since lactogen levels must be relatively high to see an effect on prolactin binding, this procedure, although not universally mandatory, is useful for the quantification of hormone receptor levels.

So far, this section has dealt primarily with prolactin receptors in rat liver. Mention has also been made of prolactin binding in other tissues of the rat as well as other species. The control of prolactin receptors in all prolactin-responsive tissues is not uniform. This point is best illustrated by the rat ventral prostate, which has abundant prolactin receptors.[89] Castration of male rats results in a reduction of prolactin receptors of the prostate,[89,90] but an increase in those of the liver, since androgens have been shown to be inhibitory to hepatic prolactin receptors.[64] On the other hand, prolactin receptors in the prostate are enhanced in animals injected with testosterone propionate or DHT[90,91] and hepatic prolactin binding is reduced.[64]

Other groups have failed to see a stimulatory effect of estrogens on mammary gland

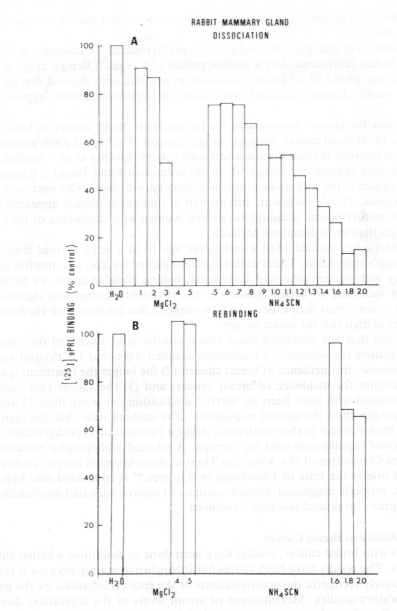

FIGURE 6.   Effect of increasing molar concentrations of magnesium chloride (MgCl₂) and ammonium thiocyanate (NH₄SCN) on (A) dissociation of [^{125}I] ovine prolactin from rabbit mammary gland receptors and (B) subsequent specific rebinding of fresh [^{125}I] ovine prolactin.

prolactin receptors,[86] whereas prolactin itself has been shown to stimulate and progesterone inhibit prolactin binding in lactating rabbit mammary glands.[92]

The need to examine the specific control mechanisms involved in the target tissue to be investigated is clear. The control of prolactin receptor levels in mammary tumors, both rat and human, is covered in a following section.

VII. PROLACTIN AND TUMORS

A. Prolactin-secreting Tumors

1. Laboratory Animal Tumors

Prolactin is produced in pituitary acidophils. Neoplastic transformation of these acidophils results in an abnormally elevated secretion of prolactin. Mammotropic tumors are one of the most frequent neoplasms in old rats, occurring in approximately 50% of both males and females 600 days of age or older.[93]

Furth[94] described the appearance of tumors in rodents which appeared after long periods of treatment with estrogenic hormones. Tranplantation of these estrogen-induced tumors indicated their prolactin secretory capacities, and they were named mammotropic tumors (MtT).[94] In subsequent transplantations, these grafts were noted to lose their initial dependence on estrogen, but still retained the ability to respond to estrogen administration. In addition, the grafts started to secrete growth hormone,[95,96] while some mammotropic tumors attained the ability to secrete adrenocorticotropic hormone (ACTH). The range of mammotropic tumors that are currently found along with their hormonal production is shown in Table 2.

2. Human Tumors

In humans, levels of plasma prolactin in excess of 200 ng/ml are a probable indicator of a prolactin-secreting tumor; however, such tumors can produce vastly differing concentrations of plasma prolactin in patients.[32] Pituitary adenomas may be caused by hypothalamic dysfunction, either overproduction of a prolactin-releasing factor or underproduction of a prolactin-inhibiting hormone or of dopamine. Hyperprolactinemia is also observed with other classes of tumors, such as craniopharyngiomas, metastases, or pituitary stalk compression.[32]

Patients with mildly or severely elevated plasma prolactin levels often have galactorrhea. This condition, characterized by milk production in nonsuckling women, ranges in severity from being almost unnoticeable to the patient to severe leakage from unstimulated breasts. In a large percentage of women with elevated prolactin, the reproductive cycles are irregular or completely absent. The various conditions identified previously by eponyms have been classified by Bohnet and Friesen[32] as "hyperprolactinemic anovulatory syndromes". Accompanying elevated prolactin levels is an absence of menstrual cycles occurring in approximately 15% of all patients with secondary amen-

TABLE 2

Hormonal Production of Various Strains of Mammotropic Tumor (MtT)

Tumor type	PRL^a (ng/ml)	GH^b (ng/ml)	ACTH^c (mU/ml)
Normal	5—200	5—200	0.06
Spontaneous (males)	132—1,820	13—330	0
DES-treated^d (females)	132—725	17—138	0
Transplanted MtT W15	3,400—23,000	15—2,510	0
Transplanted MtT W5/St	45—860	800—2,170	0
Transplanted MtT F4	50—2,900	50—790	~60

^{a} Prolactin.
^{b} Growth hormone.
^{c} Adrenocorticotropic hormone.
^{d} Diethylstilbestrol

After Furth, J., *Prolactin and Carcinogenesis: 4th Tenovus Workshop*, Boyns, A. R. and Griffiths, K., Eds., Alpha Omega Alpha, Cardiff, 1972, 137. With permission.

orrhea.[97,98] In most cases, lowering of plasma prolactin levels, either surgically by removal of the tumorous tissue or by treatment with CB-154, results in resumption of normal cycles.[99,100]

Surprisingly, galactorrhea does not occur in all patients with elevated prolactin levels, although many of these patients have a pituitary adenoma.[101] A possible explanation could involve the different circulating forms of prolactin secreted by pituitary tumors.[25,102] Since the "big-big" form of prolactin has been reported to have reduced biological activity as measured by radioreceptor assay, it could be possible to have elevated plasma prolactin as measured by radioimmunoassay with little or no prolactin activity.[32]

Finally, as discussed in Section VI, tissue sensitivity can change as a result of variation in the concentration of prolactin receptors. Some patients could be less sensitive to elevated prolactin concentrations, even if the prolactin in the circulation had full biological activity due to a deficiency of prolactin receptors in the mammary gland.

3. Ectopic Hormone Production

In addition to normal hormone production of prolactin by the pituitary and of human placental lactogen by the placenta, lactogenic hormones, as well as other hormones, can be produced at sites not normally associated with production of the hormone.

Human chorionic gonadotropin (hCG) and human placental lactogen (hPL) are normally synthesized and secreted by the syncytiotrophoblastic cells of the placenta. Secretion of hPL in the plasma of 11 of 128 patients with various forms of malignancies other than those originating in the trophoblast has been reported.[103] Recently, 10 of 72 patients with established carcinoma of the breast were found to have detectable levels of hPL in the plasma.[104] Human placental lactogen was also measured in the plasma and testicular extracts of a patient with embryonal cell carcinoma of the testicle.[105] The authors in fact propose that the hPL may be responsible for the gynecomastia observed in this patient.

The presence of hCG in the plasma of patients with breast carcinoma has also been reported to occur in approximately 15% of the samples analyzed.[104,106] The significance of the ectopically produced hCG is not known, but it is proposed that it might be useful as a possible biochemical indicator of breast cancer.

The placenta also produces a factor, human chorionic thyrotropin (hCT), which has thyroid-stimulating properties.[107,108] Attempts to study the hCT activity of human carcinoma cell lines maintained in culture or human choriocarcinoma transplanted into hamsters were unsuccessful, as the models lost their ability to secrete hCT.[109] For a detailed description of ectopic hormone production, see Chapter 5 by Samaan.

B. Prolactin-dependent Tumors

The most widely recognized prolactin-dependent tumor is the mammary carcinoma of the rodent. This tumor, and that of the human, will be covered in detail in Section VIII.

Prolactin has also been reported to affect other tumorous tissue and the following list is in good agreement with those tissues in which prolactin receptors have been identified:

1. Hypophysectomy inhibits the growth of artificially induced hepatic metastases following intraportal injection of Walker tumors cells. A marked reversal of this decline was produced by injections of ovine prolactin to hypophysectomized rats. However, the effect of exogenous prolactin in intact tumor-bearing rats was less clear.[110]

2. Prolactin has also been reported to have a suppressive effect on the growth of urethane-induced pulmonary adenomas in mice and to reduce tumor growth and increase survival of mice injected with the Maloney sarcoma virus.[111] This protective effect of prolactin on lung and muscle tumors is in contrast to the growth-promoting activity of prolactin in mammary tumors, for example. At selected periods, however, prolactin may also inhibit mammary tumor growth (see Section VIII.B).

3. An effect of prolactin at the uterine level has also been reported. An increase in the binding of [^{125}I]-labeled human prolactin to myomatous tissue was higher than binding to normal myometrium.[112]

4. In addition, a synergistic effect of estradiol and prolactin on the incidence of carcinogen-induced cervical carcinomas in mice was observed.[113] In organ cultures of cervical carcinomas from rats, prolactin stimulated [^{3}H]-thymidine incorporation.[114]

5. Finally, Fry et al.[115] have reported that increased prolactin levels induced by pituitary transplants to the kidney capsule along with injections of DES caused a marked increase in the incidence of tumors of the Harderian gland when the animals were exposed to ionizing radiation.

As the list of prolactin-responsive tissues increases, the number of reports of prolactin affecting the appearance and growth of tumors is also likely to expand.

VIII. MODELS OF HORMONE-DEPENDENT BREAST CANCER

A. Spontaneous Tumors

Several excellent reviews on prolactin and breast cancer have appeared.[93-96,116-121] Spontaneous mammary tumors appear in a high percentage of rats 24 months of age or older. These tumors are usually a single fibroadenoma.[117] Multiparous rats have been observed to have a higher incidence of spontaneous tumors than nulliparous animals.[124] The positive role of prolactin in the development of these spontaneous tumors has been clarified by several studies. Welsch et al.[123] observed that rats receiving multiple pituitary homographs, which produce elevated prolactin levels, had a greater incidence of spontaneous mammary tumors than did the control rats. The same group also showed that median-eminence hypothalamic lesions which increased plasma prolactin levels in female rats also markedly increased spontaneous tumor development.[124] The continued growth of established spontaneous mammary tumors can be rapidly reversed and regression induced by administration of ergot drugs which lower plasma prolactin levels.[125] These data indicate that the spontaneous mammary tumors of the rat are prolactin dependent, increasing in incidence with increased prolactin levels and regressing where prolactin levels decline.

Similar studies linking prolactin to mammary tumorigenesis in mice have also been reported. A number of different strains of mice which spontaneously develop mammary tumors are available. However, in the recent review by Welsch and Nagasawa,[121] the authors point out, in contrast to what occurs for the majority of mammary tumors of the rat, that "although the developmental stages of mouse mammary tumorigenesis appear to be markedly influenced by secretory levels of prolactin, the advanced spontaneous mammary tumors in most strains of mice appear to be prolactin independent."

B. Carcinogen-induced Tumors

The mammary carcinoma induced in the rat by dimethylbenzanthracene (DMBA) has been the most widely accepted model of hormone-dependent breast cancer.[126] Estrogens and prolactin have been shown to be important in the development and growth of these mammary tumors. In fact, procedures that reduce circulating levels of prolactin (hypophysectomy, ergot drugs) have been shown to reduce the number and size of these tumors.[116-121,127-129] Recently, Teller et al.[130] compared the effect of eight prolactin-inhibiting ergot alkaloids or ergoline derivatives for their ability to inhibit DMBA-induced mammary tumors. They found an arrangement of three groups of compounds in terms of antitumor activity: high (ergocryptine and Deprenon), intermediate (ergocornine, Lysenyl, Dironyl and Lergotrile), and low (CB-154 and 6605-VUFB). It should be mentioned that these data, especially for the effectiveness of CB-154, are at variance with a number of published reports[127-129] which have described this prolactin-inhibiting compound as very effective in preventing new tumor growth as well as inducing regression of established tumors.

Agents which increase plasma prolactin levels, such as adrenalectomy,[131] pregnancy,[132] pituitary homografts[133] or tumors[134] and neuroleptic agents,[116,135,136] have a positive influence in tumor growth. Tumors can also be reinitiated in hypophysectomized rats by the exogenous administration of prolactin.[116] The predominant role of prolactin in DMBA tumor growth has been shown by studies in which estrogen receptors were blocked with an antiestrogen, and tumor growth could be reinitiated by simply increasing prolactin levels.[137]

The importance of prolactin in DMBA-induced mammary tumors was confirmed by the finding that there is a direct correlation between serum prolactin levels and the susceptibility of various strains of rats to the carcinogen.[138] These data, taken together with numerous other reports correlating increased prolactin levels with enhanced tumor growth and reduced prolactin levels with an inhibition of tumor growth (see reviews), indicated a direct positive influence of prolactin on DMBA-induced mammary tumors.

Interestingly, prolactin has also been shown to have an inhibitory influence on tumor development, dependent upon the time the animals are exposed to elevated prolactin levels. Welsch et al.[133] reported that rats implanted with four pituitaries under the kidney capsule 30 days prior to the injection of DMBA failed to cause tumor growth and, in fact, led to a 27% reduction in the incidence and a 62% decline in the number of these carcinogen-induced tumors. Several other stimuli which increase prolactin secretion if given prior to DMBA treatment have an inhibitory effect on tumor development in rats.[121] In addition, agents which increase plasma prolactin levels can either have no effect or result in a reduced incidence and delayed appearance.[139,140] Therefore, although the role of prolactin is predominantly stimulatory, the specific role, either stimulatory or inhibitory, should also be taken into account when evaluating the hormonal response of a tumor.

In addition to DMBA, other chemical carcinogens have been utilized to study hormone-dependent cancer. Methycholanthrene was found to successfully induce mammary tumors in rats and these tumors were shown to be hormone dependent.[141] More recently, Gullino et al.[142] have reported the development of mammary tumors induced by nitromethylurea (NMU). These tumors seem to differ from DMBA-induced mammary tumors in that they metastasize, as do human carcinomas, and, therefore, may represent a better model to study human tumorigenesis in experimental animals.

C. In Vitro Systems

In an attempt to uniformize the methodological approach to the study of breast cancer, several groups have attempted to develop long-term cultures of mammary tumors. Cell lines have been developed for human tumors and will be discussed in Section X. For experimental tumors, reports have appeared on the use of tissue explants[143,144] of DMBA tumors which responded to prolactin in terms of an increase in estrogen receptor concentrations following exposure of the explants to prolactin in the medium.

Another group showed that DMBA-induced tumors in short-term incubations responded to both estradiol and prolactin equally by an increase in [³H]-leucine incorporation, but together the two hormones acted synergistically.[145] Chan et al.[146] reported a monolayer culture system of DMBA tumor cells. However, the response of this system to estradiol and prolactin was not the same as is observed in vivo. Similarly, organ culture of DMBA tumors yielded variable responses to estrogen and prolactin.[147] Therefore, although in vitro systems of experimental systems do exist, they are not, in their present form, the ideal model to study hormone-responsive breast cancer due to the altered tumor response to hormones compared to what occurs in the animal.

IX. HORMONAL REGULATION OF RECEPTORS IN DMBA-INDUCED MAMMARY TUMORS

A. Inhibition of DMBA-induced Tumors by RU16117

Because of the potent antiestrogenic properties of a new antiestrogenic compound, RU16117, we examined its effect on the development of DMBA-induced mammary tumors in the rat. In an attempt to correlate the tumor response to antiestrogen treatment with hormone receptor levels, the concentration of receptors for estradiol-17β, progesterone, and prolactin was determined in individual tumors[148] according to methods described.[149,150]

As illustrated in Figure 7A, tumors first appeared in control rats 53 days after DMBA administration, and the incidence of tumors increased to a maximum of 94.1% at 130 days. All treatments resulted in a delayed onset of tumor appearance. After a delay of 10 days, RU16117, at a dose of 0.5 µg/day, resulted in a curve similar to that of controls, although the incidence reached only 78.6%. When RU16117 was injected at a dose of 2 µg/day, the maximal incidence was 60% between days 99 and 106, after which the incidence fell to a value of 40% at day 130 because of the regression and disappearance of lesions in some animals. The important finding is that RU16117, at doses of either 8 or 24 µg/day, completely inhibited tumor development in all animals. Ovariectomy completely inhibited tumor appearance until day 95 when 2 out of 14 animals (14.2%) developed palpable tumors.

The average number and size of tumors were also inhibited by the lower doses of RU16117, although tumor size (Figure 7C) approached or surpassed control levels at the end of the experiment as a result of two of nine tumors in the group which became quite large.

Specific binding of [³H] estradiol, [³H]R5020, and [¹²⁵I] ovine PRL (oPRL) to DMBA-induced mammary tumors is shown in Figure 8A, B, and C, respectively. Binding of [³H]E₂ was 5.1 ± 1.0 pmol/g tissue in tumors from control animals, whereas tumors remaining in rats treated with 0.5 and 2.0 µg RU16117 have binding of 2.7 ± 0.3 and 1.9 ± 0.6 pmol/g tissue. Binding of [³H] R5020 was 8.9 ± 1.5 pmol/g tissue in the control group. The dose of 0.5 µg RU16117 was without significant effect, but lower binding (4.5 ± 0.5 pmol/g tissue) was observed in rats injected with 2 µg RU16117. In one of the tumors which developed in the ovariectomized group, the level of progesterone receptors was very low at 0.6 pmol/g tissue. RU16117 treatment caused a reduction of [¹²⁵I]oPRL binding to tumor plasma membranes from 6.2 ± 1.5% in control rats to 2.9 ± 0.6% in tumors from rats receiving 2 µg RU16117 per day (Figure 8C). In the one tumor from an ovariectomized rat, there was low binding of [¹²⁵I]oPRL (1.2%). Binding of [¹²⁵I] growth hormone was constant at 0.2 to 0.4% in all treatment groups (data not shown).

Plasma prolactin levels were slightly reduced by the 2- and 8µg doses of RU16117 and increased by the highest dose (24 µg) of antiestrogen from 21 ± 7 to 41 ± 10 ng/mℓ. Ovariectomy decreased the plasma PRL concentration, whereas treatment with RU16117 led to a progressive decrease in plasma LH levels.

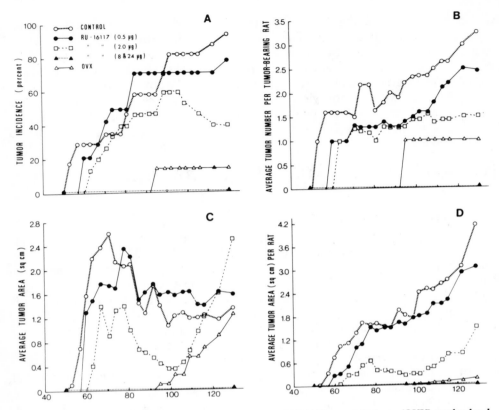

FIGURE 7.   Effect of treatment with increasing doses of RU16117 or ovariectomy (OVX) on the development of DMBA-induced mammary tumors. Injections began the day DMBA was administered and continued for the next 130 days. Animals were examined twice weekly for the presence of tumors and, when present, tumor area (length × width) was measured. (A) Tumor incidence as a function of time after DMBA, (B) average tumor number per tumor-bearing rat, (C) average tumor area (cm²), (D) average tumor area (cm²) per rat. (From Kelly, P. A., Asselin, J., Caron, M. G., Labrie, F., and Raynaud, J. P., *Cancer Res.*, 37, 76, 1977. With permission.)

These data show that the new antiestrogenic compound RU16117 at the relatively low doses of 8 and 24 μg/day is capable of completely preventing the appearance of mammary tumors after DMBA administration. This compound has weak estrogenic activity in the mouse (Rubin test—1/100 of estradiol-17β) and castrated rat (Allen Doisy test — 1/20 of estradiol-17β) and competes for uterine estradiol receptor in mouse (1/20 of estradiol-17β) and rat (1/10 of estradiol-17β).[151]

The fact that estrogens can have a dual effect on mammary carcinoma induced by DMBA is well known. Administration of estrogens stimulates tumor development in ovariectomized animals[152] whereas in animals with developed tumors, large doses of estrogens can lead to tumor regression[129] or inhibition of development.[153]

The fact that the effect of RU16117 is not due to its low estrogenic activity is indicated by the finding that doses of estradiol-17β equivalent to the estrogenic activity of the doses of RU16117 used have no marked inhibitory effect on the development of DMBA-induced tumors and a stimulatory effect on the size of tumors. Moreover, in this same system, high doses of estradiol-17β administered from the time of DMBA administration result in a delayed appearance of tumors, with approximately one half of the animals still developing tumors and the tumors that were present were at least as large as those of the controls. RU16117, on the other hand, led to complete inhibition up to at least 130 days after DMBA administration.

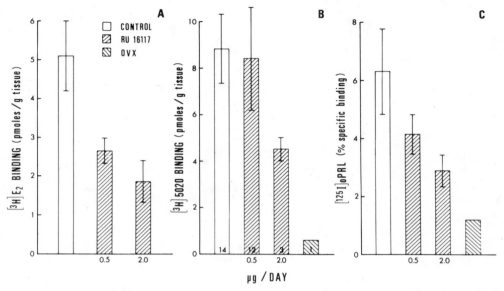

FIGURE 8. Specific binding of (A) [³H]-estradiol, (B) [³H]R5020, and (C) [¹²⁵I] ovine PRL to DMBA-induced rat mammary tumors from rats treated with increasing doses of RU16117 or ovariectomized as described in Figure 7. All tumors with an area larger than 1 cm² on the day the animals were sacrificed (day 130) were assayed. The number of tumors assayed per group is indicated in the bars in (B). (From Kelly, P. A., Asselin, J., Caron, M. G., Labrie, F., and Raynaud, J. P., *Cancer Res.*, 37, 76, 1977. With permission.)

The present data clearly show that treatment with 2 µg RU16117 led to a 40 to 60% reduction of the levels of receptors for estradiol, progesterone, and PRL in the mammary tumors. Levels of progesterone and PRL receptors were reduced to 10 to 15% of control after ovariectomy, a finding confirmed on a larger scale in subsequent experiments.[149]

B. Regression of DMBA-induced Tumors by RU16117

Since the new antiestrogen RU16117, at relatively low doses 18 to 24 µg daily), completely prevented the development of rat mammary carcinoma when administered from the day after DMBA was administered,[148] it was thought to be of interest to study the effect of this compound on the growth of DMBA tumors which were already developed and to compare the effect of such treatment with that of castration. Ovariectomy, a procedure leading to decreased levels of both estrogens and prolactin, is known to induce regression of approximately 90% of DMBA-induced tumors.[129] Once again, hormone receptor levels in tumor tissue were correlated with the response to hormonal treatment.[154]

As illustrated in Figure 9, although 4-week treatment with 2 µg of the new antiestrogen RU16117 had little effect on the growth of already established mammary tumors, doses of 8 and 24 µg led to 45 and 65% inhibition of tumor number, respectively. In control animals, a linear increase from 3.2 ± 0.6 to 4.5 ± 0.7 tumors per rat was observed during the 4 weeks of treatment. It can also be seen that ovariectomy, a treatment well known to cause tumor regression,[129] had an effect very similar to that of a daily dose of 24 µg RU16117. At the highest dose, RU16117 not only markedly decreased the number of tumors, but it also led to a marked reduction of the total tumor size. Lower doses of the antiestrogen had little or no effect on total tumor area.

In order to ascertain that the inhibitory effect of RU16117 on tumor growth was not due to any estrogenic activity of the compound, in view of the slight estrogenic activity of RU16117[151,155] and the inhibitory effect of large doses of estradiol, we ex-

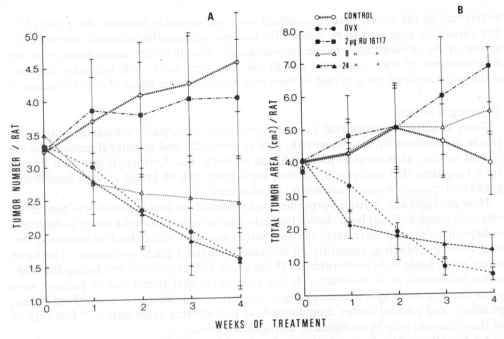

FIGURE 9.   Effect of 4-week treatment with 2, 8, or 24 μg of RU16117 daily or ovariectomy on (A) the number of established DMBA-induced mammary tumors per rat and (B) the total tumor number per animal. Treatment was started approximately 4 months after DMBA administration. (From Kelly, P. A., Asselin, J., Caron, M. G., Labrie, F., and Raynaud, J. P., *J. Natl. Cancer Inst.*, 58, 623, 1977.)

amined the effect of increasing doses of E_2 under the experimental conditions described for RU16117. Daily injections of 0.1, 0.5, 2.5, or 12.5 μg estradiol had no significant effect on the number of tumors. Although the total tumor area decreased after castration, the two low doses of estradiol induced somewhat larger tumors, whereas the two larger doses resulted in similar or slightly smaller tumor size (data not shown).

The effect of 4-week treatment with E_2, RU16117, or ovariectomy on specific binding of [³H]E_2, [³H]R5020, and [¹²⁵I]oPRL is illustrated in Figure 10. Binding of [¹²⁵I]oPRL was lower only in those animals injected with the highest dose of RU16117 and after ovariectomy. The level of progestin receptors was not markedly affected at any of the doses of E_2 or RU16117 used.

The data show that at the daily dose of 24 μg, RU16117 is as efficient as ovariectomy in inhibiting tumor growth in rats bearing DMBA-induced mammary tumors. In fact, after 4 weeks of treatment, the average number of tumors per rat and tumor size is reduced to approximately 30% of control.

These findings of low levels of hormone receptors after ovariectomy or treatment with 24 μg RU16117 may indicate that tumors unresponsive to hormonal treatment are those with low levels of receptors or that ovariectomy or RU16117 treatment causes a reduction of receptor levels. A possible mechanism of action of RU16117 in the tumor tissue could involve a decrease of the hormone receptor level, leading to relative unresponsiveness of the tissue to its hormonal environment.

Since we have found that RU16117 inhibits LH secretion[148,155] and treatment with the 24-μg dose inhibits tumor growth in the presence of increased plasma prolactin levels, it is likely that RU16117 exerts its inhibitory activity through an action at both the hypothalamic-pituitary and tumor levels.

C. Effects of Steroids and Prolactin

As already described in the foregoing sections, estrogen and prolactin play an im-

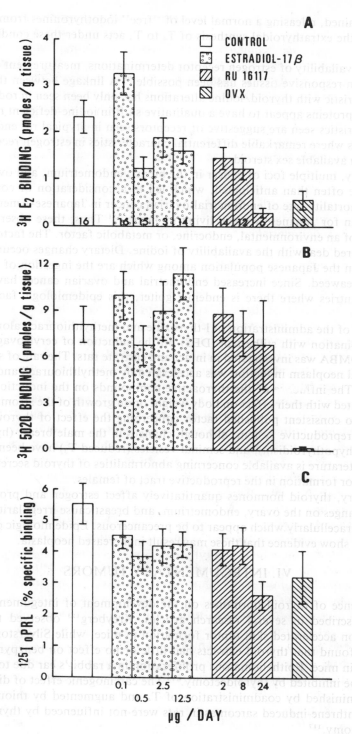

FIGURE 10. Effect of 4-week treatment with 0.1, 0.5, 2.5, or 12.5 μg of estradiol; 2, 8, or 24 μg of RU16117; or ovariectomy on the concentration of receptors for (A) [³H]estradiol, (B) [³H]R5020, or (C) [¹²⁵I]oPRL, for the tumors described in Figure 10. (From Kelly, P. A., Asselin, J., Caron, M. G., Labrie, F., and Raynaud, J. P., *J. Natl. Cancer Inst.*, 58, 623, 1977.)

portant role in the control of DMBA-induced mammary tumors. One of the difficulties with the DMBA model is that not all of the tumors are hormone dependent, and the hormone dependency may change with the age of the tumors.[156] In addition, established tumors may undergo a spontaneous regression independent of the hormonal state of the animal.[157] In fact, Bradley et al.[158] have proposed that although most DMBA tumors are dependent on estrogen and prolactin, ovariectomy and estrogen replacement alone may not accurately reflect estrogen dependency since prolactin secretion is also altered by estrogens.

Previous studies on the control of the various receptors in target itssues have shown that estrogen receptors are increased by estrogen or prolactin.[159,160] Prolactin has also been shown to stimulate the estrogen receptor in rat liver,[79] whereas the prolactin receptor in rat liver has been shown to be dependent on both estrogens[75,80] and prolactin.[81,82] It has also been well demonstrated in the uterus that estrogens stimulate the progesterone receptor.[161]

Experiments were undertaken to compare the effect of estradiol, progesterone, and prolactin given alone or in combination, on the growth of hormone-dependent tumors (those which regressed after ovariectomy) and on the levels of estrogen, progesterone, and prolactin receptors.[162] Figure 11 shows the size of five to six representative tumors following the aforementioned treatments. Tumors from intact (not ovariectomized) rats continued to grow (not shown). Following ovariectomy, there was a rapid decline in the tumor area in all groups. Progesterone treatment alone had no effect on tumor growth (Figure 11B). However, treatment with estrogen or prolactin alone increased tumor size significantly (Figure 11C and D). Combined estradiol and progesterone or estradiol and prolactin increased tumor size markedly, with some tumors reaching or exceeding the size measured before castration (Figure 11E and F).

The levels of estradiol, progesterone, and prolactin receptors are shown in Figure 12. Following castration, the levels of all three receptors were significantly reduced. Progesterone alone did not affect receptor levels, whereas estradiol injections significantly increased the level of all three receptors. Prolactin increased estrogen receptor concentration and caused a modest but nonsignificant increase in tumor prolactin recptors. Combined treatment of estradiol with either progesterone or prolactin increased the receptor levels for the three hormones to values similar to those observed with estradiol alone or in control tumors.[162,163]

Recently, DeSombre et al.[164] have proposed that a better correlation of tumor response to endocrine ablation resulted from a combination of estrogen and prolactin receptor levels than from either receptor concentration alone in the DMBA mammary tumors of the rat. For the previous study, it was of particular interest to compare the effect of hormones on tumor growth and changes of receptor levels. Combined treatment of estradiol with progesterone or prolactin resulted in enhanced tumor growth. The levels of receptors for estrogen, progesterone, and prolactin were increased to control values by these treatments, thus suggesting a correlation between the effect of hormones on the level of hormone receptors and tumor growth.[159,160]

These data confirm that the progesterone receptor in mammary tumors is dependent on estrogens. Moreover, a positive correlation between the estrogen and progesterone receptor levels in control tumors was observed ($r = 0.65$, $p < 0.01$). This demonstrated that an estrogenic control of the progesterone receptor as observed previously in the uterus[161] is also existent in the DMBA mammary tumor. However, in mammary tumors, the prolactin receptor is probably also implicated in the control of progesterone receptor since the estrogen receptor seems to be dependent on prolactin, whereas in the uterus an effect of prolactin on the estrogen receptor has not been demonstrated.

Other groups have also examined the control of prolactin receptors in rats with DMBA-induced tumors. Costlow et al.[165] found that administration of testosterone propionate induced a regression of tumor growth, as has been reported by other

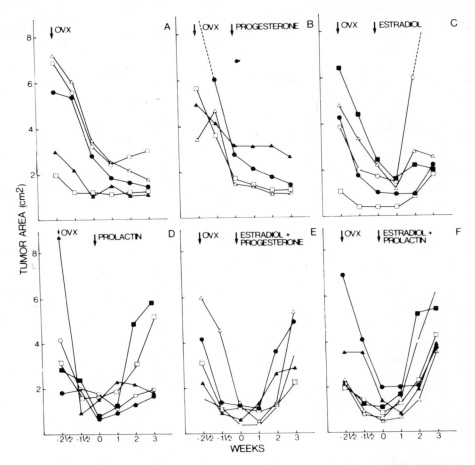

FIGURE 11. Tumor growth (area) following ovariectomy of rats with established DMBA-induced tumors. At 2½ weeks after OVX, animals received daily injections for 3 weeks of progesterone (0.5 mg), estradiol (0.5 µg), or prolactin (2 mg) or combinations of estradiol and progesterone or estradiol and prolactin. (From Asselin, J., Kelly, P. A., and Labrie, F., *Endocrinology*, 101, 1666, 1977. With permission.)

groups. They also observed that there was a 63% reduction of prolactin receptors in the tumors which responded to the androgen treatment.

In contrast to the results we have observed in DMBA-induced mammary carcinoma, an inhibitory effect of prolactin and estradiol has been reported on the binding of prolactin to mammary tumors of R3230AC rat[166] as well as those of DMBA rats.[167] Kledkiz et al.[168] correlated the inhibitory effect of estradiol benzoate on tumor growth and a reduction in prolactin binding in the mammary tumor membrane fraction of DMBA rats and suggested that a reduction in the peripheral uptake of prolactin explained the inhibitory effect on tumor growth observed with large doses of estrogen. However, doses of estradiol which inhibit tumor growth also stimulate prolactin secretion several fold, which would more than compensate for the modest loss of prolactin receptors in the target tissues.

In contrast to what occurs to prolactin binding in the liver following hypophysectomy,[75] there was only a slight reduction in prolactin receptors of tumors from hypophysectomized, DMBA-treated rats,[169] suggesting that prolactin may not have such an important role in the maintenance of its receptors in all target tissues.

Holdaway and Friesen[170] reported that it was not possible to differentiate prolactin-responsive from prolactin-dependent tumors by prolactin receptor determination of

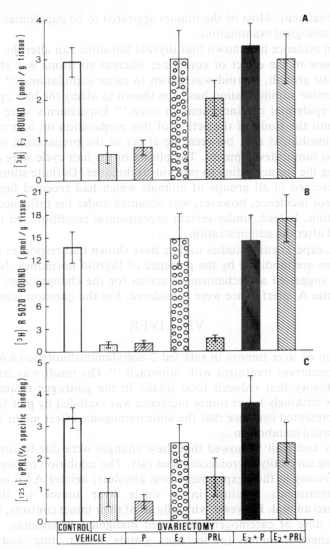

FIGURE 12.   Specific hormone receptors for estradiol, progesterone, and prolactin in the groups described in Figure 12. (From Asselin, J., Kelly, P. A., and Labrie, F., *Endocrinology*, 101, 1666, 1977. With permission.)

biopsy samples, but that following either prolactin administration or prolactin suppression, prolactin-responsive tumors had higher prolactin receptor levels. A combination of estradiol and prolactin receptor levels has been reported to more accurately predict the responsiveness to endocrine ablation.[164] We have previously reported that higher prolactin binding was observed in DMBA tumors which had shown the greater growth response to injected prolactin,[150] indicating that the level of receptor is important in determining the tissue response to the hormone.

Finally, Costlow and McGuire[171] have reported the autoradiographic localization of [125I] ovine prolactin to prolactin receptors in slices of DMBA-induced rat mammary carcinoma. Localization was restricted to tumor cells with nonspecific binding in alveolar spaces and connective tissue.

The regulation of hormone receptor levels in DMBA tumor is shown in Figure 13. Hormones can stimulate tumor growth directly, or by increasing the concentration of

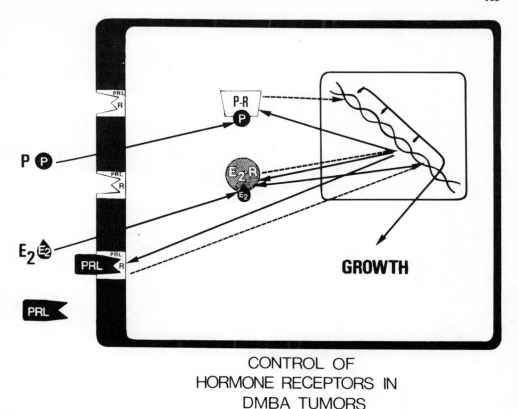

CONTROL OF
HORMONE RECEPTORS IN
DMBA TUMORS

FIGURE 13.   Hormonal control of tumor growth and hormone receptors in DMBA-induced rat mammary tumors.

specific receptors in mammary tumors of hormones which stimulate tumor growth. Prolactin increases estrogen receptor levels, as well as possibly affecting its own receptor. Estradiol stimulated progesterone receptor levels, and estrogen and progesterone, via an interaction with their respective receptors, cause the growth of DMBA tumors. Androgens, on the other hand (not shown), have been shown to have an inhibitory effect on prolactin receptors and tumor growth.

X. PROLACTIN AND HUMAN BREAST CANCER

A. Evidence for Role of Prolactin

Although the role of prolactin in the development and promotion of experimental breast cancer in rodents is well documented, it has been much more difficult to ascertain whether prolactin is involved in mammary carcinoma in humans, even after the identification and isolation of a separate human prolactin molecule. Hypophysectomy has been reported to induce clinical remission in a substantial number of patients with carcinoma of the breast,[172,173] although the role of prolactin in such remissions has been questioned.[174]

In a retrospective study, prolactin has been implicated indirectly in human breast cancer in a report by the Boston Collaborative Drug Surveillance Program, which reported an association between regular reserpine use, which is a known stimulator of prolactin secretion, and newly diagnosed breast cancer.[175] A similar correlation was found by Heinonen et al.,[176] although the association was evident only for women below 50 years of age. These findings, although not conclusive, at least suggest that a causal relationship between reserpine use and breast cancer should be considered.

There is little evidence of elevated plasma prolactin levels in the etiology of human breast cancer. Basal levels have been measured in several groups of patients with established mammary carcinoma, and these studies conclude that plasma prolactin levels are not significantly different from values observed in normal women.[177-179]

In a study reported by Kwa et al.,[180] plasma prolactin levels in breast cancer patients were similar to those of hospital-matched controls. Interestingly, however, they observed elevated prolactin levels in a large number of family members with a high risk of developing cancer (more than two first-degree relatives with a previous history of breast cancer). In a more recent study, daughters of patients with breast cancer had significantly elevated prolactin levels in the luteal phase compared to control patients.[181]

Elevated plasma prolactin levels in both pre- and postmenopausal Caucasian breast cancer patients have been observed.[182] A British group has recently reported that breast cancer patients had greater prolactin concentrations than normal controls at the follicular and periovulatory stages of the menstrual cycle, although, in general, no major differences were observed in these patients which had undergone mastectomy 3 months previously.[183] Another group reported 15 cases of advanced breast cancer in which plasma prolactin levels were consistently higher (although generally within the normal range) than control levels.[184] Finally, in patients with benign disease of the breast, prolactin concentrations were abnormally elevated, especially in women over the age of 30 years, indicating a possible involvement of prolactin in this condition.[185]

Because of possible stimulatory effects of elevated prolactin levels, L-dopa, which lowers prolactin, has been given to women with metastatic breast cancer. Minton[186] reported that 10 of 30 patients with severe bone pain became "pain free" when treated with L-dopa. Patients with low fasting prolactin levels who did not respond to L-dopa by a decrease in prolactin also had no relief of bone pain. Others have reported success with L-dopa treatment.[187] Failures with L-dopa have also been observed,[188,189] although when combined with estrogen therapy, some amelioration was observed.[189] The possiblity has even been raised that L-dopa may, in fact, act to induce remission not by its effect on plasma prolactin, but rather through a nonspecific stimulation of the immune response.[190]

A role of prolactin in breast cancer has been questioned in the report by Turkington et al.,[191] who found that pituitary stalk section in humans led to markedly elevated prolactin levels (measures by bioassay), while 8 of 11 patients showed objective remission for periods of 7 months to 12 years. The reliability of some of this bioassay data has been questioned. In fact, Diefenbach et al.[192] have reported only modest elevation in plasma prolaction to 34 ± 3 ng/ml in pituitary stalk-sectioned monkeys. However, assuming the high levels in humans are real, elevated prolactin levels could have an inhibitory effect on human breast cancer, as has been reported to be the case in experimental tumor models.[133] In fact, early pregnancy has a long-term protective effect on the development of breast cancer,[193] and the use of oral contraceptives, while not affecting the incidence of breast cancer, does protect against benign breast disease.[194] These situations are associated with increased prolactin secretion and, in the case of pregnancy, the production of a placental lactogen as well. An alteration in prolactin production occurring at the right time in terms of the development of the mammary gland or tumor may be responsible for this protective effect.

Another means of identifying whether prolactin plays a role in human breast cancer is to examine tumor response in vitro. In 1972, Salih et al.[195] described a histochemical method to determine the dehydrogenase activity of the pentose shunt of human mammary tumor biopsies in the absence and presence of ovine prolactin in the medium, thus offering a predictive tool to determine the prolactin dependency of human breast cancer. Of 50 tumors examined, 32% were prolactin dependent; for 20%, prolactin was the only hormone required. In a subsequent report, the series of patients was expanded and the percentage of prolactin-responsive tumors was similar.[196] However, recently, the reproducibility of this technique of measuring hormone responsiveness of human tumors in organ culture has been questioned.[197]

The effect of prolactin on the growth and estrogen receptor level of a cell line of human breast cancer revealed that both bovine and human prolactin could almost double the level of estrogen receptor measured in the cells, but that human prolactin was ten times more potent than ovine prolactin in this respect.[198] Another group reported that normal human breast tissue responds, in terms of mitotic index, to either insulin or human prolactin, but not to ovine prolactin, suggesting a species specificity.[199]

Welsch et al.[200] report that [³H] thymidine incorporation into DNA in human tumors in organ culture was stimulated to a degree seen in DMBA mammary tumors in only 15% of the tumors examined to which ovine prolactin had been added. If, however, all the tumors showing a greater than 20% increase in [³H]-thymidine incorporation into DNA were included, addition of prolactin to insulin and hydrocortisone treatment resulted in 40% (8/20) of the tumors which were prolactin responsive, a figure which is more in line with the previous work of Hobbs et al.[196] and also with the receptor data (*vide infra*).

B. Prolactin Receptors in Human Breast Carcinoma

If prolactin does stimulate human mammary tumors, the tissue should contain prolactin receptors, as is the case for other prolactin-responsive tissues as well as for experimental mammary tumors.[68-72] Holdaway and Friesen[201] have reported on the specific binding of prolactin to human breast tumors. Specific binding of greater than 1% of the added radioactivity (which the authors considered significant) occurred in 8 of 41 tumors (19.5%). For one tumor, enough material was present to perform a Scatchard plot, and an affinity constant (Ka) of 2.5nM^{-1} was determined, which is similar to that of other prolactin receptors.[69,74] Morgan et al.[202] have reported that 15/55 (27%) human breast tumors showed specific prolactin binding, of which 64% were prolactin dependent in culture. Prolactin binding sites in human breast tumors were also localized immunohistochemically. Of 80 cases studied, 45 were prolactin dependent in culture, whereas 30 showed positive staining for prolactin. [203] In another study of 20 tumors, 70% were described as having measurable prolactin binding.[204]

In our laboratory, we have examined 136 biopsies of human mammary carcinoma, both primary lesions and metastases. Specific prolactin binding is shown in Figure 14. Greater than 1% specific binding was observed in 24.3% of the tumors (range 1.0 to 15.8%). We feel that the values between 0.5 and 1.0% which occurred in 21.3% of the tumors also reflect the presence of receptors. Combining these two groups results in slightly under 50% of the tumors that are "prolactin responsive" in terms of possessing prolactin receptors and theoretically being able to respond to prolactin.

In contrast to what was observed by Morgan et al.,[202] we have found that human growth hormone, which has lactogenic properties, does compete with prolactin for binding. We also routinely utilized [^{125}I] ovine prolactin for the binding studies. Although there have been reports of a preferential action of human prolactin in human tumors,[198,199] ovine and human prolactin bound equally well to the tumors.

In addition to prolactin receptors in these human tumors, estrogen and progesterone receptors were also measured. There was no significant correlation of the level of prolactin receptor with that of either estrogen or progesterone.

XI. CONCLUSIONS

The physiological regulation of prolactin secretion is complex. Prolactin can circu-

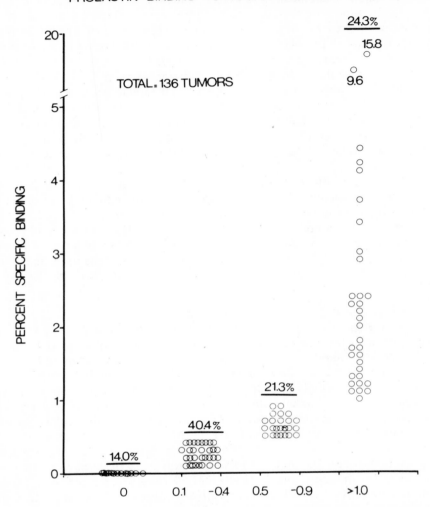

FIGURE 14.   Specific binding of [^{125}I] prolactin to biopsy specimens of human mammary carcinoma.

late in a number of molecular forms, which may have varying bioactivities or receptor activities, and the proportion of which may vary dependent on the stimulus used. The most widely accepted action of prolactin is the stimulation of mammary gland development and lactation.

A stimulatory role of both prolactin and estrogens in the development of experimental breast cancer in rodents is well documented. Estrogen has an important role as an inducer or carcinogen. Prolactin certainly acts as a promoter of many estrogen-induced cancers, as is the case also for DMBA-induced mammary tumors. However, there have also been studies in the rat which demonstrate that simply raising prolactin levels over a long period of time can induce mammary tumors. In addition, prolactin is capable of stimulating tumor growth in hypophysectomized rats, whereas estrogen has no effect. Therefore, prolactin may have a dual role, both in the development and maintenance of mammary tumors. The effects of prolactin involve an interaction with the prolactin receptor which has been quantitated in a number of prolactin-responsive tissues, including mammary tumors.

In humans, it is much more difficult to ascertain whether prolactin is involved in mammary carcinoma. In human breast carcinoma, prolactin may be implicated in the developmental states of the disease, as prolactin is an important factor controlling the normal function of the mammary gland. Recent biochemical data indicate that a certain percentage of breast cancers are prolactin responsive, but the evaluation of the definite role of prolactin as a carcinogen or cocarcinogen in human breast cancer is yet to be elucidated.

REFERENCES

1. Riddle, O., Bates, R. W., and Dykshorn, S. W., A new hormone of the anterior pituitary, *Proc. Soc. Exp. Biol. Med.,* 29, 1211, 1932.
2. Riddle, O., Bates, R. W., and Dykshorn, S. W., The preparation, identification and assay of prolactin — a hormone of the anterior pituitary, *Am. J. Physiol.,* 105, 191, 1933.
3. Forsyth, I. A., Folley, S. J., and Chadwick, A., Lactogenic and pigeon crop-stimulating activities of human pituitary growth hormone preparations, *J. Endocrinol.,* 31, 115, 1965.
4. Bewley, T. A. and Li, C. H., Primary structures of human pituitary growth hormone and sheep pituitary lactogenic hormone compared, *Science,* 168, 1361, 1970.
5. Kleinberg, D. L. and Frantz, A. G., Human prolactin: measurement in plasma by in vitro bioassay, *J. Clin. Invest.,* 50, 1557, 1971.
6. Guyda, H., Hwang, P., and Friesen, H. G., Immunologic evidence for monkey and human prolactin (MPr and HPr), *J. Clin. Endocrinol. Metab.,* 32, 120, 1971.
7. Friesen, H., Guyda, H., and Hardy, J., Biosynthesis of human growth hormone and prolactin, *J. Clin. Endocrinol. Metab.,* 31, 611, 1970.
8. Lewis, U. J., Singh, R. N. P., Sinha, Y. N., and Vanderlaan, W. P., Electrophoretic evidence for human prolactin, *J. Clin. Endocrinol. Metab.,* 33, 153, 1971.
9. Hwang, P., Guyda, H., and Friesen. H. G., Purification of human prolactin, *J. Biol. Chem.,* 247, 1955, 1972.
10. Hwang, P., Guyda, H., and Friesen, H. G., A radioimmunoassay for human prolactin, *Proc. Natl. Acad. Sci. U.S.A.,* 68, 1902, 1971.
11. Bern, H. A. and Nicoll, C. S., The comparative endocrinology of prolactin, *Rec. Prog. Horm. Res.,* 24, 681, 1968.
12. Forsyth, I. A. and Parke, L., The bioassay of human prolactin, in *Human Prolactin,* Pasteels, J. L. and Robyn, C., Eds., Excerpta Medica, Amsterdam, 1973, 71.
13. Yallow, R. S. and Berson, S. A., Assay of plasma insulin in human subjects by immunologic methods, *Nature (London),* 184, 1648, 1959.
14. Sinha, Y. N., Selby, F. W., Lewis, U. J., and Vanderlaan, W. P., A homologous radioimmunoassay for human prolactin, *J. Clin. Endocrinol. Metab.,* 36, 509, 1973.
15. Shiu, R. P. C., Kelly, P. A., and Friesen, H. G., Radioreceptor assay for prolactin and other lactogenic hormones, *Science,* 180, 968, 1973.
16. Tsushima, T., Shiu, R. P. C., Kelly, P. A., and Friesen, H. G., Radioreceptor assay for human growth hormone and lactogens: structure-function studies and clinical applications, in *Advances in Human Growth Hormone Research,* Raiti, S., Ed., U.S. Government Printing Office, Washington, D.C., 1974, 372.
17. Kelly, P. A., Tsushima, T., Shiu, R. P. C., and Friesen, H. G., Lactogenic and growth hormone like activities in pregnancy determined by radioreceptor assays, *Endocrinology,* 99, 765, 1976.
18. Kelly, P. A., Secretion and biological effects of placental lactogens, in *Proc. 5th Int. Congr. Endocrinology,* Vol. 2, James, V. H. T., Ed., Excerpta Medica, Amsterdam, 1976, 298.
19. Roth, J., Gorden, P., and Pastan, I., "Big insulin": a new component of plasma insulin detected by immunoassay, *Proc. Natl. Acad. Sci. U.S.A.,* 61, 138, 1968.
20. Berson, S. A. and Yalow, R. S., Immunologic heterogeneity of parathyroid hormone in plasma, *J. Clin. Endocrinol. Metab.,* 28, 1037, 1968.
21. Yalow, R. S. and Berson, S. A., Size and charge distinction between endogenous human plasma gastrin in peripheral blood and heptadecapeptide gastrins, *Gastroenterology,* 58, 609, 1970.
22. Yalow, R. S. and Berson, S. A., Size heterogeneity of immunoreactive human ACTH in plasma and extracts of pituitary glands and ACTH-producing thymoma, *Biochem. Biophys. Res. Commun.,* 44, 439, 1971.

23. Bala, R. M., Ferguson, K. A., and Beck, J. C., Plasma biological and immunoreactive human growth hormone-like activity, *Endocrinology,* 87, 506, 1970.
24. Suh, H. K. and Frantz, A. G., Size heterogeneity of human prolactin in plasma and pituitary extracts, *J. Clin. Endocrinol. Metab.,* 39, 928, 1974.
25. Aubert, M. L., Garnier, P. E., Kaplan, S. L., and Grumbach, M. M., Heterogeneity of circulating human prolactin (LPRL); decreased radioreceptor activity of "big" LPRL, *Endocrinology,* 96, 80A, 1975.
26. Kataoka, K., Imai, Y., and Hollander, C. S., Altered molecular heterogeneity of circulating prolactin following thyrotropin releasing hormone, *Clin. Res.,* 23, 238A, 1975.
27. Guyda, H. J., Heterogeneity of human growth hormone and prolactin secreted *in vitro:* Immunoassay and radioreceptor assay correlation, *J. Clin. Endocrinol. Metab.,* 41, 953, 1975.
28. Nicoll, C. S., Aspects of the neural control of prolactin secretion, in *Frontiers in Neuroendocrinology,* Martini, L. and Ganong, W. F., Eds., Oxford University Press, New York, 1971, 291.
29. Meites, J. and Clemens, J. A., Hypothalamic control of prolactin secretion, *Vitam. Horm. (New York),* 30, 165, 1972.
30. Clemens, J. A., Neuropharmacological aspects of the neural control of prolactin secretion, in *Hypothalamus and Endocrine Functions,* Labrie, F., Meites, J., and Pelletier, G., Eds., Plenum Press, New York, 1976, 283.
31. Friesen, H., Tolis, G., Shiu, R., and Hwang, P., Studies on human prolactin: chemistry, radioreceptor assay and clinical significance, in *Human Prolactin,* Pasteels, J. L. and Robyn, C., Eds., Excerpta Medica, Amsterdam, 1973, 11.
32. Bohnet, H. G. and Friesen, H. G., Control of prolactin secretion in man, in *Hypothalamus and Endocrine Functions,* Labrie, F., Meites, J., and Pelletier, G., Eds., Plenum Press, New York, 1976, 257.
33. Butcher, R. L., Collins, W. E., and Fugo, N. W., Plasma concentrations of LH, FSH, prolactin, progesterone and estradiol-17β throughout the 4-day estrous cycle of the rat, *Endocrinology,* 94, 1704, 1974.
34. Neill, J. D., Freeman, M. E., and Tillson, S. A., Control of the proestrous surge of prolactin and luteinizing hormone secretion by estrogens in the rat, *Endocrinology,* 89, 1448, 1971.
35. Chen, C. L. and Meites, J., Effects of estrogen and progesterone on serum and pituitary prolactin levels in ovariectomized rats, *Endocrinology,* 86, 503, 1970.
36. Lawson, D. M. and Gala, R. R., The influence of surgery, time of day, blood volume reduction and anesthetics on plasma prolactin in ovariectomized rats, *J. Endocrinol.,* 62, 75, 1974.
37. Kelly, P. A. and Labrie, F., Spontaneous diurnal prolactin peaks in estrogen-treated, ovariectomized rats, submitted.
38. Barberia, J. M., Abu-Fadil, S., Kletsky, O. A., Nakamura, R. M., and Mishell, D. R., Serum prolactin patterns in early human gestation, *Am. J. Obstet. Gynecol.,* 121, 1107, 1975.
39. Amenomari, Y., Chen, C. L., and Meites, J., Serum prolactin levels in rats during different reproductive states, *Endocrinology,* 86, 506, 1970.
40. Parker, D. C., Rossman, L. G., and Vanderlaan, E. F., Sleep-related, nyctohemeral and briefly episodic variation in human plasma prolactin concentrations, *J. Clin. Endocrinol. Metab.,* 36, 1119, 1973.
41. Koch, Y., Chow, Y. F., and Meites, J., Metabolic clearance and secretion rates of prolactin in the rat, *Endocrinology,* 89, 1303, 1971.
42. Kizer, J. S., Zivin, J. A., Jacobowitz, D. M., and Kopin, I. J., The nyctohemeral rhythm of plasma prolactin: effects of ganglionectomy, pinealectomy, constant light, constant darkness of 6-OH-dopamine administration, *Endocrinology,* 96, 1230, 1975.
43. Sassin, J. F., Frantz, A. G., Kapen, S., and Weitzman, E. D., The nocturnal rise of human prolactin is dependent on sleep, *J. Clin. Endocrinol. Metab.,* 37, 436, 1973.
44. Hwang, P., Friesen, H. G., Hardy, J., and Wilanski, D., Biosynthesis of human growth hormone and prolactin by normal pituitary glands and pituitary adenomas, *J. Clin. Endocrinol. Metab.,* 33, 1, 1971.
45. Everett, J. W., Luteotropic function of autographs of rat hypophysis, *Endocrinology,* 54, 685, 1954.
46. Chen, C. L., Amenorri, Y., Lu, K. H., Voogt, J. L., and Meites, J., Serum prolactin levels in rat with pituitary transplants or hypothalamic lesions, *Neuroendocrinology,* 6, 200, 1970.
47. Kleinberg, D. L., Noel, G. L., and Frantz, A. G., Chlorpromazine stimulation and L-Dopa suppression of plasma prolactin in man, *J. Clin. Endocrinol. Metab.,* 33, 873, 1971.
48. Burt, D. R., Creefe, I., and Snyder, F. H., Properties of [³H] dopamine associated with dopamine receptors in calf brain membranes, *Mol. Pharmacol.,* 12, 800, 1976.
49. Brown, G. N., Seeman, P., and Lee, T., Dopamine/neuroleptic receptors in basal hypothalamus and pituitary, *Endocrinology,* 99, 1407, 1976.
50. Caron, M. G., Beaulieu, M., Raymond, V., Drouin, J., Lefkowitz, R. J., and Labrie, F., Dopaminergic receptors in the anterior pituitary: correlation of [³H] dihydroergocryptine binding with dopamine inhibition in adenohypophyseal cells in primary culture, *J. Biol. Chem.,* 253, 2244, 1978.

51. Fluckiger, E., Drugs and the control of prolactin secretion, in *Prolactin and Carcinogenesis: 4th Tenovus Workshop,* Boyns, A. R. and Griffiths, K., Eds., Alpha Omega Alpha, Cardiff, 1972, 162.

52. Del Pozo, E., Brun del Re, R., Varga, L., and Friesen, H., The inhibition of prolactin secretion in man by CB-154 (2-Br-α-ergocryptine), *J. Clin. Endocrinol. Metab.,* 35, 768, 1972.

53. Tashjian, A. H., Barowski, N. J., and Jensen, D. K., Thyrotropin-releasing hormone: direct evidence for stimulation of prolactin production by pituitary cells in culture, *Biochem. Biophys. Res. Commun.,* 43, 516, 1971.

54. Convey, E. M., Tucker, H. A., Smith, V. G., and Zolman, J., Bovine prolactin, growth hormone, thyroxine and corticoid response to thyrotropin releasing hormone, *Endocrinology,* 92, 471, 1973.

55. Kelly, P. A., Bedirian, K. N., Baker, R. D., and Friesen, H. G., Effect of synthetic TRH on serum prolactin, TSH and milk production in the cow, *Endocrinology,* 92, 1289, 1973.

56. Mueller, G. P., Chen, H. J., and Meites, J., *In vivo* stimulation of prolactin release in the rat by synthetic TRH, *Proc. Soc. Exp. Biol. Med.,* 144, 613, 1973.

57. Bowers, C. Y., Friesen, H. G., Hwang, P., Guyda, H. J., and Folkers, K., Prolactin and thyrotropin release in man by synthetic proglutamyl-histidyl-prolinamide, *Biochem. Biophys. Res. Commun.,* 45, 1033, 1971.

58. Labrie, F., Barden, N., Poirier, G., and De Lean, A., Binding of thyrotropin-releasing hormone to plasma membranes of bovine anterior pituitary gland, *Proc. Natl. Acad. Sci. U.S.A.,* 69, 283, 1972.

59. De Lean, A., Ferland, L., Drouin, J., Kelly, P. A., and Labrie, F., Modulation of pituitary TRH receptor levels by estrogens and thyroid hormones, *Endocrinology,* 100, 1496, 1977.

60. De Lean, A., Garon, M., Kelly, P. A., and Labrie, F., Changes of pituitary TRH receptor level and PRL response of TRH during the rat estrous cycle, *Endocrinology,* 100, 1505, 1977.

61. Kalra, P. S., Fawcett, C. P., Krulich, L., and McCann, S. M., The effects of gonadal steroids on plasma gonadotropins and prolactin in the rat, *Endocrinology,* 92, 1256, 1973.

62. Ehara, Y., Siler, T. M., and Yen, S. S. C., Effects of large doses of estrogen on prolactin and growth hormone release, *Am. J. Obstet. Gynecol.,* 125, 455, 1976.

63. Nolin, J. M., Campbell, G. T., Nansel, D. D., and Bogdanove, E. M., Does androgen influence prolactin secretion?, *Endocrinol. Res. Commun.,* 4(1), 61, 1977.

64. Kelly, P. A., LeBlanc, G., Ferland, L., Labrie, F., and De Lean, A., Androgen inhibition of basal and estrogen-stimulated prolactin binding in rat liver, *Mol. Cell. Endocrinol.,* 9, 95, 77.

65. Nicoll, C. S. and Bern, H. A., On the actions of prolactin among the vertebrates: is there a common denominator?, in *Lactogenic Hormones,* Ciba Foundation Symp., Wolstenholme, G. E. W. and Knight, J., Eds., Churchill-Livingstone, London, 1972, 299.

66. Cowie, A. T., Hormonal factors in mammary development and lactation, in *Mammary Cancer and Neuroendocrine Therapy,* Stoll, B. A., Ed., Butterworths, London, 1974, 3.

67. Scatchard, G., The attraction of proteins for small molecules and ions, *Ann. N.Y. Acad. Sci.,* 51, 660, 1949.

68. Roth, J., Peptide hormone binding to receptors: a review of direct studies *in vitro,* Metabolism, 22, 1059, 1973.

69. Posner, B. I., Kelly, P. A., Shiu, R. P. C., and Friesen, H. G., Studies of insulin, growth hormone and prolactin binding: tissue distribution, species variation and characterization, *Endocrinology,* 96, 521, 1974.

70. Frantz, W. L., MacIndoe, J. H., and Turkington, R. W., Prolactin receptors: characteristics of the particulate fraction binding activity, *J. Endocrinol.,* 60, 485, 1974.

71. Turkington, R. W., Prolactin receptors in mammary carcinoma cells, *Cancer Res.,* 34, 758, 1974.

72. Costlow, M. E., Buschow, R. A., and McGuire, W. L., Prolactin receptors in an estrogen receptor-deficient mammary carcinoma, *Science,* 184, 85, 1974.

73. Kelly, P. A., Ferland, L., Labrie, F., and De Lean, A., Hormonal control of liver prolactin receptors, in *Hypothalamus and Endocrine Functions,* Labrie, F., Meites, J., and Pelletier, G., Eds., Plenum Press, New York, 1976, 321.

74. Kelly, P. A., Posner, B. I., Tsushima, T., and Friesen, H. G., Studies of insulin, growth hormone and prolactin binding: ontogenesis, effects of sex and pregnancy, *Endocrinology,* 96, 532, 1974.

75. Kelly, P. A., Posner, B I., and Friesen, H. G., Effects of hypophysectomy, ovariectomy and cyclo-heximide on specific binding sites for lactogenic hormones in rat liver, *Endocrinology,* 97, 1408, 1975.

76. MacLeod, R. M., Bass, M. B., Huang, S. C., and Smith, M. C., Intermediary metabolism in the liver and adipose tissue of rats with hormone-secreting pituitary tumors, *Endocrinology,* 82, 253, 1968.

77. Chen, H. W., Hamer, D. H., Heiniger, H. J., and Meier, H., Stimulation of hepatic RNA synthesis in dwarf mice by ovine prolactin, *Biochim. Biophys. Acta,* 287, 90, 1972.

78. Francis, M. J. O. and Hill, D. J., Prolactin stimulated production of somadomedin by rat liver, *Nature (London),* 255, 167, 1975.

79. Chamness, G. C., Costlow, M. E., and McGuire, W. L., Estrogen receptor in rat liver and its dependence on prolactin, *Steroids*, 26, 363, 1975.
80. Posner, B. I., Kelly, P. A., and Friesen, H. G., Induction of a lactogenic receptor in rat liver: influence of estrogen and the pituitary, *Proc. Natl. Acad. Sci. U.S.A.*, 71, 2407, 1974.
81. Posner, B. I., Kelly, P. A., and Friesen, H. G., Prolactin receptors in rat liver: possible induction by prolactin, *Science*, 187, 57, 1975.
82. Costlow, M. E., Bushcow, R. A., and McGuire, W. L., Prolactin stimulation of prolactin receptors in rat liver, *Life Sci.*, 17, 1457, 1975.
83. Posner, B. I., Regulation of lactogen specific binding sites in rat liver: studies on the role of lactogens and estrogen, *Endocrinology*, 99, 1168, 1976.
84. Auclair, C., Kelly, P. A., Labrie, F., Coy, D. H., and Schally, A. V., Inhibition of testicular luteinizing hormone receptor level by treatment with a potent luteinizing hormone-releasing hormone agonist or human chorionic gonadotropin, *Biochem. Biophys. Res. Commun.*, 76, 855, 1977.
85. Djiane, J., Durand, P., and Kelly, P. A., Evolution of prolactin receptors in rabbit mammary gland during pregnancy and lactation, *Endocrinology*, 100, 1348, 1977.
86. Holcomb, H. H., Costlow, M. E., Buschow, R. A., and McGuire, W. L., Prolactin binding in rat mammary gland during pregnancy and lactation, *Biochim. Biophys. Acta*, 428, 104, 1976.
87. Kelly, P. A. Shiu, R. P. C., Robertson, M. C., and Friesen, H. G., Characterization of rat chorionic mammotropin, *Endocrinology*, 96, 1187, 1975.
88. Holdaway, I. M., Deegan, M., and Friesen, H. G., Influence of infused prolactin on hormone binding to tissue slices, *Can. J. Physiol. Pharmacol.*, 55, 193, 1977.
89. Aragona, C. and Friesen, H. G., Specific prolactin binding sites in the prostate and testis of rats, *Endocrinology*, 97, 677, 1975.
90. Kledzik, G. S., Marshall, S., Campbell, G. A., Gelato, M., and Meites, J., Effects of castration, testosterone, estradiol, and prolactin on specific prolactin-binding activity in ventral prostate of male rats, *Endocrinology*, 98, 373, 1976.
91. Charreau, E. H., Attramadal, A., Torjesen, P. A., Calandra, R., Purvis, K., and Hansson, V., Androgen stimulation of prolactin receptors in rat prostate, *Mol. Cell. Endocrinol.*, 7, 1, 1977.
92. Djiane, J. and Durand, P., Prolactin-progesterone antagonism in self-regulation of prolactin receptors in the mammary gland, *Nature (London)*, 266, 641, 1977.
93. Furth, J., Prolactin and carcinogenesis, in *Prolactin and Carcinogenesis: 4th Tenovus Workshop*, Boyns, A. R. and Griffiths, K., Eds., Alpha Omega Alpha, Cardiff, 1972, 137.
94. Furth, J., Experimental pituitary tumors, *Recent Prog. Horm. Res.*, 11, 221, 1965.
95. Furth, J. and Clifton, K. H., Experimental pituitary tumors, in *The Pituitary Gland*, Vol. 2, Harris, G. W. and Donovan, B. T., Eds., Butterworths, London, 1966, 460.
96. Kim, U. and Furth, J., The role of prolactin in carcinogenesis, *Vitam. Horm. (N.Y.)*, 34, 107, 1976.
97. Bohnet, H. G., Duhlen, H. G., Wuttke, W., and Schneider, H. P. G., Hyperprolactinemic anovulatory syndrome, *J. Clin. Endocrinol. Metab.*, 42, 132, 1976.
98. Tyson, J. E., Anderasson, B., Huth, J., Smith, B., and Zacur, H., Neuroendocrine dysfunction in galactorrhea-ammenorrhea after contraceptive use, *Obstet. Gynecol.*, 46, 1, 1975.
99. Hardy, J., Robert, F., and Beauregard, H., Prolactin secreting pituitary adenomas: transphenoidal microsurgical treatment, in *Int. Symp. Prolactin*, Robyn, C. and Harter, M., Eds., Elsevier/North Holland Biomedical Press, Amsterdam, in press.
100. Del Pozo, E., Varga, L., Wyss, H., Tolis, G., Friesen, H. G., Wenner, R., Vetter, L., and Vettwiler, A., Clinical and hormonal response to bromocryptine (CB-154) in galactorrhea syndromes, *J. Clin. Endocrinol. Metab.*, 39, 18, 1974.
101. Fournier, P. J. R., Desjardins, P. D., and Friesen, H. G., Current understanding of human prolactin physiology and its diagnostic and therapeutic applications: a review, *Am. J. Obstet. Gynecol.*, 118, 337, 1974.
102. Gala, R. R., Van De Walle, C., and Hoffman, W. H., Alterations in serum prolactin heterogeneities by provocative tests in a patient with a pituitary tumor, *Clin. Endocrinol.*, in press.
103. Weintraub, B. D. and Rosen, S. W., Ectopic production of human chorionic somatomammotropin by non-trophoblastic cancers, *J. Clin. Endocrinol. Metab.*, 32, 94, 1971.
104. Sheth, N. A., Suraiya, J. N., Sheth, A. R., Ranadive, K. J., and Jussawalla, D. J., Ectopic production of human placental lactogen by human breast tumors, *Cancer (Philadelphia)*, 39, 1693, 1977.
105. Payne, R. A. and Ryan, R. J., Human placental lactogen in the male subject, *J. Urol.*, 107, 99, 1972.
106. Sheth, N. A., Saruiya, J. ., Ranadive, K. J., and Sheth, A. R., Ectopic production of human chorionic gonadotrophin by human breast tumors, *Br. J. Cancer*, 30, 566, 1974.
107. Hennen, G., Pierce, J. G., and Freychet, P., Human chorionic thyrotropin: further characterization and study of its secretion during pregnancy, *J. Clin. Endocrinol. Metab.*, 29, 581, 1969.
108. Hershman, J. M. and Starnes, W. R., Extraction and characterization of a thyrotopic material from human placenta, *J. Clin. Invest.*, 48, 923, 1969.

109. Ketelslegers, J. M., Nisula, B. C., and Kohler, P. E., Investigation of choriocarcinoma clonal cell lines *in vitro* and choriocarcinoma transplants in the hamster for the secretion of a thyroid-stimulating factor, *Endocrinology,* 96, 808, 1975.

110. Fisher, E. R. and Fisher, B., Antiprolactin and experimentally-induced hepatic metastases, *Proc. Soc. Exp. Biol. Med.,* 123, 364, 1966.

111. Karmali, R. A. and Horrobin, D. F., Effects of prolactin and suppression of prolactin secretion on expeimental tumors of lung and muscle in mice, *Eur. J. Cancer,* 13, 685, 1977.

112. Moodbidri, S. B., Sheth, A. R., and Rao, S. S., Binding of prolactin by myomas and normal myometrium, *Indian J. Exp. Biol.,* 12, 566, 1974.

113. Forsberg, J. G. and Breistein, L. S., A synergistic effect of oestradiol and prolactin influencing the incidence of 3-methylcholanthrene induced cervical carcinomas in mice, *Acta Pathol. Microbiol. Scand.,* 84, 384, 1976.

114. Forsberg, J. G., StrayBrestern, L., and Lingaas, E., Prolactin stimulating effect of ^{3}H-thymidine incorporation in 3-methylcholanthrene-induced cervical carcinomas in normal and estrogenized mice, *J. Natl. Cancer Inst.,* 53, 1247, 1974.

115. Fry, R. J., Garcia, A. G., Allen, K. H., Salese, A., Staffeldt, E., Tahmisian, T. H., Devine, R. L., Lombard, L. S., and Ainsworth, E. J., Effects of Pituitary Isographs on Radiation Carcinogenesis in Mammary and Harderian Glands of Mice in Biological and Environmental Effects of Low-Level Radiation, Symp. Int. Atomic Energy Agency, Vol. 7, Vienna, 1976, 213.

116. Pearson, O. H., Llerena, O., Llerena, L., Molina, A., and Butler, T., Prolactin-dependent rat mammary cancer: a model for man? *Trans. Assoc. Am. Physicians,* 82, 225, 1969.

117. Meites, J., Relation of prolactin to mammary tumorigenesis and growth in rats, in *Prolactin and Carcinogenesis: 4th Tenovus Workshop,* Boyns, A. R. and Griffiths, K., Eds., Alpha Omega Alpha, Cardiff, 1972, 54.

118. Kim, U., Pituitary function and hormonal therapy of experimental breast cancer, *Cancer Res.,* 25, 1146, 1965.

119. Pearson, O. H., Murray, R., Mozaffarian, G., and Pensky, J., Prolactin and experimental breast cancer, in *Prolactin and Carcinogenesis: 4th Tenovus Workshop,* Boyns, A. R. and Griffiths, K., Eds., Alpha Omega Alpha, Cardiff, 1972, 54.

120. Smithline, F., Sherman, L., and Kolodny, H. D., Prolactin and breast carcinoma, *N. Engl. J. Med.,* 292, 784, 1975.

121. Welsch, C. W. and Nagasawa, H., Prolactin and murine mammary tumorigenesis: a review, *Cancer Res.,* 37, 951, 1977.

122. Noble, R. L. and Cutts, J. H., Mammary tumors of the rat: a review, *Cancer Res.,* 19, 1125, 1959.

123. Welsch, C. W., Jenkins, T. W., and Meites, J., Increased incidence of mammary tumors in the female rat grafted with multiple pituitaries, *Cancer Res.,* 30, 1024, 1970.

124. Welsch, C. W., Nagasawa, H., and Meites, J., Increased incidence of spontaneous mammary tumors in female rats with induced hypothalamic lesions, *Cancer Res.,* 30, 2310, 1970.

125. Quadri, S. K. and Meites, J., Regression of spontaneous mammary tumors in rats by ergot drugs, *Proc. Soc. Exp. Biol. Med.,* 141, 359, 1972.

126. Huggins, C., Grand, L. C., and Brillantes, F. P., Mammary cancer induced by a single feeding of polynuclear hydrocarbons and its suppression, *Nature (London),* 189, 204, 1961.

127. Cassell, E., Meites, J., and Welsch, C. W., Effects of ergocornine and ergocryptine on growth of 7,12-dimethylbenzanthracene-induced mammary tumors in rats, *Cancer Res.,* 31, 1051, 1971.

128. Heuson, J. C., Waelbroeck, C., Legros, N., Gallez, G., Robyn, C., and L'Hermite, M., Inhibition of DMBA-induced mammary carcinogenesis in the rat by 2-Br-α-ergocryptine (CB-154) an inhibitor of prolactin secretion and by nafoxidine (U-11,000A), an estrogen antagonist, *Gynecol. Invest.,* 2, 130, 1971/72.

129. Quadri, S. K., Kledzik, G. S., and Meites, J., Enhanced regression of DMBA-induced mammary cancers in rats by a combination of ergocornine with ovariectomy or high doses of estrogen, *Cancer Res.,* 34, 399, 1974.

130. Teller, M. N., Stock, C. C., Hellman, L., Mountain, I. M., Bowie, M., Rosenberg, B. J., Boyar, R. M., and Budinger, J. M., Comparative effects of a series of prolactin inhibitors, 17β-estradiol and 2α-methyldihydrotestosterone propionate on growth of 7,12-dimethylbenzanthracene-induced rat mammary carcinomas, *Cancer Res.,* 37, 3932, 1977.

131. Chen, H. J., Bradley, C. J., and Meites, J., Stimulation of carcinogen-induced mammary tumor growth in rats by adrenalectomy, *Cancer Res.,* 36, 1414, 1977.

132. McCormic, G. M. and Moon, R. C., Effect of pregnancy and lactation in growth of mammary tumors induced by 7,12-dimethylbenzanthracene (DMBA), *Br. J. Cancer,* 19, 160, 1965.

133. Welsch, C. W., Clemens, J. A., and Meites, J., Effects of multiple pituitary homografts or progesterone on 7,12-dimethylbenz(a)anthracene-induced mammary tumors in rats, *J. Natl. Cancer Inst.,* 41, 465, 1968.

134. **Kim, V. and Furth, J.**, Relation of mammary tumors to mammotrophs. II. Hormone responsiveness of 3-methyl-cholanthrene-induced carcinomas, *Proc. Soc. Exp. Biol. Med.*, 103, 643, 1960.

135. **Welsch, C. W. and Meites, J.**, Effects of reserpine in development of 7,12-dimethylbenzanthracene-induced mammary tumors in female rats, *Experientia*, 26, 1133, 1970.

136. **Quadri, S. K., Clark, J. L., and Meites, J.**, Effects of LSD, pargyline and haloperidol on mammary tumor growth in rats, *Proc. Soc. Exp. Biol. Med.*, 142, 22, 1973.

137. **Manni, A., Trujillo, J. E., and Pearson, O. H.**, Predominant role of prolactin in stimulating the growth of 7,12-dimethylbenzanthracene-induced rat mammary tumors, *Cancer Res.*, 37, 1216, 1977.

138. **Boyns, A. R., Buchan, R., Cole, E. N., Forrest, A. P. M., and Griffiths, K.**, Basal prolactin blood levels in three strains of rat with differing incidence of 7,12-dimethylbenzanthracene-induced mammary tumors, *Eur. J. Cancer*, 9, 169, 1973.

139. **Feuer, G., Kellen, J. A., and Kovacs, K.**, Is there any association between elevated serum prolactin level and mammary adenocarcinoma induced by 7,12-dimethylbenz(a)anthracene?, *Res. Commun. Chem. Pathol. Pharmacol.*, 11, 435, 1975.

140. **Feuer, G., Kellen, J. A., and Kovacs, K.**, Is there any association between the pharmacologic control of prolactin release and its action on mammary carcinogenesis in the rat, *Clin. Endocrinol. (Oxford)*, 6 (Suppl.), 575, 1977.

141. **Dao, T. L., Bock, F. G., and Greiner, M. J.**, Mammary carcinogenesis by 3-methylcholanthrene. II. Inhibitory effect of pregnancy and lactation on tumor induction, *J. Natl. Cancer Inst.*, 25, 991, 1960.

142. **Gullino, P. M., Pettigrew, H. M., and Grantham, F. H.**, N-Nitromethylurea as mammary gland carcinogen in rats, *J. Natl. Cancer Inst.*, 54, 401, 1975.

143. **Leung, B. S. and Sasaki, G. H.**, Prolactin and progesterone effect on specific estradiol binding in uterine and mammary tissues *in vitro*, *Biochem. Biophys. Res. Commun.*, 55, 1180, 1973.

144. **Sasaki, G. H. and Leung, B. S.**, On the mechanism of hormone action in 7,12-dimethylbenz(a)anthracene-induced mammary tumors, *Cancer Res.*, 35, 645, 1975.

145. **Lee, C., Oyasu, R., and Chen, C.**, *In vitro* interaction of estrogen and prolactin on hormone-dependent rat mammary tumors, *Proc. Soc. Exp. Biol. Med.*, 148, 224, 1975.

146. **Chan, P. C., Tsuang, J., Head, J., and Cohen, L. A.**, Effects of estradiol and prolactin on growth of rat mammary adenocarcinoma cells in monolayer cultures (39210), *Proc. Soc. Exp. Biol. Med.*, 151, 362, 1976.

147. **Pasteels, J. L., Heuson, J. C., Heuson-Stiennon, J., and Legros, N.**, Effects of insulin, prolactin, progesterone, and estradiol on DNA synthesis in organ culture of 7,12-dimethylbenz(a)anthracene-induced rat mammary tumors, *Cancer Res.*, 36, 2162, 1976.

148. **Kelly, P. A., Asselin, J., Caron, M. G., Labrie, F., and Raynaud, J. P.**, High inhibitory activity of a new antiestrogen, RU16117 (11α-methoxyethinyl estradiol), on the development of dimethylbenz(a)anthracene-induced mammary tumors, *Cancer Res.*, 37, 76, 1977.

149. **Asselin, J., Labrie, F., Kelly, P. A., Philibert, D., and Raynaud, J. P.**, Specific progesterone receptors in dimethylbenzanthracene (DMBA)-induced mammary tumors, *Steroids*, 27, 395, 1976.

150. **Kelly, P. A., Bradley, C., Shiu, R. P. C., Meites, J., and Friesen, H. G.**, Prolactin binding to rat mammary tumor tissue, *Proc. Soc. Exp. Biol. Med.*, 146, 816, 1974.

151. **Raynaud, J. P., Bonne, C., Bouton, M. M., Moguilewsky, M., Philibert, D., and Azadian-Boulanger, G.**, Screening for antihormones by receptor studies, *J. Steroid Biochem.*, 6, 615, 1975.

152. **Leung, B. S., Sasaki, G. H., and Leung, J. S.**, Estrogen-prolactin dependency in 7,12-dimethylbenz(a)anthracene-induced tumors, *Cancer Res.*, 35, 621, 1975.

153. **Kledzik, G. S., Bradley, C. J., and Meites, J.**, Reduction of carcinogen-induced mammary cancer incidence in rats by early treatment with hormones or drugs, *Cancer Res.*, 34, 2953, 1974.

154. **Kelly, P. A., Asselin, J., Caron, M. G., Labrie, F., and Raynaud, J. P.**, Potent inhibitory effect of a new antiestrogen (RU16117) on the growth of 7,12-dimethylbenz(a)anthracene-induced rat mammary tumors, *J. Natl. Cancer Inst.*, 58, 623, 1977.

155. **Ferland, L., Labrie, F., Kelly, P. A., and Raynaud, J. P.**, Inhibitory effects of RU16117, a potent estrogen antagonist, on the estrous cycle in the rat, *Biol. Reprod.*, 18, 99, 1978.

156. **Griswald, D. P. and Green, C. H.**, Observation on the hormone sensitivity of 7,12-dimethylbenz(a)anthracene-induced mammary tumors in the Sprague-Dawley rats, *Cancer Res.*, 30, 819, 1970.

157. **Young, S. and Cowan, D. M.**, Spontaneous regression of induced mammary tumors in rats, *Br. J. Cancer*, 17, 85, 1963.

158. **Bradley, C. L., Kledzik, G. S., and Meites, J.**, Prolactin and estrogen-dependency of rat mammary cancers at early and late stages of development, *Cancer Res.*, 36, 319, 1976.

159. **Vignon, F. and Rochefort, H.**, Régulation des "récepteurs" des oestrogènes dans les tumeurs mammaires: effet de la prolactine *in vivo*, *C. R. Acad. Sci.*, 278, 103, 1974.

160. **Leung, B. and Sasaki, S.**, On the mechanism of prolactin and estrogen action in 7,12-dimethylbenz(a)anthracene-induced mammary carcinoma in the rat. II. In vivo tumor responses and estrogen receptor, *Endocrinology*, 97, 564, 1975.

161. Toft, D. O. and O'Malley, B. W., Target tissue receptor for progesterone: the influence of estrogen treatment, *Endocrinology,* 90, 1041, 1972.

162. Asselin, J., Kelly, P. A., and Labrie, F., Control of hormone receptor levels and growth of 7,12-dimethylbenz(a)anthracene-induced mammary tumors by estrogens, progesterone and prolactin, *Endocrinology,* 101, 1666, 1977.

163. Kelly, P. A., Asselin, J., Labrie, F., and Raynaud, J. P., Regulation of hormone receptor levels and growth of DMBA-induced mammary tumors by RU16117 and other steroids in the rat, in *Progesterone Receptors in Normal and Neoplastic Tissue,* McGuire, W. L., Baulieu, E. E., and Raynaud, J. P., Eds., Raven Press, New York, 1977, 85.

164. DeSombre, E. R., Kledzik, G. S., Marshall, S., and Meites, J., Estrogen and prolactin receptor concentrations in rat mammary tumors and response to endocrine ablation, *Cancer Res.,* 36, 354, 1976.

165. Costlow, M. E., Buschow, R. A., and McGuire, W. L., Prolactin receptors and androgen-induced regression of 7,12-dimethylbenz(a)anthracene-induced mammary carcinoma, *Cancer Res.,* 36, 3323, 1976.

166. Smith, R. D., Hilf, R., and Senior, A. E., Prolactin binding to R3230AC Mammary carcinoma and liver in hormone-treated and diabetic rats, *Cancer Res.,* 37, 595, 1977.

167. Smith, R. D., Hilf, R., and Senior, A. E., Prolactin binding to mammary gland, 7,12-dimethyl-benz(a)anthracene-induced mammary tumors, and liver in rats, *Cancer Res.,* 36, 3726, 1976.

168. Kledzik, G. S., Bradley, C. J., Marshall, S., Campbell, G. A., and Meites, J., Effects of high doses of estrogen on prolactin-binding activity and growth of carcinogen-induced mammary cancers in rats, *Cancer Res.,* 36, 3265, 1976.

169. Costlow, M. E., Buschow, R. A., and McGuire, W. L., Prolactin receptors in 7,12-dimethylbenz(a)anthracene-induced mammary tumors following endocrine ablation, *Cancer Res.,* 36, 3941, 1976.

170. Holdaway, I. M. and Friesen, H. G., Correlation between hormone binding and growth response of rat mammary tumor, *Cancer Res.,* 36, 1562, 1976.

171. Costlow, M. E. and McGuire, W. L., Autoradioautographic localization of prolactin receptors in 7,12-dimethylbenz(a)anthracene-induced rat mammary carcinoma, *J. Natl. Cancer Instl.,* 58, 1173, 1977.

172. Kennedy, B. J., French, L. A., and Peyton, W. T., Hypophysectomy in advanced breast cancer, *N. Engl. J. Med.,* 255, 1165, 1956.

173. Pearson, O. H. and Ray, B. S., Hypophysectomy in the treatment of metastatic mammary cancer, *Am. J. Surg.,* 99, 544, 1960.

174. McMillin, J. M., Seal, U. S., and Theologides, A., Prolactin dynamics following transphenoidal hypophysectomy for metastatic carcinoma of the breast, *Cancer (Philadelphia),* 39, 2254, 1977.

175. Boston Collaborative Drug Surveillance Program, Reserpine and breast cancer, *Lancet,* 2, 669, 1974.

176. Heinonen, O. P., Shapiro, S., Tuominen, L., and Turunen, M. I., Reserpine use in relation to breast cancer, *Lancet,* 2, 675, 1974.

177. Wilson, R. G., Buchan, R., Roberts, M. M., Forrest, A. P. M., Boyns, A. R., Cole, E. N., and Griffiths, K., Plasma prolactin and breast cancer, *Cancer (Philadelphia),* 33, 1325, 1974.

178. Sheth, N. A., Ranadive, K. J., Suraiya, J. N., and Sheth, A. R., Circulating levels of prolactin in human breast cancer, *Br. J. Cancer,* 32, 160, 1975.

179. Boyns, A. R., Cole, E. N., Griffiths, K., Roberts, M. M., Buchan, R., Wilson, R. G., and Forrest, A. P. M., Plasma prolactin in breast cancer, *Eur. J. Cancer,* 9, 99, 1973.

180. Kwa, H. G., de Jong-Bakker, M., Englesman, E., and Cleton, F. J., Plasma prolactin in human breast cancer, *Lancet,* 1, 433, 1974.

181. Kwa, H. G., Cleton, F., de Jong-Bakker, M., Bulbrook, R. D., Hayward, J. L., and Wang, D. Y., Plasma prolactin and its relationship to risk factors in human breast cancer, *Int. J. Cancer,* 17, 441, 1976.

182. Hill, P., Wynder, E. L., Kumar, H., Helman, P., Rona, G., and Kuno, K., Prolactin levels in populations at risk for breast cancer, *Cancer Res.,* 36, 4102, 1976.

183. Cole, E. N., England, P. C., Sellwood, R. A., and Griffiths, K., Serum prolactin concentrations throughout the menstrual cycle of normal women and patients with recent breast cancer, *Eur. J. Cancer,* 13, 677, 1977.

184. Rolandi, E., Barreca, T., Masturzo, P., Polleri, A., Indiveri F., and Barabino, A., Plasma prolactin in breast cancer, *Lancet,* 2, 845, 1974.

185. Cole, E. N., Seelwood, R. A., England, P. G., and Griffiths, K., Serum prolactin concentrations in benign breast disease throughout the menstrual cycle, *Eur. J. Cancer,* 13, 597, 1977.

186. Minton, J. P., The response of breast cancer patients with bone pain to L-dopa, *Cancer (Philadelphia),* 33, 358, 1974.

187. Ghozian, R., Amor, B., and Delbarre, F., L-dopa et métastases osseuses des cancers du sein, *Nouv. Presse Med.,* 3, 678, 1974.

188. **Murray, R. M., Mozaffarin, G., and Pearson, O. H.,** Prolactin levels with L-dopa treatment in metastatic breast carcinoma, in *Prolactin in Carcinogenesis: 4th Tenovus Workshop,* Boyns, A. R. and Griffiths, K., Eds., Alpha Omega Alpha, Cardiff, 1972, 158.

189. **Stoll, B. A.,** Brain catecholamines and breast cancer: a hypothesis, *Lancet,* 1, 431, 1972.

190. **Papaioannou, A. N.,** Prolactin, levodopa, and immune response in breast cancer, *Lancet,* 2, 236, 1972.

191. **Turkington, R. W., Underwood, L. E., and Wyk, J. J.,** Elevated serum prolactin levels after pituitary-stalk section in man, *N. Engl. J. Med.,* 285, 707, 1971.

192. **Diefenbach, W. P., Carmel, P. W., Frantz, A. G., and Ferin, M.,** Suppression of prolactin secretion by L-dopa in the stalk-sectioned Rhesus monkey, *J. Clin. Endocrinol. Metab.,* 43, 638, 1976.

193. **MacMahon, B., Cole, P., Lin, M., Lowe, C. R., Mirra, A. P., Ravnihar, B., Salber, E. J., Valoras, V. G., and Yvasa, S.,** Age at first birth and breast cancer risk, *Bull. WHO,* 43, 209, 1970.

194. **Vessey, M. P., Doll, R., and Jones, K.,** Oral contraceptives and breast cancer, *Lancet,* 1, 941, 1975.

195. **Salih, H., Brander, W., Flax, H., and Hobbs, J. R.,** Prolactin dependence in human breast cancers, *Lancet,* 2, 102, 1972.

196. **Hobbs, J. R., Salih, H., Flax, H., and Brander, W.,** Prolactin dependence in human breast cancer, *Proc. R. Soc. Med.,* 66, 866, 1973.

197. **Masters, J. R. W., Sangster, K., and Smith, I. I.,** Hormonal sensitivity of human breast tumors *in vitro:* pentose-shunt activity, *Cancer (Philadelphia),* 39, 1978, 1977.

198. **Shafie, S. and Brooks, S. C.,** Effect of prolactin on growth and the estrogen receptor level of human breast cancer cells (MCF-7), *Cancer Res.,* 37, 792, 1977.

199. **Diley, W. G. and Kister, S. J.,** In vitro stimulation of human breast tissue by human prolactin, *J. Natl. Cancer Inst.,* 55, 35, 1975.

200. **Welsch, C. W., De Iturri, G. C., and Brennan, M. J.,** DNA synthesis of human, mouse and rat mammary carcinomas *in vitro, Cancer (Philadelphia),* 38, 1272, 1976.

201. **Holdaway, I. M. and Friesen, H. G.,** Hormone binding by human mammary carcinoma, *Cancer Res.,* 37, p. 1946, 1977.

202. **Morgan, L., Raggatt, P. R., de Souza, I., Salih, H., and Hobbs, J. R.,** Prolactin receptors in human breast tumors, *J. Endocrinol.,* 73, 17P, 1977.

203. **De Souza, I., Hobbs, J. R., Morgan, L., and Salih, H.,** Localization of prolactin in human breast tumors, *J. Endocrinol.,* 73, 17P, 1977.

204. **Stagner, J. I., Jochimsen, P. R., and Sherman, B. M.,** Lactogenic hormone binding to human breast cancer: correlation with estrogen receptor, *Clin. Res.,* 25, 302A, 1977.

Chapter 8

HORMONES AS CARCINOGENS IN HUMANS

J. W. Meakin

TABLE OF CONTENTS

I. INTRODUCTION

Hormonal factors, endogenous and exogenous, are well established in the carcinogenesis of a variety of animal tumors, but the evidence is much less firm for human tumors. Because it is not possible to carry out definitive experiments in humans, one must make inferences from epidemiologic, pathophysiologic, and pharmacologic data of variable quality.

Considerable detail is presented in various chapters of this book regarding specific hormones and specific neoplasms. The following account is intended as an overview from the perspective of a clinician.

II. TUMORS OF THE FEMALE GENITAL TRACT

Of all human tumors, the best evidence for an association between a hormonal substance and a neoplasm is that for diethylstilbesterol (DES) and clear cell adenocarcinoma of the genital tract in young females.

Herbst and his colleagues first described the development of clear cell adenocarcinoma of the upper vagina and cervix in young females whose mothers had been treated with DES during early pregnancy.[1] By 1976 at least 333 cases of clear cell adenocarcinoma had been reported, 213 vaginal and 120 cervical.[2] In approximately two thirds of cases, documentation is sufficient to determine intrauterine exposure, prior to the 18th week, to DES or to a related nonsteroidal estrogen (dienestrol or hexestrol). The latent period was long, with an age range of cases from 7 to 27 years; 90% were older than 14 years with a peak frequency at 19 years. Herbst et al. estimate the cumulative risk of developing carcinoma in exposed females to be 0.01 to 0.1%.[3] These data must still be viewed with caution in view of a reported lack, by other authors, of an association between intrauterine exposure to estrogens and subsequent genital carcinoma in female children.[4,5] While the frequency of carcinoma in DES-exposed females is low, the majority of such patients demonstrate gross or microscopic changes in the upper vagina, cervix, uterus, or fallopian tube.[6,7]

These observations suggest that DES is teratogenic with high frequency for tissues of the Muellerian system, but that other factors may be additionally responsible for subsequent carcinogenesis at a lower frequency. Whether pubarche is related to the peak presentation of carcinoma at about 19 years is speculative. Some data suggest that oral contraceptives and pregnancy may ameliorate the nonneoplastic changes observed.[6]

Because squamous dysplasia is observed in exposed patients, there has been considerable speculation as to whether or not an increased incidence of squamous carcinoma of the genital tract will be observed, but as yet there are insufficient data.[8,9] There is now a report of abnormal sperm and anatomical abnormalities of the genital tract in young males exposed to DES in utero.[10,11]

Whether or not DES exposure in utero is carcinogenic, it is evident that exposed persons, females in particular, require careful clinical follow-up, particularly during the second and third decades. The subject has been reviewed further by Bishun et al.[12,13] and Adam et al.[14]

III. ENDOMETRIAL CARCINOMA

The incidence of carcinoma of the endometrium in the U.S. is reported to be rising.[15] The epidemiology of this neoplasm has been recently reviewed.[16] Of all the possible etiologic factors, none has generated so much controversy as that of the possible association of estrogens, particularly those of exogenous origin.

Some patients with gonadal dysgenesis, hypopituitarism, or breast cancer who have been treated for long periods with exogenous estrogens have developed endometrial carcinoma.[17-19] However, of major concern is whether or not exogenous estrogen given for contraception or to menopausal women affects the incidence in treated individuals. There is one report implicating sequential oral contraceptives with endometrial carcinoma,[20] but as yet there is no convincing evidence that combined estrogen-progestin preparations increase the risk.[21] However, several papers purport to show that exogenous estrogen, given to menopausal patients, does increase the risk of endometrial carcinoma.[22-26] These studies have been criticized for not excluding biases by Horwitz and Feinstein who find no association between exogenous estrogen and endometrial carcinoma.[27]

Endogenous estrogen excess and/or relative progestin insufficiency has also been implicated in the development of endometrial carcinoma. Estrogen-secreting tumors of the ovary[28-31] and states of hypersecretion of the ovary (either estrogen or steroid precursors of estrogen)[32-35] have been implicated in endometrial carcinoma, but the evidence is inconclusive.

Excess endogenous estrogen production has been shown to occur in women with the phenotypic characteristics associated with endometrial hyperplasia and carcinoma, namely, obesity, menopausal state, and increasing age. MacDonald and Sitteri[36] and MacDonald et al.[37] point out that even in the postmenopausal patient considerable estrone is produced in extraglandular sites from androstenedione of adrenal and ovarian origin; this conversion is increased in obesity, with advancing age, and in the presence of liver disease. Relative progestin deficiency in this age group may compound the effects of excess estrogen.

Therefore, while the evidence for a significant role for exogenous or endogenous estrogen in the development of endometrial carcinoma remains inconclusive, it would appear prudent for the clinician to use estrogen-progestin combinations only when indicated for contraception and for replacement therapy in ovarian deficiency states.

IV. BREAST CARCINOMA

The epidemiology of breast cancer is replete with data suggesting hormonal elements in the pathogenesis of these neoplasms. This is summarized as follows.

Menstrual activity — Early menarche[38] and late menopause[39] have been reported to be associated with an increased risk of developing breast cancer. In addition to the duration of ovarian activity, there has been some evidence adduced that anovulatory cycles or short luteal-phase cycles increase the risk of breast cancer.[40,41] This has been interpreted to mean that progestins may inhibit the carcinogenic affects of estrogens.

Pregnancy — The younger a woman experiences her first full-term pregnancy, the less likely she is to develop breast cancer.[42] This observation has caused considerable speculation concerning the mechanisms involved. Whether exposure of the breast to pregnancy-associated increases in prolactin, estriol, estetrol, or some other factor remains a matter of speculation.

Endogenous estrogen — The quality and quantity of endogenous estrogen have long been implicated in the development of breast cancer. There are anecdotal reports of the absence of breast carcinoma in patients with gonadal dysgenesis unless they receive estrogen replacement therapy. Ovarian activity in normal menstrual activity has already been discussed. In addition, two other areas merit further comment. As for carcinoma of the endometrium, the peripheral conversion of adrenal precursors (e.g., androstenedione) to estrogens (e.g., estrone) may be the explanation for the increased risk of breast cancer with increasing weight and height.[43] The hypothesis that the quantitative relationship of estriol to other estrogens (especially estrone and estradiol) is important has long been promoted and criticized.[44] With the demonstration of quantitatively significant amounts of other endogenous estrogen metabolites (e.g., 2-hydroxy and 2-methoxy estrogens generally, and 15-α-OH estriol, estetrol, in pregnancy), it is apparent that epidemiologic studies of the interaction of estriol, estrone, and estradiol may have been based on too limited an assessment of estrogen metabolism.[45]

Exogenous estrogen — In males, there are anecdotal reports of breast carcinoma induced by prolonged estrogen administration. However, the matter is a more serious one in females because of the high frequency of the disease. There is an ever increasing literature suggesting that estrogen therapy is associated with an increased risk of breast cancer, but other data do not support such a conclusion.[46-50,70] However, if the estrogen is combined with a progestin, as in oral contraceptives, the increased risk would appear to be eliminated.[51,52] An exception to this statement is the patient with an increased risk of harboring an occult carcinoma (e.g., benign breast disease) whose lesion may be stimulated to the level of clinical detection by exogenous estrogen-progestin combinations.[53,54]

Antiestrogens — A recent report of synchronous, bilateral breast cancer in young women given the antiestrogen clomiphene for infertility may be fortuitous or provide a clue to hormonal mechanisms in mammary carcinogenesis.[55]

Androgens — There are considerable data to suggest that androgen metabolites (particularly a reduction in their amount) may increase the risk of breast cancer.[45,56]

Thyroid hormones — There is also a considerable literature linking thyroid disease and thyroid replacement therapy with breast cancer, which has been recently reviewed.[57] Presently, no firm conclusions can be drawn.

V. LIVER NEOPLASMS

Benign — A number of reports in the literature associate the use of hormonal, oral contraceptives with liver adenomas and nodular hyperplasia,[58-60] but others do not.[61] No firm conclusions can be drawn, but the low frequency of these associations suggests that it is not a major health problem.

Malignant — Hepatocellular carcinoma has been reported in association with the use of androgens and anabolic steroids[62-68] usually, but not exclusively, in patients with aplastic anemia or Fanconi's anemia. A possible association may exist for oral contraceptives,[69] but probably does not.[61] The major concern in this area for the future relates to the ever-increasing use of anabolic steroids in athletes.

REFERENCES

1. Herbst, A. L., Ulfedler, H., and Poskanger, D. C., Adenocarcinoma of the vagina: association of maternal stilbesterol therapy with tumor appearances in young women, *N. Engl. J. Med.*, 284, 878, 1971.
2. Herbst, A. L., Registry for Research on Hormonal Transplacental Carcinogenesis Newsletter Chicago, 1977.
3. Herbst, A. L., Cole, P., Colton, T., Robboy, S. J., and Scully, R. E., Age-incidence and risk of diethylstilbesterol-related clear cell adenocarcinoma of the vagina and cervix, *Am. J. Obstet. Gynecol.*, 128, 43, 1977.
4. Lanier, A. P., Noller, K. L., Decker, D. G., Elveback, L. R., and Kurland, L. T., Cancer and stilbestrol, *Mayo Clin. Proc.*, 48, 793, 1973.
5. Kinlen, L. J., A survey of the use of oestrogens during pregnancy in the United Kingdom and of genito-urinary cancer mortality and incidence rates in young people in England and Wales, *J. Obstet. Gynecol. Brit. Comm.*, 81, 849, 1974.
6. Herbst, A. L., Poskanzer, D. C., Robboy, S. J., Friedlander, L., and Scully, R. E., Prenatal exposure to stilbesterol. A prospective comparison of exposed female offspring with unexposed controls, *N. Engl. J. Med.*, 292, 334, 1975.
7. Kaufman, R. H., Binder, G. L., Gray, P. M., and Adam, E., Upper genital tract changes associated with exposure in utero to diethylstilbestrol, *Am. J. Obstet. Gynecol.*, 128, 51, 1977.
8. Robboy, S. J., Prat, J., Welch, W. R., and Barnes, A. B., Squamous cell neoplasia controversy in the female exposed to diethylstilbesterol, *Hum. Pathol.*, 8, 483, 1977.
9. Lamb, E. J., Invasive squamous cell carcinoma of the cervix in a diethylstilbesterol offspring, *Am. J. Obstet. Gynecol.*, 129, 924, 1977.
10. Gill, W. B., Schumacher, G. F. B., and Bibbo, M., Pathological semen and anatomical abnormalities of the genital tract in human male subjects exposed to diethylstilbestrol in utero, *J. Urol.*, 117, 477, 1977.
11. Bibbo, M., Gill, W. B., Azizi, F., Blough, R., Fang, D. S., Rosenfield, R. L., Schumacher, G. F. B., Sleeper, K., Souek, M. G., and Wied, G. L., Follow-up study of male and female offspring of DES-exposed mothers, *Obstet. Gynecol.*, 49, 1, 1977.
12. Bishun, N. P., Smith, N. S., and Williams, D. C., Stilbestrol and human cancer, *Clin. Oncol.*, 3, 75, 1977.
13. Bishun, N. P., Smith, N. S., Williams, D. C., and Raven, R. W., Carcinogenic and possible mutagenic effects of stilbestrol in offspring exposed in utero, *J. Surg. Oncol.*, 9, 293, 1977.
14. Adam, E., Decker, D. G., Herbst, A. L., Noller, K. L., Tilley, B. D., and Townsend, D. E., Vaginal and cervical cancers and other abnormalities associated with exposure in utero to diethylstilbestrol and related synthetic hormones, *Cancer Res.*, 37, 1249, 1977.
15. Weiss, N. S., Szekely, D. R., and Austin, D. F., Increasing incidence of endometrial cancer in the United States, *N. Engl. J. Med.*, 294, 1259, 1976.
16. Elwood, J. M., Cole, P., Rothman, K. J., and Kaplan, S. D., Epidemiology of endometrial cancer, *J. Natl. Cancer Inst.*, 59, 1055, 1977.
17. Scully, R. E., Estrogens and endometrial carcinoma, *Hum. Pathol.*, 8, 481, 1977.
18. Cutler, B. S., Forbes, A. P., Ingersoll, F. M., and Scully, R. E., Endometrial carcinoma after stilbestrol therapy in gonadal dysgenesis, *N. Engl. J. Med.*, 287, 629, 1972.
19. Hoover, R., Everson, R., Fraumeni, J. F., Jr., and Myers, M. H., Cancer of the uterine corpus after hormonal treatment for breast cancer, *Lancet*, 1, 885, 1976.
20. Silverberg, S. G. and Makowski, E. L., Endometrial carcinoma in young women taking oral contraceptive agents, *Obstet. Gynecol.*, 46, 503, 1975.
21. Moghissi, K. S., Oral contraceptives, *J. Toxicol. Environ. Health*, 3, 243, 1977.
22. Ziel, H. K. and Finkle, W. D., Increased risk of endometrial carcinoma among users of conjugated estrogens, *N. Engl. J. Med.*, 293, 1167, 1975.

23. Smith, D. C., Prentice, R., Thompson, D. J., and Henman, W. L., Association of exogenous estrogen and endometrial carcinoma, *N. Engl. J. Med.*, 293, 1164, 1975.

24. Mack, T. M., Pike, M. C., Henderson, B. E., Pfeffer, R. I., Gerkins, V. R., Arthur, M., and Brown, S. E., Estrogens and endometrial cancer in a retirement community, *N. Engl. J. Med.*, 294, 1262, 1976.

25. McDonald, T. W., Annegers, J. F., O'Fallow, W. M., Dockerty, M. B., Malkasian, G. D., and Kurland, L. T., Exogenous estrogen and endometrial carcinoma: case-control and incidence study, *Am. J. Obstet. Gynecol.*, 127, 572, 1977.

26. Gordon, J., Reagan, J. W., Finkle, W. D., and Ziel, H. K., Estrogen and endometrial carcinoma, *N. Engl. J. Med.*, 297, 570, 1977.

27. Horwitz, R. I. and Feinstein, A. R., New methods of sampling and analysis to remove bias in case-control research: no association found for estrogens and endometrial cancer, *Clin. Res.*, 25, 459A, 1977.

28. Diddle, A. W., Granulosa and theca-cell ovarian tumours: prognosis, *Cancer (Philadelphia)*, 5, 215, 1952.

29. Sjostedt, S. and Wahlen, T., Prognosis of granulosa cell tumours, *Acta Obstet. Gynecol. Scand. Suppl.*, 40, 6, 1961.

30. Gusberg, S. B. and Kardon, P., Proliferative endometrial response to theca-granulosa cell tumors, *Am. J. Obstet. Gynecol.*, 111, 633, 1971.

31. Greene, R. R., Feminizing tumors of the ovary and carcinoma of the endometrium, *Obstet. Gynecol. Ann.*, 2, 393, 1973.

32. Sommers, S. C., Hertig, A. T., and Bengloff, H., Genesis of endometrial carcinoma. II. Cases 19 to 35 years old, *Cancer (Philadelphia)*, 2, 957, 1949.

33. Jackson, R. L. and Dockerty, M. B., The Stein-Leventhal syndrome: analysis of 43 cases with special reference to association with endometrial carcinoma, *Am. J. Obstet. Gynecol.*, 73, 161, 1957.

34. Peterson, E. P., Endometrial carcinoma in young women. A clinic profile, *Obstet. Gynecol.*, 31, 702, 1968.

35. Fechner, R. E. and Kaufman, R. H., Endometrial adenocarcinoma in Stein-Leventhal syndrome, *Cancer (Philadelphia)*, 34, 444, 1974.

36. MacDonald, P. C. and Siiteri, P. K., The relationship between the extraglandular production of estrone and the occurrence of endometrial neoplasia, *Gynecol. Oncol.*, 2, 259, 1974.

37. MacDonald, P. C., Crodin, J. M., Edman, C. D., Vellias, F., and Siiteri, P. K., Origin of estrogen in a postmenopausal woman with a nonendocrine tumor of the ovary and endometrial hyperplasia, *Obstet. Gynecol.*, 47, 644, 1976.

38. Staszewski, J., Age at menarche and breast cancer, *J. Natl. Cancer Inst.*, 47, 934, 1971.

39. Trichopoulos, D., MacMahon, B., and Cole, P., Menopause and breast cancer risk, *J. Natl. Cancer Inst.*, 48, 605, 1972.

40. MacMahon, B., Cole, P., and Brown, J., Etiology of human breast cancer: a review, *J. Natl. Cancer Inst.*, 50, 21, 1973.

41. Ketcham, A. S. and Sindelar, W. F., Risk factors in breast cancer, *Prog. Clin. Canc.*, 6, 99, 1975.

42. MacMahon, B., Cole, P., Lin, T. M., Lowe, C. R., Mirra, A. P., Ravnihar, B., Salber, E. J., Valaoras, V. G., and Yuasa, S., Age at first birth and breast cancer risk, *Bull. W.H.O.*, 43, 209, 1970.

43. DeWaard, F., Cornelis, J. P., Aoki, K., and Yoshida, M., Breast cancer incidence according to weight and height in two cities of the Netherlands and in Aichi prefecture, Japan, *Cancer (Philadelphia)*, 40, 1269, 1977.

44. Cole, P., Brown, J. B., and MacMahon, B., Oestrogen profiles of parous and nulliparous women, *Lancet*, 2, 596, 1976.

45. Zumoff, B., Fishman, J., Bradlow, H. L., and Hellman, L., Hormone profiles in hormone-dependent cancers, *Cancer Res.*, 35, 3365, 1975.

46. Henderson, B. E., Powell, D., Rosario, I., Keys, C., Hanisch, R., Young, M., Casagrande, J. Gerkins, V., and Pike, M. C., An epidemiologic study of breast cancer, *J. Natl. Cancer Inst.*, 53, 609, 1974.

47. Casagrande, J., Gerkins, V., and Henderson, B. E., Exogenous estrogens and breast cancer in women with natural menopause, *J. Natl. Cancer Inst.*, 56, 839, 1976.

48. Hoover, R., Gray, L. A., Cole, P., and MacMahon, B., Menopausal estrogens and breast cancer, *N. Engl. J. Med.*, 295, 401, 1976.

49. Lipsett, M. B., Estrogen use and cancer risk, *JAMA*, 237, 1112, 1977.

50. Bibbo, M., Haenszel, W. M., Wied, G. L., Hubby, M., and Herbst, A. L., A twenty-five year follow-up study of women exposed to diethylstilbestrol during pregnancy, *N. Engl. J. Med.*, 298, 763, 1978.

51. Vessey, M. P., Doll, R., and Jones, K., Oral contraceptives and breast cancer, *Lancet*, 1, 941, 1975.

52. Ory, H., Cole, P., MacMahon, B., and Hoover, R., Oral contraceptives and reduced risk of benign breast diseases, *N. Engl. J. Med.*, 294, 419, 1976.

53. Fasal, E. and Paffenbarger, R. S., Jr., Oral contraceptives as related to cancer and benign lesions of the breast, *J. Natl. Cancer Inst.*, 55, 767, 1975.
54. Paffenbarger, R. S., Fasal, E., Simmons, M. E., and Kampert, J. B., Cancer risk as related to use of oral contraceptives during fertile years, *Cancer (Philadelphia)*, 39, 1887, 1977.
55. Bolton, P. M., Bilateral breast cancer associated with clomiphene, *Lancet*, 2, 1176, 1977.
56. Bulbrook, R. D., Hayward, J. L., and Spicer, C. C., Relation between urinary androgen and corticoid excretion and subsequent breast cancer, *Lancet*, 3, 395, 1971.
57. Gorman, C. A., Becker, D. V., Greenspan, F. S., Levy, R. P., Oppenheimer, J. H., Rivlin, R. S., Robbins, J., and van der Laan, W. P., American Thyroid Association statement on breast cancer and thyroid hormone therapy, *Am. J. Surg.*, 134, 622, 1977.
58. Edmonson, H. A., Henderson, B., and Benton, B., Liver-cell adenomas associated with use of oral contraceptives, *N. Engl. J. Med.*, 294, 470, (and correction p. 1070), 1976.
59. Moesner, J., Baunsgaard, P., Starklint, H., and Thommesen, N., Focal nodular hyperplasia of the liver, *Acta Pathol. Microbiol. Scand. Sect. A*, 85, 113, 1977.
60. Lough, J., Kinch, R., Spellman, S., and Shaffer, E., Oral contraceptives, smoking and nodular hyperplasia of the liver, *Can. Med. Assoc. J.*, 118, 403, 1978.
61. Vessey, M. P., Kay, C. R., Baldwin, J. A., Clarke, J. A., and MacLeod, I. B., Oral contraceptives and benign liver tumours, *Br. Med. J.*, 1, 1064, 1977.
62. Bernstein, M. S., Hunter, R. L., and Yacknin, S., Hepatoma and peliosis hepatis developing in a patient with Fanconi's anemia, *N. Engl. J. Med.*, 284, 1135, 1971.
63. Johnson, F. L., Feagler, J. R., Lerner, K. G., Majerus, P. W., Siegel, M., Hartman, J. R., and Thomas, O. D., Association of androgenic-anabolic steroid therapy with development of hepatocellular carcinoma, *Lancet*, 2, 1273, 1972.
64. Guy, J. T. and Auslander, M. O., Androgenic steroids and hepatocellular carcinoma, *Lancet*, 1, 148, 1973.
65. Ziegenfuss, J. and Carabasi, R., Androgens and hepatocellular carcinoma, *Lancet*, 2, 262, 1973.
66. Henderson, J. T., Richmond, J., and Sumerling, M. D., Androgenic-anabolic steroid therapy and hepatocellular carcinoma, *Lancet*, 1, 934, 1973.
67. Meadows, A. T., Naiman, J. L., and Valdeo-Dapena, M., Hepatoma associated with androgen therapy for aplastic anemia, *J. Pediatr.*, 84, 109, 1974.
68. Farrell, G. C., Joshua, D. F., Uren, R. F., Baird, P. J., Perkins, K. W., and Kronenberg, H., Androgen-induced hepatoma, *Lancet*, 1, 430, 1975.
69. Klatskin, G., Hepatic tumors: possible relationship to use of oral contraceptives, *Gastorenterology*, 73, 386, 1977.
70. Sartwell, P. E., Arthes, F. G., and Tonascia, J. A., Exogenous hormones, reproductive history, and breast cancer, *J. Natl. Cancer Inst.*, 59, 1589, 1977.

C

production of hormones by, see Hormones
protein kinase activity in, I: 74—78
Nervous system, fetal, role of thyroid hormones
in metabolism, II: 135
Norepinephrine
inhibition of prolactin secretion, I: 119
receptors, I: 117
stimulation of growth hormone release, I: 126
suppression of corticotrophin-releasing factor
secretion, I: 129
synthesis, I: 116, 117
Norethynodrel, study of effects on breast cancers,
I: 139
North American women, breast cancer in, II: 122

O

Obesity, role in breast cancer, II: 122
Oral contraceptives
as protection against benign breast disease,
II:184
association with endometrial cancer, II: 196
association with liver neoplasms, II: 197, 198
effect on breast cancer, studies of, I: 139, 140
effect on endometrium, II: 56
hormones used in, I: 138
mechanism of action, II: 51
role in cervical disorders, I: 141—144
role in endometrial cancer studied, I: 145, 146
role in hepatic tumors studied, I: 147—150
role in hepatoma increase, I: 8
role in mammary neoplasia, II: 64—72
role in tumorigenesis, II: 61—72
Ovaries
activity, role of thyroid hormones in, II: 147
cancer of
effect of dietary iodine on incidence, II: 148
hormone receptors in, I: 36
role of estrogen in, II: 33
role of thyroid hormones in, II: 147
effect on of progestins, II: 52
effect on of prolactin, II: 163
metabolism of progesterone in, II: 48, 59
production of progesterone, II: 46, 59
prolactin binding in, II: 164
tumors, role of progestins in, II: 62
Ovulation
effect on of progesterone, II: 50
inhibition of
by progestins, II: 52
in contraceptive action, II: 51
role of melatonin in, I: 156
Oxytocin, effect on progesterone production,
II:59

P

Parathyroid adenomas, adenylate cyclase activity
in, I: 67, 72

Parathyroid hormone, ectopic production, I: 98,
101
Parkinson's disease, effect on of melatonin, I:157
Peliosis hepatitis, association with androgen-
anabolic steroid preparations, II: 7
Pesticides, risk-benefit ratio in use, I: 5
PgR, see Progesterone, receptors
Pharyngolaryngeal epithelioma, hormone
receptors in, I: 36
Phenobarbital, role in tumor development, II: 17
Phosphate, role in lymphoma treatment, II: 89
Photoperiod influencing DMBA-induced tumors,
I: 158
Pima Indians, diabetes in, II: 122
Pineal gland
antagonism to of hypophysis, I: 156
as endocrine organ, I: 156
association with Parkinson's disease, I: 157
association with Tay-Sachs disease, I: 157
chemical carcinogenesis in pinealectomized
animals, I: 158
early studies, I: 155, 156
effect of pinealectomy on tumors, I: 159
effect on of light, I: 156, 157
effect on transplantable tumors, I: 158
enzyme studies, I: 157
extracts
treatment of schizophrenia, I: 157
treatment of tumors in mice, I: 159
function, I: 156
hyperplasia, relationship to malignancy, I: 158
morphologic changes in, relationship to
malignancies, I: 158
postnatal transformation, I: 157
role in mental retardation, I: 157
therapy in cancer patients, effects of, I: 159
tumors
induction, attempted, I: 158
malignant, relationship to, I: 157
pinealomas, types of, I: 160, 161
precocious puberty associated with, I: 156
weight
in malignancies, I: 157
relationship to age and sex, I: 158
Pinealomas, types of, I: 160, 161
Pituitary
acidophils, production of prolactin in, II: 171
adenomas caused by hypothalamic dysfunction,
II: 171
control of thyroid development, II: 131
dopamine receptors in, II: 162
hormone receptors, I: 27
hormones
effect on of progestins and progesterone, II:
51
secretion, effect on of hypothalamus, I: 116
metabolism of progesterone in, II: 47
regulation of thyroid activity, II: 133, 134
role in maintaining prolactin binding sites,
II:165
transplants, prolactin concentration of, I: 120
tumors
in Cushing's disease, I: 130